Disorders of the Nervous System

DATE DUE		
DEC. 16. 1981		
FEB. -3. 1982		
JUL. 16. 1982		
JUL. 29. 1982		
FEB. 21. 1983		
MAR. 17. 1984		
OCT. -1 1984		
OCT. 22. 1984		
JUL. -8. 1985		

```
WL          Reeves, Alexander
100
R33d        Disorders of the nervous
1981        system
```

INTERNAL MEDICINE SERIES

Coordinating Editors

JACK D. MYERS, M.D.
University Professor of Medicine, University of Pittsburgh

DAVID E. ROGERS, M.D.
President, The Robert Wood Johnson Foundation
Princeton, New Jersey

RESPIRATORY INSUFFICIENCY
Benjamin Burrows, M.D., Ronald J. Knudson, M.D.,
and Louis J. Kettel, M.D.

ENDOCRINE DISORDERS: A Pathophysiologic Approach
Will G. Ryan, M.D.

GASTROINTESTINAL DISORDERS: A Pathophysiologic Approach
Norton J. Greenberger, M.D.

FUNDAMENTALS OF HEMATOLOGY
Richard A. Rifkind, M.D., Arthur Bank, M.D., Paul A. Marks, M.D.,
Hymie L. Nossel, M.D., Rose Ruth Ellison, M.D.,
and John Lindenbaum, M.D.

CARDIOLOGY: A Clinical Approach
Ron J. Vanden Belt, M.D., James A. Ronan, Jr., M.D.,
and Julius L. Bedynek, Jr., M.D., Ph.D.

DISORDERS OF THE NERVOUS SYSTEM: A Primer
Alexander G. Reeves, M.D., Edward Valenstein, M.D.,
José L. Ochoa, M.D., and John E. Woodford, M.D.

DISORDERS OF THE NERVOUS SYSTEM
A Primer

ALEXANDER G. REEVES, M.D.
Professor of Medicine (Neurology) and Anatomy
Dartmouth-Hitchcock Medical Center
Hanover, New Hampshire

With contributions by

EDWARD VALENSTEIN, M.D.
Associate Professor of Neurology
University of Florida Medical School
Gainesville, Florida

JOSÉ L. OCHOA, M.D.
Associate Professor of Medicine (Neurology)
Dartmouth-Hitchcock Medical Center
Hanover, New Hampshire

JOHN E. WOODFORD, M.D.
Staff Neurosurgeon
Dean Clinic
Madison, Wisconsin

YEAR BOOK MEDICAL PUBLISHERS, INC.
CHICAGO • LONDON

Library of Congress Cataloging in Publication Data

Reeves, Alexander G
  Disorders of the nervous system.

  (Internal medicine series)
  Includes bibliographies and index.
  1. Nervous system—Diseases. I. Title. [DNLM:
1. Nervous system diseases. WL100 R33d]
RC341.R38   616.8   80-24086
ISBN 0-8151-7136-6

To
Wilbur D. Hagamen,
Teacher Supreme,
model for all who
would teach neural sciences

Preface

THIS BOOK is not comprehensive in scope. It is meant to be a preliminary clinical neurology text for medical students. It is the compilation of eight years' experience teaching introductory neurology to second-year medical students at Dartmouth. General references for further reading are given at the end of each chapter and it is assumed that, as at Dartmouth, faculty will supplement the students' reading with current journal and textual materials when appropriate. A basic course in neural sciences has been a prerequisite and neuropathology and physical diagnosis are taught in parallel. A clerkship on the neurology wards has traditionally followed.

There are two basic divisions in the text. The first six chapters constitute an introduction to neurologic diagnostic concepts. An attempt is made to introduce a basis for the neurologic evaluation and, to a lesser degree, the methods. These can be taught in parallel or subsequently in physical diagnosis courses. The remaining fourteen chapters deal with selected aspects of neurologic symptoms and disease. Well-defined principles are introduced, but there are frequent speculative constructs in neurologic pathophysiology that, it is hoped, will stimulate discussion and further reading.

We are indebted to many people who have assisted in the production of this book: to our neurology residents and colleagues and many generations of medical students who have given incalculable and critical input during evolution of the text and neurology teaching at Dartmouth; to Joan Clifford and Judy Murphy for their secretarial and copyreading expertise; to the Sandoz Foundation and Dr. Craig Burrell for their timely support and advice during the preparation of the manuscript; to Drs. Louis Caplan and Laurence Levitt for their critical and constructive review of the manuscript; and, finally, to Fred Rogers and Edward Quigley and the staff at Year Book for their editorial assistance and patient encouragement.

ALEXANDER G. REEVES

Table of Contents

PART II SYMPTOMS, SYSTEMS, AND DISEASES

Part I

Evaluation of the Nervous System

1

General Physical Examination

IN THIS CHAPTER we consider some aspects of the general physical examination that are especially pertinent to neurologic evaluation. In later chapters we discuss other aspects of the neurologic examination and the involvement of specific disease processes and systems.

Vital Signs

Of particular importance is evaluation of the *respiratory rate and pattern* in patients with depressed consciousness. This topic will be elaborated on in the section on the evaluation of coma in chapter 19. Segmental involvement of the brain stem from the diencephalon through the medulla may be associated with characteristic and therefore localizing patterns of respiration at each level of involvement as long as there is *bilateral* dysfunction. Unilateral dysfunction is usually not reflected by respiratory abnormalities. The abnormal patterns of breathing most likely represent loss of higher control of the primary medullary respiratory center. Suppression of medullary function by metabolic or direct mechanical involvement results in apnea; an apneic patient will be asphyxiated if respiratory support is not supplied.

Figure 1–1 is a schematic of respiratory patterns elicited by bilateral lesions at various levels in the brain stem.

Though relatively nonspecific and of little value in localizing, *blood pressure* is frequently elevated considerably above pre-

morbid levels when there is increased intracranial pressure and then drops when intracranial pressure is lowered. Blood pressure drops to very low levels following loss of medullary function; however, for therapeutic purposes severely depressed blood pressure should be assumed secondary to blood loss until proved otherwise. For a person with peripheral nervous system dysfunction (called *peripheral neuropathy*), which may be the result of many factors (i.e., diabetes, alcoholism, or malnutrition), symptomatic hypotension may occur on assuming the erect position (orthostatic hypotension). This can be related to involvement of the peripheral autonomic nervous system with loss of peripheral vasomotor tone. Isolated central or peripheral autonomic failure secondary to drug ingestion and metabolic or degenerative disease processes is also a frequent cause of orthostatic hypotension and other autonomic dysfunction. Orthostatic hypotension can be elicited most easily by having the patient exercise prior to testing; this causes a reactive peripheral vasodilatation that slowly returns to normal when the person is at rest.

The *pulse rate* may be slowed (bradycardia) or hastened (tachycardia) with increased intracranial pressure, and therefore any change must be suspect in a person with central nervous system involvement. Arrhythmias, particularly sinus arrhythmias, and nonspecific ST-T wave changes are frequently seen on electrocardiograms of per-

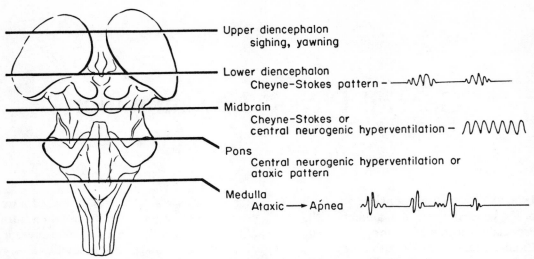

Fig 1-1.—Patterns of breathing associated with various levels of bilateral brain stem involvement (see also chap. 19).

sons who have had either hemorrhagic or ischemic strokes. If auricular fibrillation is present, systemic embolization of thrombus formed in the nonpulsatile left atrium should be considered the likely cause of a stroke.

Head

Changes in the *shape* and *size* of the cranium frequently reflect changes in the intracranial contents.

In children younger than the age of closure of skull sutures, increased intracranial pressure is reflected in widened suture lines that are frequently palpable and quite visible in radiographs. If the pressure is prolonged, a mottled decalcification or beaten silver appearance of the skull and demineralization of the dorsum sellae may appear on x-rays. Bulging of the anterior fontanelle in the erect or seated infant is a reliable sign of increased intracranial pressure or contents. Progressively enlarging ventricles, hydrocephalus, causes enlargement of the skull, which can be observed easily. Early diagnosis of hydrocephalus is possible by measuring the cranial circumference on standard well-baby checkups and comparing it with standard charts. Subdural fluid effusions, usually associated with meningitis and subdural or epidural

hematomas, also cause excessive skull enlargement in infants and toddlers who have nonfused suture lines. Premature closure of sutures causes characteristic distortions that should be recognized early because associated restriction of brain expansion may result in neuronal damage and mental retardation (Fig 1-2).

In adults, the shape and size of the cranium are less often revealing. The presence of asymmetric bony prominences contralateral to sensorimotor deficits or in a person with focal seizures suggests an underlying meningioma, a benign tumor that occasionally causes secondary osteoblastic activity in proximate parts of the skull.

In both adults and children who have a history of head trauma or in persons who are stuporous or comatose for unknown reason, the skull should be gingerly palpated for soft-tissue swelling, which suggests head trauma and possible underlying fracture. Ecchymoses around the eyes or over the mastoid region suggest recent head trauma. Natural lymphatic drainage of blood breakdown products in the scalp collects in these areas.

When the head is gingerly rotated from side to side, the brain, which is essentially floating in the subarachnoid cerebrospinal fluid and is tethered to the dura and contig-

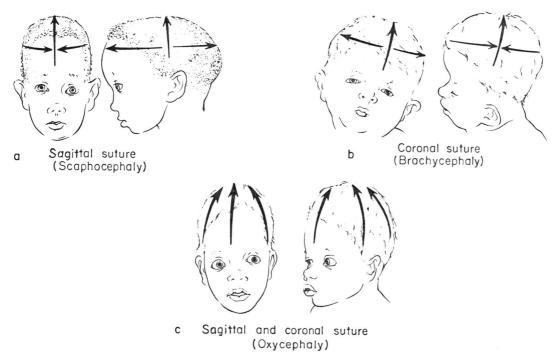

a Sagittal suture
(Scaphocephaly)

b Coronal suture
(Brachycephaly)

c Sagittal and coronal suture
(Oxycephaly)

Fig 1–2.—Head shapes associated with premature closure of sutures.
a, sagittal; **b,** coronal; and **c,** both.

uous skull by cranial nerves, blood vessels, and arachnoid membranes, is relatively resistant to the movement. The movement stretches the cranial nerves, the larger blood vessels, and the dura. Under normal circumstances, no significant discomfort is caused by this stress. However, when the surface blood vessels or dura, which are sensitive to pain, are already swollen from a mass lesion or from inflammatory edema as with migraine or arteritis, pain may be increased or experienced for the first time on shearing. The patient frequently can point to the area of involvement.

Auscultation of the cranium (with the bell of the stethoscope) over the mastoid region, temporal region, forehead, closed eyes, and in bald individuals more extensively is carried out in attempt to identify a vascular bruit arising from an arteriovenous malformation over the brain surface. The bruit is caused by the increased flow in the arteriovenous short-circuit that makes up the malformation.

Physicians do not routinely listen to patients' heads. Indeed, if all the examinations that we have described and will describe were carried out on all patients, it would be difficult to see more than several patients a day. An efficient diagnostic approach demands careful evaluation and utilization of historical data in a problem-oriented fashion. This demands that the physician focus on those parts of the physical examination that are pertinent to the specific problem or problems elicited by history or by basic screening.

Whose head should be auscultated? The person with a history suggesting an arteriovenous malformation is one candidate. Episodic headaches always restricted to the same side of the head are usually migraine; however, most migraine sufferers claim occasional contralateral headaches. Arteriovenous malformation headaches are almost always limited to the side of the head with the abnormality, and for this reason physicians should listen to the heads of patients who have headaches that always occur on the same side. Most of these patients have migraine, but an occasional one has a malformation. Focal or generalized seizures in a person with unilateral headache suggest brain tumor first but also arteriovenous malformation; this demands auscultation. On occasion the person with arteriovenous malformation hears the bruit, particularly at night when distractions are at a minimum.

The small child or infant with a congenital arteriovenous malformation in the area of the internal cerebral veins and the vein of Galen has a bruit that is audible over the whole head. He may have congestive heart failure from the high flow demands of the shunt, and also an enlarging head, the result of a communicating hydrocephalus. This is caused by the high pressure in the sagittal sinus and therefore increased resistance to absorption of cerebrospinal fluid through the arachnoid granulations. Compression of the aqueduct of Sylvius by the vein of Galen enlargement may also be the cause of the hydrocephalus.

The infant with meningitis and diffuse cerebral vasodilatation and the infant or child with severe anemia may have diffuse cranial bruits caused by high flow through the cerebral or diploic vasculature. These bruits are usually inaudible in the older child or adult whose skull is thicker and thus dampens the sound.

Eyes

We restrict our discussion of the eyes to two phenomena, papilledema and subhyaloid hemorrhage. Increased intracranial pressure occurs when the contents of the cranium exceed the capacity of the intracranial physiologic mechanisms and anatomy to accommodate additional space-occupying processes. The major accommodating factors are the cerebrospinal fluid space and its ability to be drained by the venous sinuses, the venous space and its collapsibility, the ability of sutures to spread in infants and toddlers, the ability of brain tissue to be compressed and

lose substance, the ability of the foramen magnum (and to a lesser degree other foramina) to transmit pressure to the extracranial spaces, and, finally, the possibility of decreased production of cerebrospinal fluid from the choroid plexi when intracranial pressure rises to high levels. The major causes of increased intracranial pressure are cerebral edema, acute hydrocephalus (blockage of cerebrospinal fluid [CSF] absorption, relative or absolute), mass lesions (e.g., neoplasm, abscess, hemorrhage), and venous occlusion (e.g., sagittal or lateral sinus thrombosis).

Papilledema or edema of the optic disk usually indicates increased intracranial pressure. When it is fully developed, recognition is not difficult; swollen and elevated disk edges, engorged and pulseless veins, and increased vascularity of the disk margins are the obvious signs. With further development, hemorrhage (both superficial and deep) and exudates appear. If the process is chronic, filmy white strands of glia proliferate in and around the disk. It is at this late stage that the patient may complain of episodic obscured vision. This precedes final occlusion of the retinal arterial supply and infarction of the retina with permanent blindness. Recognition of this possibility in its early symptomatic stages demands appropriate intracranial medical and/or surgical decompression procedures.

The early, subtle signs of intracranial hypertension should be learned. Prior to well-established and easily recognizable papilledema, the usually present (approximately 75% of population) or easily elicited (approximately 25%) *venous pulsations* disappear. These are best seen in the normal fundus where the veins disappear into the substance of the disk. They reflect the arterial pulse pressure superimposed on a baseline intraocular pressure; the veins partially collapse during systole and expand during diastole. If the pulsations are not spontaneously present, a minimal amount of pressure on the globe brings them out in almost all persons who do not have increased intracranial pressure (less than 200 mm of CSF). The minimal compression partially collapses the veins and allows them to expand during diastole. If intracranial pressure is 200 mm of CSF or greater, venous pulsation usually is not present but sometimes can be elicited by firm pressure on the globe. The mechanism for loss of venous pulsations is presumed to be an increase in venous backpressure subsequent to intracranial hypertension. However, venous pulsations may be lost or suppressed with a depression of intraocular pressure (e.g., immediately following removal of the lens for cataracts), and if the low global pressure is sustained, full-fledged papilledema occasionally develops. Therefore, it can be assumed that papilledema is a function of the ratio of intracranial pressure to intraocular pressure; elevation of the former or depression of the latter is adequate to elicit edema of the disk. For practical purposes, papilledema is almost always the result of increased intracranial pressure. Increased intraocular pressure (glaucoma) should delay the appearance of papilledema, and this is so; it can be the source of some diagnostic confusion.

The retina is very sensitive to mechanical pressure. You may demonstrate this by pressing very lightly on the lateral side of one of your eyes. The depolarization block caused by minimal compression of the retina creates a blind spot (scotoma) in the contralateral field (i.e., next to your nose). In like manner, early and poorly visible swelling of the disk margin depolarizes and blocks the proximate retina and enlarges the physiologic blind spot. The blind spot represents the retina-deficient optic disk and is routinely plotted and of fairly uniform size when formal visual fields are studied with a tangent screen or perimeter (see chap. 3).

Papillitis or inflammatory edema of the disk is not easily differentiated from papilledema by fundoscopy. Indeed, in most cases they are identical. Papillitis is most often caused by demyelinating processes in young and middle-aged persons and by optic nerve arterial involvement in older individuals. It is not associated with increased intracranial pressure or decreased orbital pressure. As opposed to papilledema, however, it is almost always unilateral. The visual field loss associated with papillitis is almost invariably central, because the macular or cone vision fibers are primarily affected. A central scotoma (blind area) is present and thus visual acuity is severely and uncorrectably limited (see chap. 3). Additionally, because of the disk margin edema, the blind spot is enlarged. No loss of visual acuity occurs with papilledema until quite late when the arterial supply is compromised by compression. This visual loss usually starts at the periphery, with central vision preserved until late.

Subhyaloid hemorrhage is a collection of extravasated blood just beneath the inner limiting membrane of the retina (Fig 1–3). Most retinal hemorrhages occur in the vascular layer of the retina in or deep to the nerve fiber layer. If the hemorrhage is large, it may tear through the nerve fiber layer but then is stopped from diffusing into the vitreous by the inner limiting membrane; or if a hemorrhage is from one of the major retinal veins that lie superficial to the nerve fiber layer, it also pools directly beneath the inner limiting membrane. In persons with long-standing diabetes mellitus or systemic hypertension, these blot-like hemorrhages may be present but are usually associated with other abnormalities of the retina, including hemorrhages of the nerve fiber layer (flame-shaped or striated), narrowing and atherosclerotic distortion of the arteries, exudates, capillary aneurysms, and vascular proliferation (neovascularization). With an acute, catastrophic rise in intracranial pressure, almost invariably caused by intracranial arterial hemorrhage (subarachnoid or intracerebral), or head trauma with hemorrhage and brain contusion or laceration, subhyaloid hemorrhages are frequently observed close to the disk margins. They appear almost immediately and frequently on

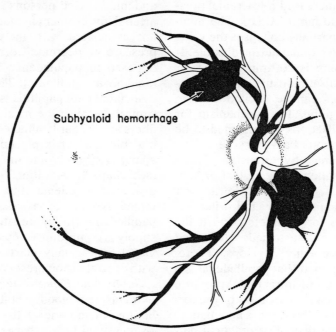

Subhyaloid hemorrhage

Fig 1–3.—Subhyaloid hemorrhages following an acute and catastrophic rise of intracranial pressure. With the patient seated or standing, one may see the formation of a meniscus in these superficial collections of blood.

the background of a relatively normal-appearing retina. They are presumably caused by a rapid and excessive rise in the central retinal venous pressure, which leads to rupture of the small venular radicals near the disk. Papilledema may follow within several hours. On a normal background the hemorrhages are diagnostic and should allow the physician to avoid lumbar puncture, which, in the presence of cerebral hemorrhage or cerebral contusion or laceration, could further predispose the patient to brain herniation (see chaps. 18 and 19).

Acute central retinal vein thrombosis, frequently associated with long-standing diabetes mellitus, causes subhyaloid hemorrhages. It is almost always unilateral, however, and usually massively distributed throughout the retina or in the segmental distribution of one or several central venous branches. The patient does not appear otherwise ill and complains only of loss of vision in the involved eye. The visual loss may be surprisingly minimal.

Ears

In bacterial meningitis, particularly in children, one of the most frequent portals of entry for bacteria is the chronically or acutely infected middle ear. The presence of otitis media is readily visible on otoscopic examination as an opaque, bulging, erythematous tympanic membrane and should be looked for in all persons who are suspected of having meningitis. Successful care of the meningitis may depend on eradication of the otitis, which may necessitate puncturing the ear drum (myringotomy) for drainage in addition to administering appropriate antibiotics.

The patient who is unconscious and has no history or obvious signs of etiologic significance should be suspected of having head trauma. In addition to palpation of the cranium for evidence of fracture and observation for ecchymoses, the physician should look for a bulging, blue-red tympanic membrane. If present, it indicates hemorrhage into the middle ear and is pathognomonic for severe head trauma. Basilar skull fracture with dissection through the middle ear is considered the cause; however, severe shearing of the ossicles may be enough to cause tears in blood vessels and hemorrhage.

The external ear will be important in the person with hearing loss, especially if it is of the conduction type (see chap. 3).

Neck

The spinal cord and cervical roots are stretched slightly when the head is flexed onto the chest. This ordinarily can be done without any discomfort; however, this is not so when the meningeal sheaths of the roots are inflamed. Pain and reflex stiffening of the nuchal muscles are elicited when meningitis is present. Because the spinal cord is pulled by this maneuver and moved upward slightly in the spinal canal, the lower lumbosacral roots are also stretched and pain is frequently experienced in the low back and legs as well as the neck. Occasionally, spontaneous flexion of the legs and hips occurs on neck flexion. This is a reflex attempt to put some slack in the stretched lumbosacral roots. This is accomplished because, with the legs in the flexed position, the femoral and sciatic nerves and therefore their roots of origin are slackened. It is usually not symptomatically successful; however, it is a reliable indicator of meningitis and other causes of root irritation (Brudzinski's sign).

A majority of the population by age 65 to 70 have x-ray evidence of degenerative disease of the cervical spine. This osteoarthritic change, frequently referred to as *cervical spondylosis,* appears to be a quirk of evolu-

tion. The degeneration is possibly caused by the constant trauma of the weight of the oversized human head on the neck. The solution may be to evolve to loss of the neck entirely with the head swiveling on the shoulders, to fuse all the cervical vertebrae into an inflexible tubular structure thus sacrificing mobility, or to develop a smaller head. The first and the last seem unlikely, and to some degree fusion already occurs as part of the degenerative process, unfortunately occurring after the fact, that is, as a result of the potentially damaging hypertrophic degenerative process. It would be most profitable to understand why some of the aged do not develop spondylosis.

Despite the appearance of severe cervical osteoarthritis on x-rays, disabling symptoms do not occur in the majority of people with cervical spondylosis. On passive or active movement of the head and neck posteriorly and laterally, to a lesser degree anteriorly, limitation of movement is easily observed though frequently not volunteered initially as a problem by the patient. This is because the process of restriction has been so gradual (over many years usually) that psychological compensation for loss of function has occurred and it is ignored.

The major symptoms and signs caused by spondylosis result from irritation or destruction of the cervical roots and/or the spinal cord by the hypertrophic degenerative disks. Root involvement gives segmental signs of positive or negative character (e.g., pain and paresthesias, loss of sensation and power, or both), whereas similar segmental and also long-tract motor and sensory difficulties are caused by cord impingement.

A remarkable symptom, "electric shocks" radiating from the posterior nuchal region into the arms, trunk, and legs separately or in combination, can be elicited by having the patient rapidly extend his head; flexion also may be effective. Lhermitte's symptom (or Lhermitte's sign) signals cervical spinal cord involvement and is probably caused by rapid distortion of the cervical cord and associated depolarization in irritable dorsal and/or ventrolateral sensory columns. During extension of the neck, the spinal canal is narrowed in its anterior-posterior diameter by anterior buckling of the posterior-lying ligamentum flavum. In persons with cervical osteoarthritis, the ligamentum flavum is hypertrophied and the vertebral canal is narrowed more than normally on neck extension; in combination with the canal narrowing caused by posterior intervertebral disk protrusion, this may be enough to cause transient concussion of the ventral or dorsal surface of the cord. Lhermitte's symptoms presumably are caused by traumatic depolarization of the sensory tracts. Lhermitte initially described this symptom in patients who had multiple sclerosis involving the cervical spinal cord. In this situation neck flexion that stretches the spinal cord probably causes symptomatic depolarization in the dorsal column or spinothalamic tracts made irritable by a demyelinating placque or other lesion (e.g., neoplasm and syrinx). In general, a physician should suspect an extramedullary lesion if Lhermitte's symptom is elicited by extension of the neck and an intramedullary lesion if elicited by flexion.

A useful maneuver for corroborating your suspicions of root irritation by posterior lateral protrusion of degenerated disk material is for you to extend the patient's neck and then press his head firmly downward, thus narrowing already narrowed spinal foramina. Frequently this elicits the patient's symptoms and thus corroborates suspicions. More marked foraminal narrowing can be elicited by extending the head and then flexing it to left or right. On pressing the head inferiorly (Spurling's maneuver), further foraminal occlusion occurs on the side to

Fig 1-4.—Spurling's maneuver. With the neck extended and flexed to the side, downward pressure causes narrowing of the spinal foramina on the flexed side. No symptoms of root compression occur unless one or more foramina are already compromised (e.g., by degenerative disease or tumor).

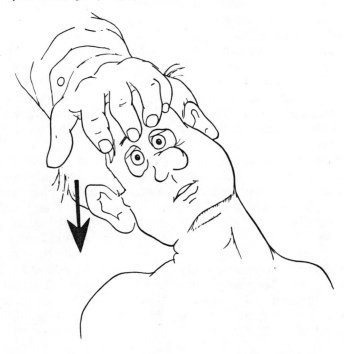

which the head is flexed (Fig 1–4). Direct pressure on the posterior lateral part of the neck with the thumb or index finger may also produce discomfort over the involved roots.

Extremities

Straight leg raising, passive flexion of the straightened leg on the hip, or the reverse, extension of the leg on the hip, is used to indicate the presence or absence of irritative or destructive lesions involving the lumbosacral plexus and roots. When the leg is flexed on the hip, the posterior-lying sciatic nerve, which originates in the lower lumbar and up-

per sacral roots (L4–S2), is stretched and therefore also stretches to some degree the plexus and roots (Fig 1–5,A). Extension of the leg on the hip (the patient is lying on the side or prone) stretches the anterior-lying femoral nerve, which originates from the middle lumbar roots (L2–L4) (Fig 1–5,B).

Any mass or inflammatory process impinging on the nerve, plexus, or roots is likely to bind or irritate these structures and cause pain in the peripheral distribution of the nerve. The pain can be exacerbated by straight leg raising. Most often the pain is in the muscle and bone distribution of the nerves as opposed to the skin or dermatomal

Fig 1–5.—Straight leg raising test. **a,** sciatic nerve (L4–S2) stretch. **b,** femoral nerve (L2–L4) stretch.

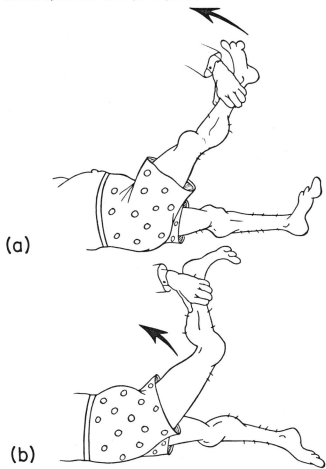

(a)

(b)

distribution. Buttock, posterior thigh, calf, and heel discomforts are characteristic of sciatic system involvement, whereas groin and anterior thigh pains are characteristic of femoral system involvement. If there is skin involvement, loss of sensation occurs in appropriate dermatomes or peripheral nerve distribution if the lesion is destructive. Paresthesias, pins-and-needles sensations, are more common symptoms of dermatomal involvement than pain. A symptomatic irritative lesion may not cause any loss of nerve function.

Low-back pain with or without radiation to the leg or legs is the most common cue for the physician to do the straight leg raising test. The most common cause of low-back pain is very likely lumbosacral disk disease, and if pain radiates into the leg, a herniated disk is usually the cause. Ninety-five percent of involved disks are between the L4–5 or L5–S1 vertebral bodies. Therefore, because the L5 and S1 roots exit at these spaces, straight leg raising with the patient supine, causing sciatic stretch, is the maneuver of choice. Four percent of lower spine disk problems occur at L3–4 or L2–3, whereas the remaining 1% incidence is shared by L1–2 and the thoracic disks. With the higher lumbar protrusions, femoral stretching is the maneuver of choice. Positive test results reproduce or increase the patient's complaints

of leg and back pain. Negative test results cause pain only from stretching tendons: this is especially notable in the hamstring and gastrocnemius tendons on sciatic straight leg raising.

Acute or chronic arthritis of the hip on occasion causes referred pain in the knee and less commonly in the foot. Straight leg raising distorts the hip joint and increases the symptoms and therefore may be misleading. This can be avoided by rotating the femor on the hip while the knee and hip are flexed, which puts slack on the sciatic and femoral nerves (Fig 1–6). Pain caused or increased by this maneuver (Patrick's maneuver) suggests hip disease, and appropriate x-rays can confirm this suspicion.

Flexion of the head on the chest (chin on chest) pulls the spinal cord upward and stretches the lumbosacral roots somewhat. Lumbosacral root irritation may therefore be increased, causing reproduction or exacerbation of the patient's low-back and leg pain. This maneuver does not change the symptoms of hip disease.

Meningitis manifests itself throughout the subarachnoid space, and therefore straight leg raising has positive results because the lumbosacral roots and investments are inflamed. This can easily be inferred from our earlier discussion of Brudzinski's sign.

Fig 1–6.—Patrick's maneuver. Rotation of the leg on the hip with heel on knee does not stretch the sciatic or femoral nerves. Pain elicited should be considered to be of musculoskeletal origin and not caused by root or plexus involvement.

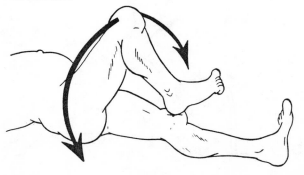

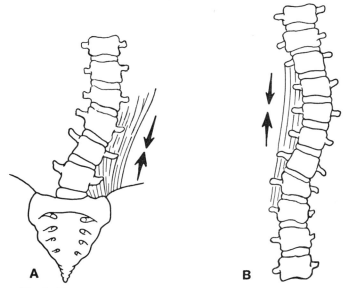

Fig 1–7.—Curvature of vertebral column associated with unilateral paraspinal muscle spasm. A, lumbosacral; B, cervical, dorsal, dorsolumbar.

Spine

Pathologic processes (degenerative, neoplastic, or inflammatory) in or near the spinal column frequently give rise to local muscle spasm and pain. If the process is unilateral, muscle spasm, presumably the result of direct or indirect irritation of the dorsal sensory and/or motor branches to the paraspinal muscles, causes characteristic distortion of the spine in addition to palpable firmness and tenderness. When the paraspinal muscles contract unilaterally, they bow the spine laterally; the concave side of the bow appears on the side of increased muscle tension (Fig 1–7,B). This lateral bowing is called *scoliosis* and can be observed most easily when the patient is erect. Observation is further facilitated by making a mark with a pen on the palpable top of the dorsal spinous processes of the vertebrae. The only exception to the rule of contralateral bowing occurs at the lumbosacral junction where the paraspinal muscles are broadly attached to the sacrum and the ilium. The bowing occurs to the side of the spasm in this instance (Fig 1–7,A).

Percussion of the spine to elicit point tenderness is routinely carried out with the hypothenar portion of the fist. Because a large area is covered with each blow to the spine and there is diffusion to several vertebral segments, it is more reasonable to use a percussion hammer and tap each spinous process. Often this accurately localizes the segments involved.

Pelvis and Rectum

Every general medical evaluation should include examinations of the pelvis and rectum. However, on neurologic evaluation these examinations are not called for unless the patient cues them by certain complaints. The most common cue is the complaint of low-back pain with or without radiation into the legs. Even though disk and spine or paraspinous disorders are the usual cause of this complaint, several common pelvic neoplastic disorders give rise to very similar complaints and may be associated with positive straight leg raising. Carcinoma of the cervix is the most common form of female pelvic neoplasm. It spreads by local extension and therefore (by invading the pelvic [lumbosacral] plexus) may first become symptomatic as low-back and/or leg pain. Carcinoma of the prostate is the most common male pelvic tumor and also spreads by local extension. Low-back and/or leg pain may be the symptom that brings a patient for medical attention. Rectal carcinoma occasionally gives rise to low-back pain because of spread to and enlargement of local lymph nodes. Rectal and pelvic examinations are mandatory when low-back pain is a complaint.

When urinary or fecal incontinence is present or a complaint, rectal examination is indicated to evaluate both reflex and voluntary anal sphincter function.

2

Hemispheric Function

EDWARD VALENSTEIN

ALTHOUGH GREAT functional specificity has always been attributed to structures in the brain stem and spinal cord, the cerebral hemispheres have often been thought to function as a whole. Damage to a portion of the hemisphere would affect all hemispheric function, to a degree proportional to the volume of brain destroyed. While this concept remains unproved for any human intellectual function, exceptions are easy to find. Persons with bilateral hippocampal lesions have defective memory but otherwise normal intellectual capacity. Persons with selective damage to the language areas in the dominant hemisphere are aphasic; tasks not related to language may be performed well.

In this chapter we comment on the value of a variety of clinical findings in the diagnosis and localization of disease in the cerebral hemispheres.

Regressive Reflexes

These are a group of reflexes normally present in an infant. They are inhibited by neocortical development but may reappear in persons with cortical lesions. They include feeding reflexes (rooting, sucking, or biting in response to tactile or visual stimuli) and forced grasping with hands (palmar grasp) or feet (plantar grasp). These reflexes are usually seen in persons with lesions in the fron-

tal lobes, and they provide unequivocal evidence of organic disease in patients who might otherwise be misdiagnosed as depressed or psychotic.

Certain other reflexes are also commonly seen in demented patients, but they are not so specific because they can also be seen in nondemented persons who have subcortical lesions. These include the oculocephalic (doll's eye, see chap. 3) and nuchocephalic* reflexes, the glabellar reflex (persistent blinking in response to repetitive tapping between the eyebrows), and the snout reflex (elicited by tapping the lips, which pucker in response).

Signs of Frontal Lobe Disease

The absence of specific cognitive deficits may well be the best evidence that a demented patient has disease primarily in the frontal lobes. When tested for memory, language, calculations, and perceptual skills, these patients may perform normally; however, in real life they display poor judgment, inadequate planning, and little motivation. With more advanced disease, they may become inappropriately jocular ("Witzelsucht") and irritable and lose their social graces. It has

---

*The patient is stood or seated with eyes closed in front of the examiner. The examiner rotates the patient's shoulders. The uninhibited response consists of the patient's head remaining straight.

been proposed that the frontal lobes are anatomically situated (in terms of their connections) between the perceptual-motor systems of the hemispheres and the limbic system and that lesions in the frontal lobes might then divorce perception and action from motivation.

Other persons with lesions primarily in the medial aspects of the frontal lobes display a marked paucity of movement (akinesia), which in its extreme is akinetic mutism. This suggests that there is some functional specialization within the frontal lobes; however, this has not yet been worked out.

Gegenhalten (paratonia) and perseveration are often seen in persons with frontal lobe lesions but are by no means specific for this location. *Gegenhalten* refers to an increase in tone; instead of relaxing, the patient either resists or tries to help when the examiner attempts to move the limbs passively. *Perseveration* refers to the repetition of a response when it is no longer appropriate. A person may raise his hand on command, for example, and then continue to raise his hand when asked to point to the floor or touch his nose. Verbal responses can similarly demonstrate perseveration. Perseveration may occur for a variety of reasons: inability to make the correct response, failure to check the response against the question, or lack of attention to the task. However, it also may be an inability to terminate or change ongoing motor activity or postures. This has been considered more likely to occur with loss of the inhibitory influences of the frontal lobes.

A number of tests have proved sensitive to the akinesia of patients with frontal lobe disease, and to their tendency to persist in incorrect behavior even when they know they are wrong. A test of word fluency can easily be given at the bedside. The patient is asked to produce in one minute as many words as he can (excluding proper nouns) beginning with a given letter. Normals can produce 14, ± 5, words using the letters A, F, or S. Patients with left frontal lobe lesions produce fewer words, and often repeat words or persist in using proper nouns. Psychologists can administer the Wisconsin Card-Sorting Test, which is also sensitive to frontal lobe deficits.

Functions of the Left ("Dominant") Hemisphere

LANGUAGE AND CEREBRAL DOMINANCE

In most people the left hemisphere is proficient in language functions. The right hemisphere is usually not devoid of linguistic ability; however, in most right-handers this ability is slight, whereas it is likely to be better in left-handers. Stated another way, the vast majority (more than 99%) of right-handers have control of language primarily in the left hemisphere; left-handers may have language control mostly in the left hemisphere or in both hemispheres, but rarely is it only on the right. Because of this dramatic asymmetry and because language is such an important function, cerebral "dominance" is usually equated with language dominance. As will be seen, however, there are hemispheric asymmetries for other functions as well, so one should not refer to a hemisphere as being "dominant" unless a specific function (such as language, handedness, or visuospatial skill) is specified.

Recent studies demonstrate a possible anatomical basis for language dominance: In two thirds of brains the supratemporal plane including Wernicke's area (a major language center) is larger on the left side, whereas it is larger on the right in only 11% of brains. This asymmetry is apparent from birth.

APHASIA

Our knowledge about the organization of language function in the brain comes in large part from the study of aphasic patients. The classification used here is based on the classical formulations of Karl Wernicke and others and on modern interpretations by

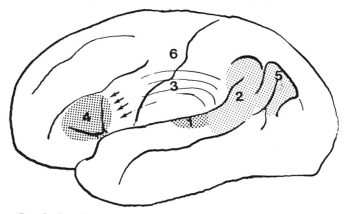

Fig 2–1.—Diagrammatic representation of major left cortical regions associated with verbal language functions. Key: *1*, Heschl's gyrus (auditory cortex); *2*, Wernicke's area; *3*, arcuate fasciculus; *4*, Broca's area; *5*, angular gyrus; *6*, motor cortex.

Geschwind and others. We present a simplified scheme.

Figure 2–1 illustrates the major language areas in the left hemisphere. Heschl's gyrus (1) is the primary auditory receiving area of the cortex. Adjacent to it lies Wernicke's area (2), which is the major auditory association area. This is connected via the arcuate fasciculus (3) to Broca's area (4), which is just anterior to the face areas on the motor strip. This peri-Sylvian region is thus well situated to receive and analyze auditory input and to produce verbal output (via the motor cortex). The functions of these peri-

Sylvian speech areas are best demonstrated by persons in whom the surrounding brain is destroyed, leaving these regions connected only to subcortical structures (Fig 2–2). Such persons with "isolation of the speech area" have little spontaneous speech but tend to repeat what is spoken to them (echolalia). They may correct grammatical errors in sentences they are given to repeat, and they can often complete rote phrases—for example, when told "roses are red . . ." they might say "violets are blue. . . ." They show little or no comprehension, even of language they can repeat perfectly. These

Fig 2–2.—Zone of left cortical destruction causing isolation of the speech area.

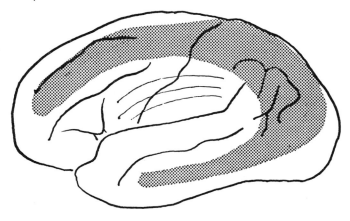

TABLE 2-1.—CLASSIFICATION OF APHASIA

TYPE OF APHASIA	SPONTANEOUS SPEECH	COMPRE-HENSION	REPETITION	NAMING	ASSOCIATED SIGNS
Transcortical					
Sensory, severe	Fluent, echolalic	Poor	Good	Poor	Variable (signs of "watershed" infarction)
Mild (anomic aphasia)	Fluent, circum-locutions	Good	Good	Poor	± Gerstmann's syndrome
Motor	Nonfluent except when repeating	Good	Good	Can be good	± Right hemiparesis
Mixed (sensory + motor), "isolation of the speech area"	Nonfluent	Poor	Good	Poor	Signs of watershed lesion (weakness in proximal upper extremity, etc.)
Wernicke's	Fluent, paraphasic	Poor	Poor	Poor	May be normal; may see visual field defect or cortical sensory loss; may have mild hemiparesis
Broca's	Nonfluent	Good	Poor (but can be better than sponta-neous speech)	Poor	Right hemiparesis
Conduction	Fluent, paraphasic	Good	Poor	Poor	Variable, often cortical sensory loss or loss of pain perception on right side
Global (Wernicke's + Broca's)	Nonfluent	Poor	Poor	Poor	Right hemiparesis

peri-Sylvian language areas can thus be re-garded as a repetition machine, with some knowledge of the rules of grammar and some ability to remember and learn language by rote. For language to be understood, these areas must be connected to other regions of the cortex, in particular to the angular gyrus (5). The angular gyrus is connected not only to the auditory association area but also to visual and somatosensory association areas, and is thus well situated to associate data from the different sensory areas. This may be crucial in the development of language: The angular gyrus is phylogenetically a recent development and is poorly developed in sub-human primates.

Aphasia of the isolated speech area is the most severe of a group of aphasias that spare the peri-Sylvian region and in which, there-fore, repetition is normal. These are the "transcortical" aphasias in Table 2-1. When only the anterior region is affected (see Fig

2-2) the only deficit is the inability of the person to initiate speech. Comprehension is normal and repetition is performed fluently. This is called *transcortical motor aphasia*. When the lesion is restricted to the posterior region (the angular gyrus), spontaneous speech, although vacuous, is fluent but lan-guage comprehension is poor (*transcortical sensory aphasia*). Anomic aphasia can be considered a mild form of transcortical sen-sory aphasia in which comprehension is nearly normal. Spontaneous speech is fluent and conveys meaning, but the person has trouble finding words and may give a defini-tion instead (for example, "that's the thing you write with" for "pencil").

Conversely, when the peri-Sylvian lan-guage areas are involved in a lesion, the re-sulting aphasia is characterized by faulty repetition. In severe cases persons may have trouble repeating single words; in mild cases they may have trouble only with complex grammatical sentences (such as "if he were here she would go" or "no ifs ands or buts"). Within this category, three distinct syndromes are recognized: Wernicke's aphasia, Broca's aphasia, and conduction aphasia (see Table 2–1).

When Wernicke's area is destroyed, there is usually a severe disruption of language comprehension, because most verbal input must travel through Wernicke's area. The fact that patients with Wernicke's aphasia fail to understand written as well as spoken language indicates that phonetic (visual-auditory) associations are required for reading. Spontaneous speech is fluent and copious; it appears that Broca's area, when left on its own, is quite loquacious. The language is vacuous, however, containing many meaningless "filler" phrases, paraphasias (incorrect words or syllables), and very few nouns.

Lesions in Broca's area for the most part spare comprehension, because Wernicke's area and its connections to the rest of the brain are intact. Speech is sparse (at the extreme, these patients are mute) and is produced with a great deal of effort.

A lesion that disconnects Wernicke's and Broca's areas (a lesion of the arcuate fasciculus) produces another distinctive type of aphasia: conduction aphasia. Here, spontaneous speech is fluent and paraphasic (since, as in Wernicke's aphasia, Broca's area is left on its own). Because Wernicke's area and its major posterior connections are intact, comprehension is relatively spared. Repetition, of course, is poor. To complicate matters, some patients with conduction aphasias actually have lesions in Wernicke's area. It is postulated that these patients have enough language function in the right hemisphere to subserve comprehension but that the right hemisphere is not proficient enough to repeat normally.

When both Broca's and Wernicke's areas are destroyed (as in a complete middle cerebral artery territory infarction), the patient is nonfluent (often mute) and has poor comprehension. This is called "global" aphasia.

Certain elementary neurologic findings may accompany the different types of aphasia and aid in the localization of the lesion. As would be expected from the proximity of Broca's area to the motor strip, Broca's aphasia is almost always accompanied by right hemiparesis. Patients with Wernicke's aphasia may show no elementary neurologic findings, or they may have a visual field deficit (frequently a homonymous superior quadrantanopia from interruption of the temporal optic radiations). Patients with conduction aphasia may have a sensory deficit, which in some cases is restricted to a deficit in pain sensation (the parietal operculum contains the secondary sensory area, which may be a cortical region for the appreciation of pain).

Examination of the aphasic patient should yield information about each of the categories listed in Table 2–1. *Spontaneous speech* should be described: Is it fluent (produced without effort, with groups of words or phrases) or nonfluent? Does it contain paraphasias or circumlocutions? *Comprehension* should be tested by having the person point to objects that you name (avoid gesturing) or by simple yes-no responses. It must first be ascertained whether yes-no answering is reliable: A patient with conduction aphasia may have good comprehension, but his verbal output may be unreliable so he could say yes for no. *Repetition* should be tested by having the patient repeat a complex grammatical phrase; if he fails, simpler phrases or single words can be tried. *Naming* can be tested by confrontation with the object or by verbal definitions. *Writing* is always abnormal in a true aphasic because aphasia involves a disturbance of language, not just of speech. Although a patient may be able to write his name or a single word, he is unable to produce linguistically correct sentences.

Aphasia should be differentiated from nonaphasic disorders of speech. *Dysarthria* refers to poor pronunciation. Although some aphasic patients are also dysarthric, most dysarthric patients produce normal language (if it can be understood). *Muteness* sometimes occurs acutely in persons with Broca's aphasia or global aphasia, but often mute patients do not have lesions in the cortical language areas. Muteness can be produced by bulbar or pseudobulbar paralysis or by severe akinesia (akinetic mutism—see chap. 20). If the mute patient is not aphasic, his writing (if it can be tested) is normal.

Recovery from aphasia probably results from resolution of the pathologic process (see chap. 7) and from takeover of language function by the right hemisphere. The more bilateral the speech representation, the less severe the aphasia and the more rapid the recovery. Aphasias therefore tend to be milder and of shorter duration in left-handers, who are likely to have bilateral speech representation. In addition, the ability of the right hemisphere to adopt language function decreases with age (probably as a result of the general decrease in "plasticity" of the nervous system), so that the prognosis for recovery from aphasia becomes increasingly worse with age. Left-hemisphere damage in childhood is generally well compensated.

GERSTMANN'S SYNDROME

Some persons do not have severe aphasia but nevertheless have difficulty with language-related tasks. The well-known Gerstmann's syndrome consists of deficits in four such tasks: writing, arithmetic, finger-naming, and right-left orientation (again, to verbal command or with verbal identification). As usually stated, the syndrome consists of agraphia, acalculia, finger agnosia, and right-left disorientation. Often there is mild anomic aphasia as well. When most or all of these signs are present in relative isolation, the lesion is most likely in the left hemisphere, in the region of the supramarginal and angular gyri.

APRAXIA

The term *apraxia* is commonly applied to so many different types of situations that its meaning has become diluted. We limit our discussion to one well-defined type of aprax-

ia (ideomotor apraxia), which is commonly seen in clinical practice.

Ideomotor apraxia is defined as the inability to follow a (verbal) command despite understanding the command and having the ability to perform the action other than to command. For example, if one says to a patient, "show me how you would blow out a match" and the patient says "puff," he has demonstrated comprehension of the command, but has produced an inadequate response. If you then present him with a lighted match, he may blow it out promptly, demonstrating that he has the capacity to perform the movements correctly but failed on command.

Persons with conduction aphasia commonly have ideomotor apraxia. This can be easily understood: The patient is able to comprehend the command (Wernicke's area and posterior connections are intact), but the direct pathways to the motor strip are interrupted, so that the patient must use inadequate alternate pathways to effect the movement. As a result, a poor imitation of the movement is made. With the direct sensory stimulus (that is, seeing the match burning), the appropriate motor response can be evoked by other pathways.

For similar reasons, persons with Broca's aphasia are usually apraxic with their left hands. Other examples of apraxic responses are given in Table 2–2.

TABLE 2–2.— EXAMPLES OF
IDEOMOTOR APRAXIA

COMMAND	APRAXIC RESPONSE
Show me how you would:	
Blow out a match	Says "puff" or makes inadequate blowing movements
Cough	Clears throat, etc., but does not cough properly
Brush your teeth	Uses finger as toothbrush instead of pretending to hold toothbrush
Use a hammer	Uses fist as hammer instead of pretending to hold hammer

Lesions of the Corpus Callosum and Disconnection Syndromes

A lesion can disrupt the connections between two cortical areas without interfering with the independent functioning of these areas. Functions that require transfer of information between these areas will then be deficient. Conduction aphasia and ideomotor apraxia are examples of disconnection syndromes. Another group of disconnection syndromes involve lesions of the corpus callosum. These syndromes all depend on language usually being largely restricted to the left hemisphere. The callosal lesions prevent the left hemisphere from receiving information from certain parts of the right hemisphere, and consequently the patient's verbal responses concerning this information are deficient.

Fig 2–3.—Left visual cortex and splenium infarction causing alexia without agraphia (pure word blindness). Words seen only in the left visual field cannot be transmitted from the right occipital cortex via the interrupted callosal pathway to the verbal language regions on the left.

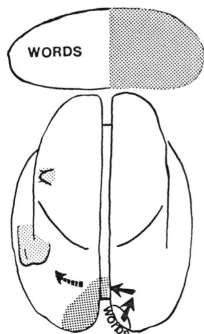

ALEXIA WITHOUT AGRAPHIA, OR PURE WORD BLINDNESS

This syndrome is most commonly caused by infarction of the left occipital cortex and the splenium (posterior fifth) of the corpus callosum (Fig 2–3). Both areas are in the territory of the posterior cerebral artery. The patient has a right homonymous hemianopia, but in addition, visual information that reaches the right occipital lobe cannot cross through the splenium of the corpus callosum to reach the language areas of the left hemisphere. The patient is therefore not able to read. Although some patients also cannot name objects that are presented visually (visual agnosia), in most persons (for reasons that are not clear) visual agnosia is restricted to color-naming. In contrast with the patient's inability to read, he is not aphasic and can write normally. If given enough time to forget what he has written, he is unable to read that also!

PURE WORD DEAFNESS

This syndrome is analogous to pure word blindness. The lesion usually destroys the left primary auditory cortex and also the callosal connections of the left auditory association area (Wernicke's area), but it does not involve Wernicke's area or the other speech areas (Fig 2–4). The person can hear (using Heschl's gyrus on the right side) but cannot understand spoken language. He may recognize the ring of the telephone, but when he answers it he hears "noise" instead of language and hangs up. His own speech is normal, and he can read and write normally. In contrast to pure word blindness (alexia without agraphia), which is caused by infarction in the territory of one vessel and is therefore quite common, pure word deafness is caused by a lesion or lesions in areas that are not usually affected selectively by vascular disease, and the syndrome is therefore very rare. When it does occur it is likely to be diagnosed as a psychiatric problem.

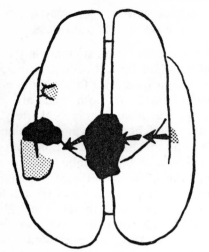

Fig 2–4.—Metastatic tumor destroying the left auditory cortex and callosal connections of right auditory cortex to Wernicke's area, causing pure word deafness.

SECTIONS OF THE CORPUS CALLOSUM

The entire corpus callosum and anterior commissure have been sectioned for the treatment of intractable epilepsy (to prevent the spread of seizure discharges). Surprisingly, patients who were treated functioned quite well and were initially thought to be normal. When tested carefully, however, typical deficits were detected: The patients were alexic in their left visual field, they could not name objects placed in their left hands, they could not write with their left hands (something all normal persons can do even though their handwriting may be bad), they were apraxic with their left hands, and they could not transfer visual or tactile information from one hemisphere to the other. Because in nonexperimental settings visual information is not confined to one half-field (the eyes move) and information can be transferred from one hand to the other in many ways (visual, transferring the object, making a sound with the object, and so on), these deficits are not bothersome to the patients. Occasionally, however, they complain of strange things happening. One patient told

his physician that he had tried to hit his wife without knowing why. Even though he was right-handed, he had tried to hit her with his left hand. Of course, in a sense, the "patient" who was talking to the physician was not the same "patient" who hit his wife; the talking patient—that is, the patient's left hemisphere—did not know why his own right hemisphere directed his left hand to hit his wife. It appears, then, that callosally sectioned patients actually have two relatively independent "identities"; however, the continuity of experience usually suffices to prevent overt conflict.

Functions of the Right Hemisphere

The right hemisphere, although relatively aphasic, has skills of its own. Precise definition of these skills has proved difficult, but evidence is now good that the right hemisphere is dominant for complex visuospatial analysis. When a person with a callosal section is presented complex nonverbal, visual stimuli, he can recognize and recall stimuli presented to the left half-field accurately and without effort, whereas the same sort of figures presented to the right half-field are recognized (often inaccurately) only after extensive (often verbal) analysis. Patients with right hemisphere lesions may have difficulty in drawing maps (or placing cities correctly on maps) or in finding their way about the hospital ward.

There is also some evidence that musical abilities are more severely impaired by lesions in the right hemisphere. Persons with right temporal lobectomies have more difficulty remembering melodies than those with left temporal lobectomies who have more difficulty with verbal memory, although the more posterior language areas are intact.

Denial of illness and neglect of the left side are the most striking and common problems encountered in persons with right hemisphere disease. Denial of illness may vary from explicit denial of all disability to (usually implausible) minimization of a disability ("Oh, that's my lazy left side again"). One severely affected patient, when turned on his right side for a lumbar puncture, complained that someone was lying on top of him; the "other person" was his left side! The patient usually fails to orient to stimuli on the left side, whether visual, auditory, or tactile. Mild forms of left-sided neglect may have to be elicited by double simultaneous stimulation; a stimulus to the normal (right) side prevents the appreciation of a stimulus to the left side ("extinction").

These findings can in large part be explained by considering two aspects of behavior that are impaired in these persons: attention and emotional behavior. In animals, attention to the contralateral half of space can be diminished by unilateral lesions in certain regions of the frontal and parietal lobes, the cingulate gyrus, the thalamic intralaminar nuclei, and the brain stem (midbrain) reticular activating system. It has been postulated that these regions (among others) are part of a system by which the cortex, having processed information it deems novel or significant for the organism, can arouse the hemisphere via midbrain and thalamic activating systems. The neglect seen in animals with lesions in these areas is similar to that in humans with right hemisphere lesions. If this proposal is correct, one would expect (since these systems are bilateral) to see similar neglect in persons with left hemisphere lesions. In fact, we do, but the neglect is usually much less severe. This suggests that there is an important hemispheric asymmetry in attentional mechanisms. It has been proposed that the right hemisphere normally is able to mediate attention to either side, and thus partially to compensate for attentional deficits caused by left hemisphere lesions. The left hemisphere can only mediate attention to the right, and therefore right hemisphere lesions result in severe bilateral attentional deficits, with some ability to orient to right-sided stimuli preserved by function of the left hemisphere.

Patients with right hemisphere lesions also have striking abnormalities in emotional behavior. They are emotionally flat. They rarely get upset by their disability and they rarely appear deeply depressed. They have difficulty understanding emotional inflection and they are unable to imitate emotional inflection in their own speech. Further evidence to support the importance of the right hemisphere in emotional behavior comes from studies showing that electric shock administered to the right hemisphere is more effective in relieving depression than shocks to the left hemisphere.

Memory

Memory is a complex function, and it is likely that "memories" are "stored" in many areas of the brain. The laying down of memories, however, appears to be a function of restricted areas of the limbic system and thalamus, including the hippocampi, the dorsomedial thalamic nucleus, and possibly the mammillary bodies and fornix. Bilateral lesions of these structures result in an amnesic state. Although there are variations in the clinical presentation, the overall pattern of memory loss is remarkably uniform regardless of the type of pathology.

The amnesic syndrome consists of (1) anterograde amnesia (failure to learn new material), (2) retrograde amnesia (failure to retrieve memories acquired prior to the onset of the lesion), and (3) relative sparing of remote memories.

Charlie Q., 28 years old and recently married, flew off his motorcycle and hit a tree with his head. He was unconscious for three days and over the next week gradually became communicative. At that time, he failed to recognize his physicians, even though they saw him every day and always told him who they were. He knew his parents but failed to recognize his wife. He thought it was 1967 (it was actually 1974) and that Johnson was President. After two months he began to improve. His retrograde amnesia began to shrink, events in the past (late 1960s) generally recovering before more recent events, although events of great significance (such as his marriage) tended to recover sooner. When he was again able to remember new material (loss of the anterograde amnesia), his retrograde amnesia had shrunk to a few days prior to the motorcycle accident.

To explain these findings, the following have been postulated: (1) because anterograde amnesia is always accompanied by retrograde amnesia, it is likely that the mechanism used for encoding memories is the same as, or closely related to, the mechanism used for retrieval of recent memories; and (2) retrieval of remote memories is achieved by a different mechanism. We may suppose that normally memories decay if not reinforced. Reinforcement may take place by repetition or may only require that the memories have significance to the person. On the average, recent memories are less well reinforced than remote memories simply because remote information that was not reinforced is already lost. If well-reinforced memories were stored differently from poorly reinforced memories (for example, if they were represented more diffusely in the hemispheres), they might be retrieved more easily and therefore might not require the special mechanism needed for the retrieval of poorly reinforced memories.

Immediate memory (called "short-term memory" by some), as tested by the ability to repeat information without any intervening distraction, is not involved in classical amnesic syndromes in humans. For this reason, tests of immediate memory (such as the digit span test) should be regarded as tests of attention. Obviously, immediate or short-term memory is a prerequisite for the acquisition of "long-term" (what we have called "recent" and "remote") memories. Memory should be tested by giving a person something to remember, asking him to repeat it immediately (to be sure he is attentive), distracting him by giving other tests, and after three to five minutes asking him to remember (test of memorization or recent memory). Recent memory can be tested further by checking orientation to place and time and by asking about current events and recent

presidents. Remote memory can be tested by asking about well-known events during a person's youth.

The Mental Status Examination

An outline of a brief mental status examination is given in Table 2–3. The preliminary assessment, requiring only observation during conversation plus a few questions regarding thought content, helps to rule out deficits that might invalidate further testing.

TABLE 2–3.—BRIEF MENTAL STATUS EXAMINATION

A. Preliminary observations
  1. State of consciousness (comatose, drowsy, alert)
  2. Attentiveness
  3. Mood and affect (?depressed, euphoric, indifferent, etc.)
  4. Thought content (?hallucinations, paranoia, etc.)
  5. Behavior (inappropriate jocularity, rudeness, etc.)
B. Memory
  1. Orientation to time and place
  2. Digit span (a test of attentiveness)
  3. Give patient three items to remember; require recall three minutes after distraction
  4. Other tests of recent memory: current events, presidents, etc.
  5. Remote memory (old news events, childhood memories, etc.)
C. Manipulation of knowledge (reasoning)
  1. Proverb interpretations
  2. Similarities (what is the same about a chair and a table, etc.)
D. Left-hemisphere function
  1. Gerstmann's syndrome
    a. Calculations
    b. Writing
    c. Right-left orientation
    d. Finger identification ("show me your ring finger," etc.)
  2. Aphasia testing: listen to spontaneous speech; test naming. If both are normal and the patient comprehends language well, no further testing is needed. If not, proceed to a more thorough evaluation, as outlined in the section on aphasia.
E. Right-hemisphere function
  1. Map localization
  2. Constructional apraxia (see text—this actually also tests left-hemisphere function)
  3. Observe for dressing apraxia, etc.
F. Further testing if indicated

In addition, if a person is obviously aphasic, specific aphasia testing (to define the limits of language comprehension and expressive abilities) should be done before any attempt is made to complete the routine mental status examination.

Memory should be tested as outlined in the previous section. Interpretation of proverbs and similarities tests the patient's reasoning abilities. Although deficits in these functions may not be localizing, they may at times be the most striking evidence for dementia. It is wise to remember that memory may be entirely normal in the demented patient so long as the hippocampi and the other structures needed for the acquisition of memories are spared.

The screening examination should include tests for the components of Gerstmann's syndrome and a simple test or two for right-hemisphere function; map localization is easily tested. The ability to copy a cube (a test for constructional apraxia) is lost with disease in either hemisphere and is therefore a reasonably good screening test for hemispheric disease. Performance on a mental status examination (and especially on tests of proverb interpretation, arithmetic, and similar skills) must be evaluated in light of the patient's education, social background, and level of cooperation and motivation.

More extensive testing may be necessary if deficits are found. This testing may be based on the ideas set forth in this chapter or it may be designed to test other ideas. It is always wise to be flexible in examining these functions: The information obtained depends, to a great extent, on the questions asked. Although some clinicians are particularly knowledgeable and skilled in testing higher mental functions, there is no final authority. The examination of a patient with deficits in higher integrative functions is, at best, an experiment designed to further our knowledge about the function of the human brain.

REFERENCES

Benson, D. F.: *Aphasia, Alexia, and Agraphia.* New York, Churchill Livingstone, 1979.

Geschwind, N.: *Selected Papers on Language and the Brain.* Boston, Reidel, 1974.

Vinken, P. J., Bruyn, F. W. (eds.): Disorders of speech, perception and symbolic behavior, in *Handbook of Clinical Neurology,* vol. 4. New York, John Wiley & Sons, 1969.

3

Cranial Nerve Evaluation

IN THIS CHAPTER, the cranial nerves and their testing are discussed along with examples of disease states that involve individual nerves. Cranial nerves are more often involved singly or in groups as part of a complex syndrome of dysfunction in which many elements of the nervous system are affected. There is great value in careful evaluation and recognition of involvement of the cranial nerves because this frequently allows a close anatomical definition of pathology. Recognition of involvement of the long-tract systems, motor and sensory, is less helpful in localizing because they extend from the hemisphere through the spinal cord.

I. Olfaction

Unilateral depression or loss of olfaction occurs only when destructive or occluding processes affect the olfactory pathway at or rostral to the olfactory trigone (Fig 3–1). Dysfunction must be in the olfactory tract, bulbs, nerve filaments, or olfactory mucosa in the roof of the nasal passages.

The olfactory pathway divides in front of the anterior perforated substance to travel via (1) the lateral olfactory stria to the primary olfactory cortex (prepyriform-pyriform) in the ipsilateral temporal lobe and (2) the anterior limb or stria (not the medial stria) that dives into the anterior perforated substance to join the anterior commissure, which carries it to the contralateral olfactory cortex. Destruction of olfactory cortex or olfactory pathways distal to the trigone must be bilat-

eral to depress olfactory function. Potentially irritative lesions (tumor, posttraumatic or ischemic scarring, arteriovenous abnormalities, etc.) in the olfactory cortical regions may be the source of epileptiform activity and cause olfactory symptoms; that is, the patient may complain of hallucinations of smell. Typically, these olfactory hallucinations are described as acrid and unpleasant and are not lateralized by the patient.

Olfaction is tested by having a patient with eyes closed, sniff a relatively familiar odor from a small vial, occluding the nares alternately to test each side separately. Substances such as acetic acid and ammonia should not be used for testing because they cause strong trigeminal stimulation and can therefore be sensed by an anosmic person. Coffee grounds are popular because they are recognized by approximately 80% of normal individuals and cause minimal trigeminal stimulation. Three distinct levels of function can be determined: (1) cannot smell, (2) can smell something, (3) recognizes coffee. In addition, a person may recognize an asymmetry of sensitivity despite an inability to recognize the substance. Lack of recognition is not significant if the patient responds by saying he smells a substance bilaterally; recognition on one side suggests contralateral hyposmia if the patient claims to smell something only on the opposite side.

Examples of disease processes that cause or are associated with decreased or otherwise abnormal smell are as follows:

1. Mechanical.

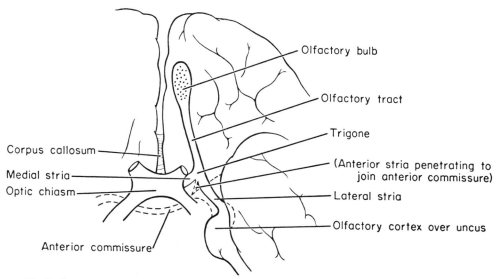

Fig 3–1.—Basal view of cerebral hemispheres showing the olfactory system. Lesions of the trigone, tract, bulb, olfactory filaments (schematically represented by dots on olfactory bulb), and olfactory epithelium cause unilateral loss of olfaction. Unilateral lesions of the lateral stria or olfactory cortex do not cause loss of olfaction because of the bilateral temporal lobe distribution of each olfactory apparatus through the anterior stria and anterior commissure.

a. Common cold with occlusion of nasal passages (most common cause of hyposmia).

b. Unilateral occlusion by deviated nasal septum.

c. Occipital head trauma with shearing effect on olfactory nerve filaments passing through cribriform plate (Fig 3–2).

d. Frontal head trauma, if it results in a fracture line through the cribriform plate, causes anosmia by tearing the fine olfactory nerve filaments. (In the absence of fracture, frontal head trauma is less likely to cause hyposmia.)

e. Tumors (most commonly meningioma) on the mid portion of the sphenoid ridge or in the olfactory groove, both capable of pressing on the olfactory tract. If the tumor is on the sphenoid ridge so that, in addition to pushing on the olfactory tract, it compresses down on the optic nerve, it causes the syndrome of ipsilateral anosmia, optic atrophy, and possibly also contralateral papilledema because of increased intracranial pressure (Foster-Kennedy syndrome).

2. Metabolic.

a. Pernicious anemia (vitamin B_{12} deficiency) is frequently associated with bilateral decreased olfaction.

b. Vitamin A deficiency is associated with hyposmia and dysosmia (odors are unpleasant), possibly the result of nasal mucosal abnormalities.

c. Zinc deficiency has recently been associated with hyposmia and dysosmia.

d. Diabetes mellitus. Presumably this hyposmia is secondary to demyelination in the olfactory tracts or loss of the peripheral olfactory neuron.

e. Multiple sclerosis is a rare cause of hyposmia, presumably on the basis of olfactory tract demyelination.

f. Herpes simplex encephalitis, which tends to localize in the temporal lobes

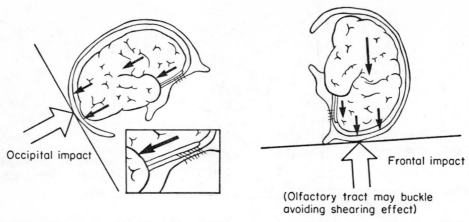

Occipital impact

Frontal impact

(Olfactory tract may buckle avoiding shearing effect)

Fig 3–2.—Shearing of olfactory nerve filaments with occipital trauma; it is less prominent with frontal trauma.

and cause severe hemorrhagic necrotic destruction, may cause anosmia secondary to bilateral olfactory cortex destruction or alternatively, because the virus may enter the nervous system via the olfactory mucosa, may destroy one or both olfactory nerves and bulbs in the process. The presentation of acute-onset anosmia and a severe memory-encoding deficit (the latter secondary to bilateral mesial temporal lobe destruction) in a person who is febrile suggests the possibility of herpes simplex encephalitis, a potentially treatable disorder.

g. Hepatic disease, particularly acute hepatitis, is frequently associated with an unpleasantness of odors (dysosmia).

Unilateral destructive or compressing (mass) lesions in the anterior temporal lobe may cause olfactory hallucinations, a focal epileptiform discharge that often spreads to involve other portions of the limbic system and neocortex (see chap. 9).

II. Vision

For a more detailed elaboration of visual system anatomy and function, refer to a neuroanatomy text. Figure 3–3 shows diagrammatic representations of the visual pathway including expected abnormalities of vision caused by lesions of its various parts.

Unilateral lesions of the retina and optic nerves cause monocular defects. Lesions from the chiasm back give rise to binocular field defects because of crossing of the nasal half of the retinal fibers from each eye. An exception to this rule occurs when there is involvement of the fibers representing the nasal retinal (temporal field) peripheral crescents. The fibers from this portion of the retina have no homonymous counterpart in the opposite peripheral temporal retina (nasal field). Peripheral crescents, therefore, remain monocular in representation from the retina to the visual cortex (Figs 3 – 3 to 3 – 5).

Formal testing of vision divides this function into two basic aspects: (1) central or cone vision and (2) peripheral or rod vision. Peripheral vision is the greatest part of the visual field, whereas central vision represents a relatively small segment of the projected visual world. Nevertheless, it is mainly with central vision that we interpret our lighted environment with the cones being the substrate for accurate as well as color vision. Peripheral visual awareness serves a major orienting function of directing central vision by visual-oculomotor responses toward peripheral stimuli. The more peripheral the field, the less capable of form or figure perception it becomes, which is in keeping with the centrifugal thinning out of the population of peripheral field receptors (rods) in the retina. At the far periphery one is capable of perceiving only moving objects, and at the borders of the field only retinal-oculomotor reflexes remain (the eyes are reflexively turned toward a moving stimulus, which is not consciously perceived). Rods have a very low threshold for activation (pigment bleaching) by light as compared with cones and are thus more suited for night vision. The cones, with a high threshold for pigment bleaching by light, are relatively useless in the dark.

Visual acuity is first tested by having a person read a chart containing standard-sized figures (numbers, letters, or other forms) as perceived at a standard distance. The notation 20/20 vision means that at 20 ft a size 20 object can be perceived, 20/70 that a size 70 object can be perceived at 20 ft, and so on. This type of testing is not practical at the bedside, so charts have been developed to be presented at 14 in. (Fig 3–6). These give an extrapolated visual acuity in terms of 20 ft and determine neurologic visual dysfunction but may miss refraction errors, particularly nearsightedness (myopia). For quick screening it is useful to know that recognition of small-case newsprint at 14 in. is equivalent to 20/30 vision.

Visual acuity can be depressed by ocular media changes, that is, changes in the ocular structures anterior to the retina. Before we can make any conclusion concerning possible neurologic depression of visual acuity, it is necessary to rule out these anterior causes of difficulty. If a person customarily wears glasses, he should be tested with them on. If difficulties still exist, then acuity testing should be supplemented. Occlusive processes (e.g., cataracts) can usually be seen on ophthalmoscopic examination, and refraction errors can be corrected with a series of lenses or, more simply, at the bedside by attempting to correct acuity loss with a pinhole that neatly corrects most refraction errors (Fig 3–7). It does this by allowing parallel rays to pass only through the central nonrefracting portion of the ocular apparatus, thus simulating with the globe a pinhole camera capable of the infinite focus of an image on the retina. Pinholes would make inexpensive but impractical glasses, however, because peripheral vision, most central vision, and a great amount of light are eliminated.

A further way to test refractive errors, which is particularly useful in the uncooperative patient, is to determine the diopters (e.g., +3, −3) of ophthalmoscope adjustment necessary to focus on the macula or optic nerve head. This assumes 0 to be equivalent to normal acuity.

After determining that the acuity deficit is not a refraction or occlusive problem and therefore, by default, is a dysfunction in the neural visual apparatus, it is necessary to determine visual field integrity to discover the locus of involvement. Visual field loss tends not to be an all-or-nothing phenomenon. The patient frequently has a partial deficit, particularly in the central field, and can see larger objects persisting after small objects are no longer perceived. Small objects are therefore best used in attempting to find deficits.

Central fields are tested formally by using a large tangent screen 3 m from the subject who is asked to fixate on a central target. Various sized objects are projected onto or moved in front of the screen, and the patient's capabilities with each eye are mapped (Fig 3–8).

At the bedside, the method of confrontation is used and can be quite accurate if carefully done. One eye (e.g., the left) is covered and the person is asked to fix his vision on the examiner's pupil (i.e., the right) at a distance of approximately 1.5 ft. A small, colored object (3 mm red—a match is adequate) is moved into the central field halfway between the patient and the examiner, and the patient is asked to indicate when he sees the object turn red and whether it disappears or loses its color anywhere in the field. This technique allows the examiner to compare

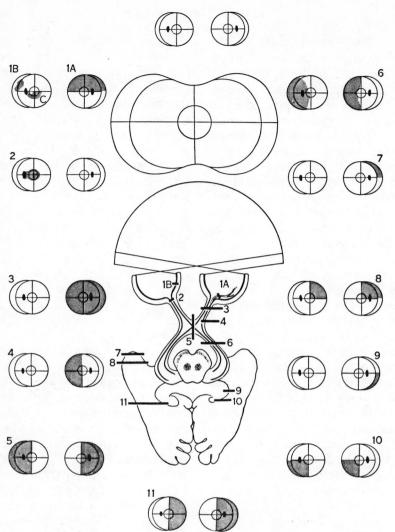

Fig 3–3.—1, retinal lesions (scotomata): (a) Vascular—ischemic, hemorrhagic. Typical and pathognomonic altitudinal defect is seen with branch arterial occlusion; appropriate for altitudinal distribution of renal arteries. Complete blindness occurs and is associated with central retinal artery occlusion by atherosclerosis, embolism, arteritis, or the arterial compression of severe papilledema. (b) Inflammatory—choroiditis, granuloma; neoplastic—primary or metastatic; mechanical—retinal tear or detachment. (c) Glaucoma—frequent selective nerve fiber bundle loss causing a crescent scotoma. 2, loss of central (macular) visual bundle (central scotoma): (a) Demyelination—multiple sclerosis, isolated optic neuritis. (b) Ischemia of optic nerve. (c) Metabolic—vitamin B_{12} deficiency; alcoholic—nutritional amblyopia. 3, transection of optic nerve (monocular blindness): (a) Tumor—subfrontal (sphenoid wing) meningioma, optic glioma. (b) Trauma—laceration. 4, loss of lateral portion of optic chiasma (nasal

hemianopia): Mechanical compression by enlarged, atherosclerotic carotid artery; can be unilateral or bilateral. 5, loss of medial portion of chiasma (bitemporal hemianopia): (a) Tumor—pituitary neoplasm, most often chromophobe adenoma with suprasellar extensions, or suprasellar neoplasm such as craniopharyngioma. (b) Hydrocephalus with ballooning of floor of third ventricle. 6, optic tract or lateral geniculate loss (contralateral homonymous hemianopia—frequently incongruous): Vascular—infarction in distribution of anterior choroidal artery. 7, monocular crescent bundle (contralateral superior monocular crescent defect): Tumor, infarction, or hemorrhage in anterior temporal lobe or potentially also with involvement of anterior inferior calcarine cortex. 8, loss of temporal radiations, i.e., Meyer's loop (contralateral homonymous superior quadrantanopia): Tumor, infarction, or hemorrhage in temporal lobe. 9, loss of upper monocular crescent bundle (contralateral inferior monocular crescentic defect): Tumor, infarction, or hemorrhage

30

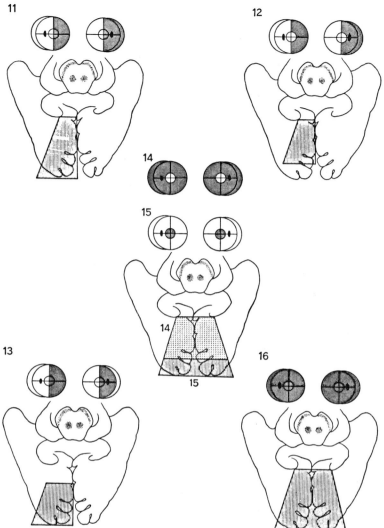

in parietal lobe or anterior superior calcarine cortex. 10, loss of parietal radiations (contralateral homonymous inferior quadrantanopia): Tumor, infarction, or hemorrhage in lower parietal region or upper calcarine cortex. 11, loss of total optic radiation (contralateral homonymous hemianopia, usually congruous): Tumor, infarction, or hemorrhage, temporal-parietal junction. 12, loss of anterior and middle calcarine cortex (contralateral homonymous hemianopia with macular sparing): Macular sparing occurs when calcarine infarction is caused by posterior cerebral artery occlusion if the middle cerebral artery supplies the posterior calcarine cortex. 13, loss of middle and posterior calcarine cortex (contralateral homonymous hemianopia with monocular crescent sparing): Tumor, infarction, or hemorrhage unilaterally in calcarine cortex. 14, loss of anterior and middle calcarine cortex bilaterally (loss of all peripheral vision with sparing of central vision—keyhole vision): Parasagittal tumor bilaterally compressing both anterior and middle portions

of calcarine cortex; this type of defect is more commonly seen with bilateral peripheral retinal encroachment such as progressive retinitis pigmentosa and occasionally chronic papilledema. Bilateral posterior cerebral artery occlusion may leave a similar field if middle cerebral artery collateral is adequate posteriorly. 15, bilateral loss of posterior calcarine cortex (bilateral central visual field loss): Parasagittal tumor bilaterally compressing posterior calcarine cortex; this type of defect is more commonly seen following bilateral optic nerve involvement (see 2). 16, bilateral complete loss of calcarine cortex (cortical blindness): Bilateral posterior cerebral artery occlusion, usually at or near bifurcation from basilar artery. This type of blindness is frequently associated with denial of visual loss (Anton's syndrome), presumably a result of bilateral mesial temporal lobe ischemia-infarction. Parasagittal tumor and trauma with extensive mesial occipital calcarine compression or contusion are less common causes of cortical blindness.

31

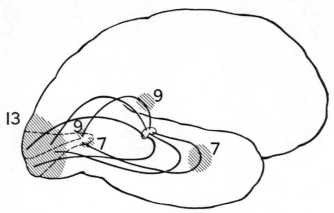

Fig 3—4.—Lateral view of right visual radiations. See Figure 3—3 for details of lesions 7, 9, and 13.

the patient's vision with his own (presumably normal) and, additionally, he can observe whether the patient is fixating on the central object (examiner's pupil) during the examination. This latter observation cannot be made during the tangent screen testing. A colored object is used because it defines the major extent of cone vision and because, on occasion, a partial loss of central vision manifests itself more as a depression of color perception than as depression of visual acuity. The subject reports any change in color or loss of color of the object within the central field (a chromatopsic defect).

Also, if central visual loss has existed for a long time (two weeks or more), examination of the appropriate fundus with an ophthalmoscope may reveal evidence of atrophy of the temporal portion of the optic nerve head (optic disk), which contains the macular or central fibers. Atrophy causes the disk to become pale owing to gradual loss of its blood supply along with loss of functional nervous tissue. Comparison with the opposite disk is useful in borderline cases when changes are minimal and the problem is monocular.

In the temporal portion of the visual field, a well-delineated oval scotoma or blind spot is always present (see Fig 3—8). This repre-

Fig 3—5.—Schematic representation of visual fields.

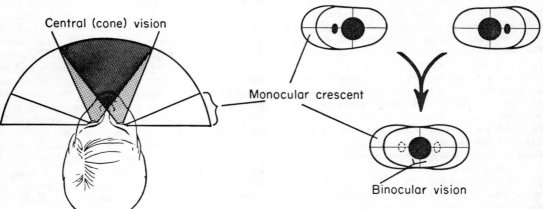

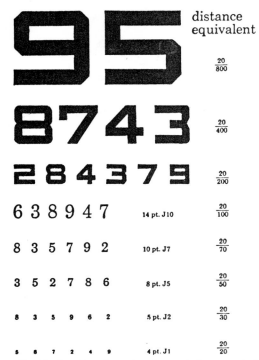

distance equivalent

$\frac{20}{800}$

$\frac{20}{400}$

$\frac{20}{200}$

6 3 8 9 4 7   14 pt. J10 $\frac{20}{100}$

8 3 5 7 9 2   10 pt. J7 $\frac{20}{70}$

3 5 2 7 8 6   8 pt. J5 $\frac{20}{50}$

8 3 5 9 6 2   5 pt. J2 $\frac{20}{30}$

5 8 7 2 4 9   4 pt. J1 $\frac{20}{20}$

Fig 3–6.—Visual acuity chart of the actual size used to determine visual acuity at 14 in.

sents the nerve head of the optic fundus (the disk), which is not covered by receptive retinal tissue. When a 3-mm object is passed over this area, a person usually says it disappears. Because the presence of a blind spot in the visual field is occasionally denied on con-

frontation, it is necessary to suggest to the patient that the object will likely disappear in some part of the visual field. If the object is moving midway between the examiner and the patient and both are fixating on each others' pupils, their blind spots should be superimposed. If, when the examiner loses the object in his blind spot, the patient does not do the same, the confrontation field examination is not reliable. Checking the reliability of the examination is the main reason for seeking the blind spot at the bedside. Tangent screen testing allows accurate mapping of the blind spot. An early sign of edema or swelling of the optic disk (papilledema) is enlargement of the blind spot. This is because the retina is extremely sensitive to mechanical pressure, and minimal, unobservable edema of the optic nerve head causes significant dysfunction in the bordering receptive retina and therefore enlargement of the blind spot.

Peripheral visual fields are formally tested using the tangent screen (Fig 3–8) and more completely using a perimeter (Fig 3–9), which takes into account that the total visual field is an arc (see Fig 3–5). A tangent screen is flat and so cannot demonstrate the total extent of the peripheral visual field. A relatively large, white (color is not useful with rod vision testing) object (approximately 10 mm in diameter) is moved along the perime-

Fig 3–7.—Use of pinhole to correct for abnormalities of visual refraction when measuring visual acuity.

Plastic spoon with pinholes 4 mm. apart (made with heated pin)

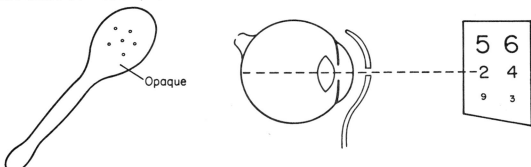

Opaque

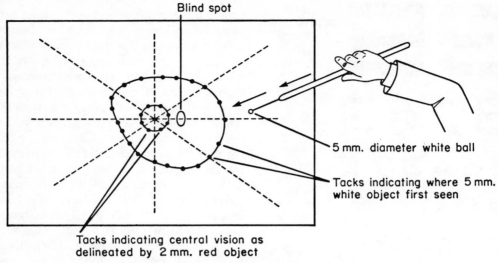

Blind spot

5 mm. diameter white ball

Tacks indicating where 5 mm. white object first seen

Tacks indicating central vision as delineated by 2 mm. red object

Fig 3—8. — Tangent screen examination of visual field.

ter from the outside in and the peripheral field is mapped out in degrees. The outside limits represent where the patient, while fixing on a central target, first sees the moving object. A simple and more practical technique is used at the bedside. The patient is asked to fixate on the examiner's pupil as in testing central vision, and a large object, frequently the examiner's index finger, tip first, is moved into the patient's visual field from a position lateral to the patient's head. The

peripheral fields are thus approximated within a few moments (Fig 3 – 10).

It is useful at the bedside to use tachystoscopic double simultaneous stimulation (TDSS) of the visual fields. This entails the rapid momentary presentation of two objects simultaneously into opposite fields. In practice a momentary movement of the tip of the index finger in both fields is suitable (see Fig 3 – 10). Screening to test all peripheral quadrants with both of the patient's eyes open and

Fig 3—9. — Perimetric examination to determine complete visual field. In the example, only peripheral vision is measured. To measure central vision, a small (e.g., 2 mm), colored object is used.

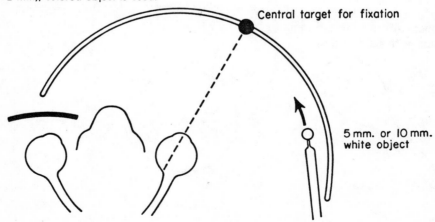

Central target for fixation

5 mm. or 10 mm. white object

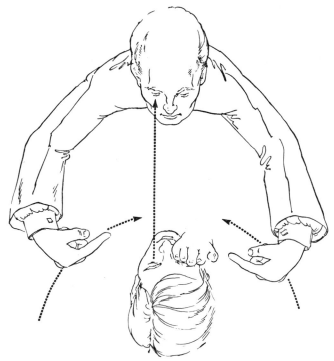

Fig 3–10.—Technique for confrontation examination of visual fields.

fixating on the examiner's nose reveals all peripheral defects except the rare nasal hemianopias and hemianopias with temporal crescent sparing (see Fig 3–4). Monocular testing does not miss any peripheral defects but takes twice as long. TDSS testing is advantageous because minor partial field deficits, which may not be picked up on unilateral stimulation, become apparent; the object in the abnormal field is extinguished. A rapid single excursion of the examiner's index fingers in the peripheral fields is adequate (see Fig 3–10). Double simultaneous stimulation with red match heads (3-mm object) is useful for central field testing; the subject is asked to respond whether he sees one or two *red* objects, which are moved rapidly in and out of the central fields. Extinction in the visual field may represent either a partial dysfunction in the visual pathways or an inattention phenomenon. This difficulty is usu-

ally part of a broader syndrome of hemispatial inattention, usually resulting from contralateral telencephalic lesions, particularly in the cortex, which are often parietal but occasionally frontal in location.

III, IV, VI. Ocular Motility

Oculomotor function can be divided into two categories: (1) *extraocular muscle function*, which is represented by the medial, inferior, and superior recti, the inferior oblique, and levator palpebrae muscles, all innervated by the oculomotor nerve (III); the superior oblique muscle innervated by the trochlear nerve (IV); and the lateral rectus muscle innervated by the abducens nerve (VI); and (2) *intrinsic ocular muscles,* which are innervated by the autonomic systems and include the iris sphincter and the ciliary apparatus of accommodation, innervated by the parasympathetic component of cranial nerve III, and the radial pupillodilator muscles, innervated by the ascending cervical sympathetic system with its spinal origin from segments T1 through T3.

EXTRAOCULAR MUSCLE FUNCTION

Figure 3–11 illustrates the correct eye positions for testing the extraocular muscles in relative isolation. As can be seen in Figures 3–11 and 3–12, a lateral position of the eyeball is necessary for testing the inferior and superior recti, whereas a medial position is necessary for testing the inferior and superior oblique muscles. In the position of lateral gaze, the superior and inferior rectus muscles lie in line with the axis of the globe; in the nasal or medial gaze position, the obliques become nearly parallel to the axis of the globe and are, therefore, the prime muscles for vertical gaze. Vertical gaze from the neutral position (Fig 3–11) tests both the vertical rectus and to a lesser degree the oblique muscles. It is necessary to evaluate vertical movements from the neutral position

to determine the presence of vertical nystagmus, a sign of brain stem as opposed to peripheral vestibular system involvement (for further information, refer to the section on cranial nerve VIII), and to determine the integrity of the supranuclear function vertical gaze, which may be defective despite adequate individual muscle activity. Figure 3–13 illustrates the expected findings with isolated loss of function of cranial nerves III, IV, and VI. The broken vector lines show which versions are lost. The solid vector lines indicate the resting tonus of the remaining extraocular muscles. Following denervation, as a rule, the eye at rest lies in the direction of the now-unopposed antagonist muscles. The afflicted person frequently adjusts his head in an attempt to ameliorate the double vision caused by the muscle imbalance. This may be successful if cranial nerve IV or VI is involved but only when the eyes are at rest in the ideal compensatory position. When cranial nerve III is involved, the imbalance is usually too great to be accommodated.

The person with an extraocular muscle

Fig 3–11. — Eye positions for testing extraocular muscle function.

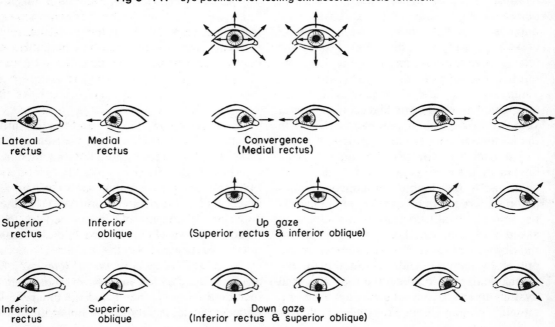

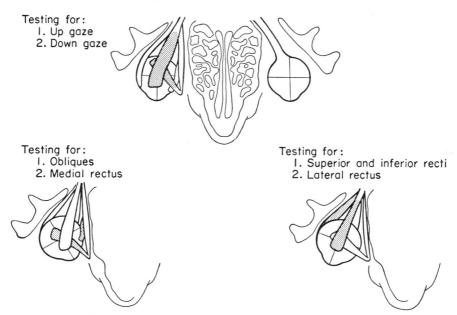

Testing for:
1. Up gaze
2. Down gaze

Testing for:
1. Obliques
2. Medial rectus

Testing for:
1. Superior and inferior recti
2. Lateral rectus

Fig 3–12.—Appropriate eye positions for initiating oblique and vertical rectus muscle versions in relative isolation and for testing up and down gaze.

defect of recent onset usually complains of double vision (diplopia). This results from the inability to fuse the macular regions (central vision) of both eyes on an object. The weak muscle is unable to focus the object on the macula; the image falls on an area peripheral to the macula and the person sees the object in the field appropriate to the new retinal position (i.e., always farther out in the field of attempted gaze) and therefore it appears to the brain as a second image. Additionally, because the image falls on a lesser density of cones, it is less distinct, and the person may compare it to the ghost images seen on maladjusted television sets. One can delineate which extraocular muscle or muscles are defective by determining which eye sees the abnormal image (the image farthest out in the field of gaze and blurred). This can be done by placing a transparent red piece of plastic or glass in front of one eye and asking the patient (who is observing a small light source such as a penlight or white object) which image is red, the inside or outside, lower or upper, depending on whether the diplopia is maximum in the vertical or lateral field of gaze. Figure 3–14 demonstrates the findings in one patient with medial rectus dysfunction and in one with lateral rectus dysfunction. The abnormal image in both cases is lateral in the field of gaze (having reviewed the visual field representation of various parts of the retina, you should be able to determine why this is so) and blurred, even though different eyes are involved in each case. The cover test, which asks the patient to identify which image disappears on covering one eye, is based on the same principles but is more difficult for the patient than the red glass test in which both images remain for the patient to contrast. The red glass and cover tests are particularly useful in delineating minimal muscle dysfunction, in which it is frequently difficult to determine which muscles are involved by observation on primary muscle testing.

It is worthwhile at this point to review the anatomy of the central pathways of the oculomotor system. Figures 3–15 and 3–16 schematically outline the major central path-

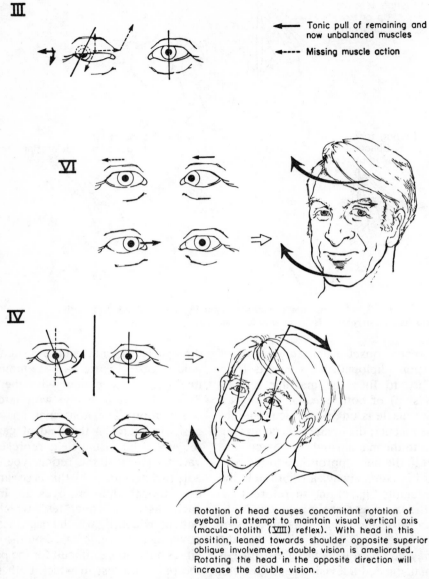

Tonic pull of remaining and now unbalanced muscles

Missing muscle action

Rotation of head causes concomitant rotation of eyeball in attempt to maintain visual vertical axis (macula-otolith (VIII) reflex). With head in this position, leaned towards shoulder opposite superior oblique involvement, double vision is ameliorated. Rotating the head in the opposite direction will increase the double vision.

Fig 3–13.—Eye findings with isolated unilateral loss of function of cranial nerves III, IV, and VI. Broken arrows represent lost function; solid arrows represent tone in unaffected muscles. Compensatory head adjustments frequently are seen with loss of IV and VI.

ways that are important to conjugate lateral gaze, conjugate vertical gaze, and convergence. Additionally, the deficits caused by destructive lesions in various parts of these systems are diagrammed.

PUPILLARY FUNCTION

The iris is subserved by two autonomic motor systems: (1) the sympathetic, which innervates the radial iris dilator muscles, and (2) the parasympathetic, which innervates

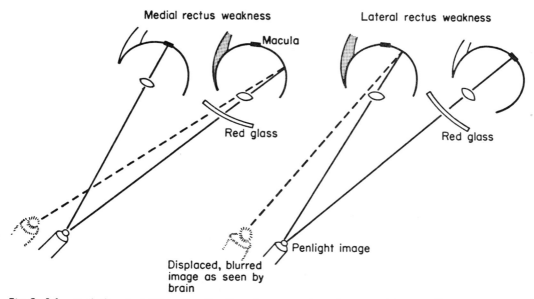

Medial rectus weakness Lateral rectus weakness

Macula

Red glass Red glass

Penlight image

Displaced, blurred image as seen by brain

Fig 3-14.—Red glass test. When the direction of gaze uses the weak muscle, the image is always displaced away from the macula of the retina so that the brain interprets the abnormal, blurred (off-macula) image as being farther out in the field of gaze than the normal image. The examiner needs only to determine which eye sees the farthest displaced image to determine the abnormal side. Blurring is less useful because it is usually minimal and not noticed by the patient.

the circular sphincter (iris constrictor) muscles and the ciliary apparatus for lens accommodation. Figures 3-17 and 3-18 show the origins and courses of these two systems.

During the normal waking state the two systems are tonically and reflexively active, depending in part on emotionality and darkness, which increase sympathetic tone and therefore pupillodilation, and on brightness, visual accommodation, and ocular convergence, which cause increased parasympathetic tone and therefore pupilloconstriction. During sleep sympathetic tone is depressed and the pupils are small. This is presumed to be caused by active suppression of the diencephalic reticular activating system and the origins of the sympathetic system therein. Normal waking pupil size with average ambient illumination is 2 to 6 mm. With age, the average size of the pupil decreases. Approximately 25% of individuals have asymmetric pupils (anisocoria), with a difference of usually less than 0.5 mm in diameter. This

must be kept in mind when attributing asymmetry to disease, particularly if there are no other signs of neurologic dysfunction.

At the bedside, the first step in evaluating pupil dysfunction is observation of the resting state. A small pupil suggests sympathetic dysfunction; a large pupil, parasympathetic dysfunction. Loss of both systems would leave one with a nonreactive, midposition pupil, 4-7 mm in diameter, with the size varying from individual to individual. This is seen most often in persons with lesions that destroy the midbrain (see chap. 19).

Next, the integrity of the pupillary reflexes is evaluated. Parasympathetic function is tested by having the patient accommodate, first looking at a distant object, which tends to dilate the pupils, and then quickly looking at a close object, which should cause the pupils to constrict. Additionally, the pupils constrict when the patient is asked to converge, which is most easily done by having him look at his nose. Convergence-pupillo-

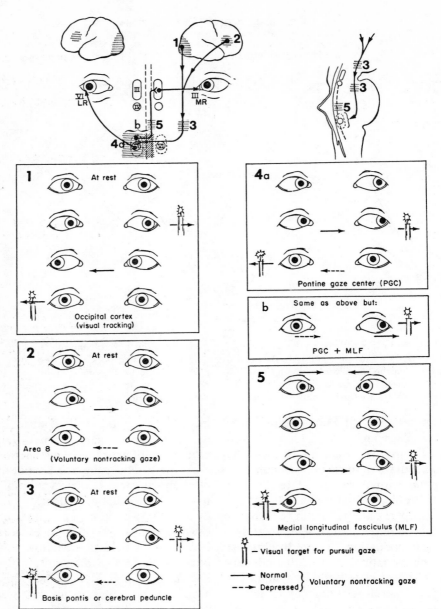

1 — Visual target for pursuit gaze

→ Normal
- -→ Depressed } Voluntary nontracking gaze

Fig 3–15. — Pathways for conjugate horizontal gaze with schematic representation of eye-movement abnormalities occurring with lesions *(shaded areas)* in various parts of this system. **1**, occipital cortical lesion associated with depression of contralateral visual pursuit gaze (this may be variable, with some test parameters indicating difficulty with gaze toward the side of the lesion). **2**, premotor frontal lobe lesion encompassing area 8, associated with depression of contralateral voluntary nontracking gaze. **3**, basis pontis or cerebral peduncle lesion associated with depression of contralateral pursuit and voluntary gaze. **4a**, paramedian pontine reticular (pontine gaze center) lesion associated with loss of ipsilateral gaze. **4b**, lesion also encompasses medial longitudinal fasciculus, causing loss of contralateral adduction. This combination of ipsilateral horizontal gaze deficiency with medial longitudinal fasciculus involvement is aptly called the one-and-one-half syndrome. **5**, lesion in medial longitudinal fasciculus (MLF) between abducens and oculomotor nuclei associated with loss of adduction of ipsilateral eye on contralateral horizontal gaze. However, convergence is intact because it is controlled through the upper pons and pretectal region of the midbrain using the intact oculomotor nucleus and nerve. The name for this isolated medial rectus weakness is internuclear ophthalmoplegia.

40

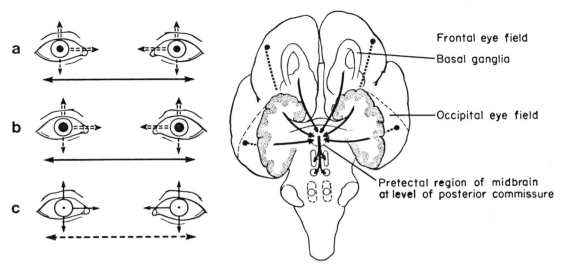

Frontal eye field

Basal ganglia

Occipital eye field

Pretectal region of midbrain at level of posterior commissure

Fig 3–16.—Diagrammatic representation of the major regions involved with conjugate vertical and convergent gaze and eye opening. Eye findings with lesions in different regions are illustrated. Broken arrows represent loss of function; solid arrows represent normal function. (a) Diffuse bilateral cerebral cortex disease or severe bilateral involvement of the basal ganglia (as in parkinsonism) is associated with difficulty in upward gaze, convergence, and later downward gaze, essentially a deafferentation of the pretectal vertical gaze zone. Unilateral cortical or basal ganglia disease does not cause clinically apparent problems with vertical or convergent gaze. (b) Pretectal destruction (e.g., compression by pineal tumor) causes more severe difficulty with vertical up gaze and convergence to complete loss of these functions. Deeper involvement in the region medial to the red nucleus is necessary to cause significant loss of down gaze. Involvement of the pupillary light reflex region in the pretectum and also the descending sympathetic pathways results in midposition, fixed-to-light pupils, frequently beginning with small reactive pupils because the sympathetic pathways are more dorsal and possibly more sensitive to compression. Lesions, usually ischemic, restricted to the periaqueductal region of the midbrain, cause similar abnormalities and, in addition, a peculiar nystagmus that is convergent or involves all the eye muscles simultaneously and causes a jerky retraction of the eyes into the orbit (nystagmus retractorius) on attempted voluntary gaze. (c) A central lesion in the lower pons transecting both the basis pontis and the tegmentum (most often infarction or hemorrhage) leaves a person quadriplegic and mute with loss of all horizontal gaze function. Vertical gaze and convergence (also eye opening) are the only remaining means of communication. If this goes unrecognized, the patient will be essentially locked in. A higher bilateral lesion (e.g., midpons) interrupts the reticular formation necessary for the maintenance of consciousness and causes coma. Lesions that transect the basis pontis or the basis pendunculi, sparing the tegmentum, do not depress consciousness but leave the patient quadriplegic with no voluntary horizontal gaze (see Fig 3–15, lesion 3); reflex vestibular-oculomotor connections are preserved because they are located entirely within the tegmentum, and therefore caloric irrigations or the oculocephalic maneuver gives reflex conjugate horizontal and vertical gaze of the eyes (see the section on nerve VIII).

constriction and accommodation-pupilloconstriction can be functionally separated, and on rare occasions with lesions in the pretectal region, only one may be dysfunctional. More common is loss of the light reflex with preservation of accommodation and convergence pupilloconstriction. This may be caused by lesions in the peripheral autonomic nervous system or lesions in the pretectal regions of the midbrain. Variable amounts of sympathetic involvement are usually present, leaving the pupil small in the resting state. Commonly associated with tertiary syphilis in the past, this type of pupil (the Argyll-Robertson pupil) is seen most often today associated with diabetes mellitus.

The light reflex is tested by illuminating first one eye and then the other; both the di-

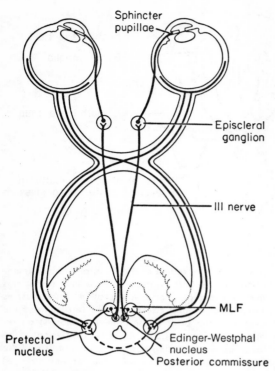

Fig 3-17.—Parasympathetic innervation of the iris with afferent pathway for light reflex. Note the bilateral distribution of each retinal input to the pretectal region and therefore the Edinger-Westphal nucleus.

rect reaction (constriction in the illuminated eye) and the consensual reaction (constriction in the opposite eye) are observed. The direct and consensual responses are equal in intensity because of equal bilateral input to the pretectal region and Edinger-Westphal nuclei from each retina (see Fig 3-17).

Pupillodilation, which is tested by darkening the room or simply shading the eye, is an active sympathetic function with associated parasympathetic inhibition. A sudden noxious stimulus, such as a pinch, particularly to the neck or upper thorax, causes active bilateral pupillodilation. This is called the ciliospinal reflex and depends predominantly on the integrity of the appropriate segmental somatic afferents, the upper thoracic sympathetic motor column (T1-T3 ventrolateral horn), and the ascending cervical sympathetic pupillodilator system (see Fig 3-18). Interruption of the descending sympathetic pathways in the brain stem frequently has no effect on the reflex. Therefore, if the patient has a constricted pupil presumed secondary to loss of sympathetic tone, absence of the ciliospinal reflex suggests peripheral sympathetic denervation or, if other neurologic signs are present, upper thoracic cord damage. Presence of the reflex despite depressed resting sympathetic tone suggests central denervation above the thoracic cord.

A constellation of signs is caused by lesions in the sympathetic system. Sweating is depressed in the face on the side of the denervation, the upper lid becomes slightly ptotic, and the lower lid is slightly elevated due to denervation of Müller's muscles (the smooth muscles that cause a small amount of lid-opening tone during alertness). Vasodilation is transiently seen over the ipsilateral face, and increased facial temperature can be perceived. These abnormalities, in addition to pupilloconstriction, are seen in conjunction with peripheral cervical sympathetic system damage and together constitute Horner's syndrome. The same picture occurs with spinal root lesions that transect the sympathetic outflow (T1, T2, T3); however, sweating is also depressed over the ipsilateral arm and neck. With spinal cord and brain stem lesions as high as the posterior hypothalamus, the syndrome is the same with the exception of sweating defects, which are present over all the body ipsilateral to the lesion in addition to the face, neck, and upper extremities.

The final neuron in the cervicocranial sympathetic pathway arises in the superior cervical ganglion and sends axons to the head as plexuses surrounding the internal and external carotid arteries. Lesions involving the internal carotid artery plexus (as in the middle-ear region) cause miosis and ptosis and loss of sweating only in the forehead region—the area of the face supplied by the internal carotid system. Lesions of the supe-

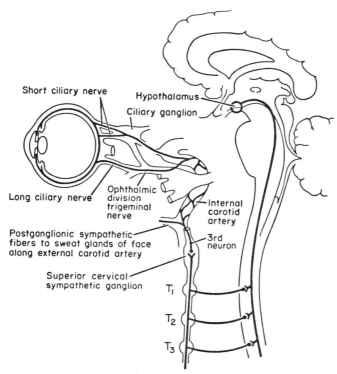

Fig 3–18.—Sympathetic innervation of the iris and sweat glands of the face.

rior cervical ganglion cause the same problems, but loss of sweating occurs over the whole face. Destruction of the external carotid plexus causes only sweating loss over the face except for the forehead. Lesions of the lower portion of the cervical sympathetic chain (e.g., carcinoma of thyroid) cause loss of sweating in the face and neck and, if the lesion is at the thoracic outlet, loss of sweating over the upper extremity. Lesions of the brain stem and cervical spinal cord descending sympathetic pathways cause depression of sweating over the whole side of the body. Lesions of the spinal cord below $T1-T3$ cause a loss of sweating below the level of the lesion. Testing for sweating defects can therefore be very useful in localization of the lesion. A simple method is to warm the patient and watch for sweating loss or asymmetry. This is made more obvious by painting the parts to be tested with an iodine preparation (e.g., forehead, cheek, neck, hand, and foot) and then when they are dry, dusting the areas with starch. When the patient sweats after being warmed with blankets (covering the tested areas with plastic is useful), the iodine runs into the starch and blackens it. Asymmetries are relatively easy to observe.

V. Trigeminal Nerve

The three divisions of the fifth nerve (ophthalmic, maxillary, and mandibular) are the source of somatesthetic perception for the entire face (Figs 3–19 and 3–20), the oral cavity, and the nasal passages.

Facial sensation can be tested simply at the bedside by having the patient close his eyes and respond affirmatively to touch with a light wisp of cotton over the three divisions of the trigeminal nerve. He should compare

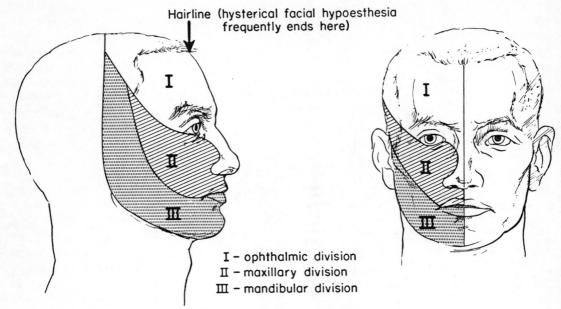

Hairline (hysterical facial hypoesthesia frequently ends here)

I – ophthalmic division
II – maxillary division
III – mandibular division

Fig 3–19. — Trigeminal innervation of facial sensation.

Fig 3–20. — Dorsal view of trigeminal system in the brain stem, showing acoustic tumor compressing the lateral aspect of the brain stem and the spinal tract and nucleus of the fifth nerve. The most superficial fibers of the tract are from the ophthalmic division, thus explaining the early loss of the corneal reflex.

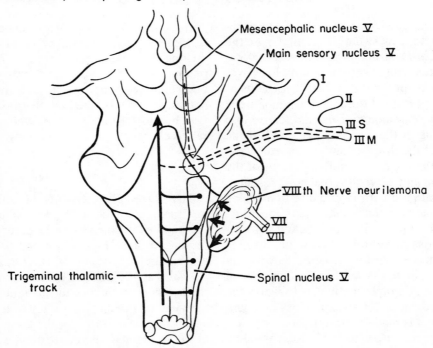

Mesencephalic nucleus V
Main sensory nucleus V
I
II
III S
III M
VIIIth Nerve neurilemoma
VII
VIII
Spinal nucleus V
Trigeminal thalamic track

or contrast perception on one side versus the other. Pain perception as tested by a pin should be similarly checked. In sensory testing, with the exception of reflexes, which allow observation of a motor response, the examiner depends largely on the reliability of the subject. Patterns of hypo- or hypersensitivity appropriate for classical sensory nerve distributions are useful clues to the reliability of the findings. The patient with hysterical or feigned sensory loss in the face frequently has bizarre perceptive patterns such as a hairline or perfect midline demarcation of hyposensitivity, neither of which can be explained on the basis of central or peripheral damage to trigeminal structures (see Fig 3–19).

The temporalis, masseter, and pterygoid muscles are supplied by the motor division of the mandibular branch of cranial nerve V and subserve jaw closing and opening. Supranuclear innervation of these muscles (hemispheric and brain stem pyramidal and extrapyramidal systems) is essentially symmetrically bilateral. A unilateral lesion above the level of the fifth-nerve motor nucleus,

therefore, does not cause any obvious defect of jaw function. Large bilateral lesions of the hemispheres or brain stem above the fifth-nerve nucleus cause bilateral depression of voluntary jaw function. If the bilateral involvement lies above the brain stem, very basic brain stem-mediated chewing reflexes may remain and actually become hyperactive. The jaw jerk, a V/V stretch reflex elicited by tapping the jaw downward, is also hyperactive (see chap. 6).

The paired temporalis and masseter muscles function in jaw closure, whereas the two pairs of pterygoid muscles open, protrude, and move the mandible from side to side. Observation of temporal region asymmetry and palpation of the symmetry of bulk and tension in tight jaw closure test the temporalis and masseter muscles. The pterygoids open the jaw in concert with a downward and opposing inward motion (Fig 3–21).

When the pterygoids are weak on one side, the jaw deviates toward the weak side on opening, with the inward vector of the opposite pterygoid being unopposed (Fig 3–22).

The corneal reflex, a bilateral blink re-

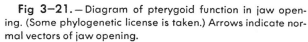

Fig 3–21.—Diagram of pterygoid function in jaw opening. (Some phylogenetic license is taken.) Arrows indicate normal vectors of jaw opening.

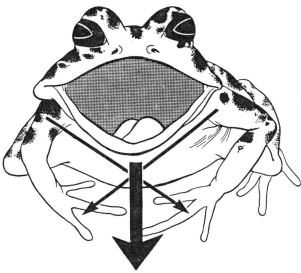

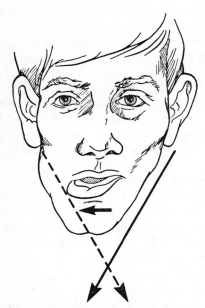

Fig 3–22.—Deviation of jaw on opening to side of weakened pterygoid muscles. Broken arrow represents loss of right pterygoid strength.

sponse to stimulation of the cornea, is a useful and objective test for evaluating simultaneously the ophthalmic division of the fifth-nerve (the afferent limb) and the seventh-nerve motor innervation of the orbicularis oculi (the efferent limb). A wisp of cotton is touched lightly to the lateral aspects of the cornea, with the examiner approaching from laterally and behind the patient's field of vision to avoid a visually evoked blink response. Both the eye stimulated and the opposite eye are observed in the direct and normally equal consensual responses. In the routine screening neurologic examination, the corneal reflex should be tested because it is a sensitive and objective indicator of fifth- and seventh-nerve dysfunction. A good example of dysfunction occurs with eighth-nerve neurilemomas, which comprise approximately 5% of all intracranial tumors. Patients are frequently seen first for their unilateral deafness, and on routine neurologic evaluation the only other indication of involvement may be depression of the ipsilateral direct and contralateral consensual cor-

neal reflex, presumably because of pressure by the tumor, which lies in the angle between the cerebellum and pons, on the superficially positioned descending tract and nucleus of the trigeminal nerve (see Fig 3–20). If the depression of the reflex were secondary to seventh-nerve hypofunction, only the direct response would be depressed; the contralateral consensual response would be full because the afferent arc (V) would be intact.

An instructive example of trigeminal nerve dysfunction is tic douloureux or trigeminal neuralgia, an irritative phenomenon of unknown etiology. This process causes severe paroxysmal pains in one or more divisions of the trigeminal nerve, with the maxillary division being most often affected and the ophthalmic least. In the past, surgical section of the various peripheral branches or the trigeminal root itself was frequently done for alleviation of the condition. Because of nerve regeneration and return of pain some months following branch destruction, complete root section became a popular form of permanent cure. A great difficulty with both these procedures is the frequently objectionable complete anesthesia of the divisions involved or of the entire face with root section and, additionally, the loss of the corneal reflex. This is an important response to foreign material that touches the cornea, and if absent, ulceration and subsequent opacification of the cornea may impair vision. Unfortunately, this is not an uncommon sequel to root section. Subsequently, a technique has been developed that spares the motor division, which runs on the lower surface of the trigeminal root and ganglion and contains enough sensory fibers to preserve a small amount of facial sensation and the corneal reflex, but not enough to interfere with the amelioration of neuralgia.

Knowledge of the central functional anatomy of the trigeminal system suggested another solution to this problem. Pain and temperature perception is predominantly localized in the lower two thirds of the spinal nucleus of the fifth nerve, so it was postulated that section of the spinal tract input to this portion of the nucleus might relieve the pain of tic douloureux and leave enough sensation subserved by the upper third of the spinal nucleus, the main sensory nucleus, and the mesencephalic root to have a tolerably mild hypoesthesia and preserved corneal reflex. Indeed, this turned out to be true and confirmed the experimentally established anatomical distribution of pain, temperature, and general sensation in the nucleus of the fifth nerve. Unfortunately, the operation is not simple because the approach is in a very vascular area and the dangers of destructive hemorrhage or vascular occlusion and infarction of the brain stem are always present. The possibility of these complications, which, in fact, did occur in a certain percentage of patients, became too high a price to pay for relief of the neuralgia and the operation was abandoned by most neurosurgeons.

Fortunately, we now have an antiepileptic drug (carbamazepine) that is quite successful in relieving tic in many persons for long periods of time. Sensory root section is reserved for intractable cases.

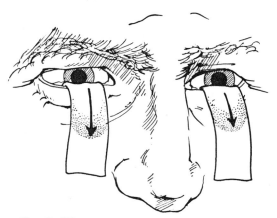

Fig 3–23.—Filter paper test for symmetry of lacrimal secretion. The length of paper soaking in a set time period is measured.

small sheet of filter paper partially under the lower lid (Fig 3–23). The length of soaking of the filter paper in a set period of time (15–20 minutes) can be measured and compared. Because of variable sympathetic coinnervation of lacrimation, loss of function is unpredictable and may not occur at all. The means of evaluating the remaining major functions of the nerve are more simple and useful.

VII. Facial Nerve

Most of the facial nerve subserves facial expression. In addition, the facial nerve contains fibers that are involved in a multiplicity of other functions, including taste perception from the anterior two thirds of the tongue, perception of cutaneous stimuli in the external auditory canal and over part of the pinna and mastoid region, innervation of the stapedius muscle in the middle ear, and innervation of the lacrimal gland and the submaxillary and submandibular salivary glands.

It is difficult to test routinely the secretory gland functions of the facial nerve, partly because of the frequent partial nature of its functional contribution but more because of the difficulty in quantitating lacrimation and salivation. Lacrimation can be tested semiquantitatively at the bedside by placing a

FACIAL EXPRESSION

There is more than one source of supranuclear innervation of the facial motor nucleus in the lower pons. Pyramidal innervation, the major source of voluntary facial movement, arises primarily from the precentral gyrus in the lower portion of the cerebral convexity (Fig 3–24). It is important to recall that the whole face, as is the case with most of the axial musculature, is bilaterally innervated by the supranuclear hemispheric motor systems. This bilateral innervation is not even, however. Although either side of the upper face (the frontalis muscles) has almost 50/50 ipsilateral versus contralateral balance of supranuclear innervation, the lower regions of the face as a general rule have, in descending order, a greater and greater contralateral innervation. A lesion involving the right motor cortex (e.g., carotid-middle cerebral

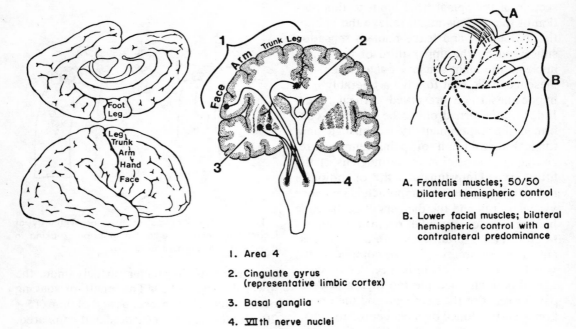

A. Frontalis muscles; 50/50 bilateral hemispheric control

B. Lower facial muscles; bilateral hemispheric control with a contralateral predominance

1. Area 4

2. Cingulate gyrus (representative limbic cortex)

3. Basal ganglia

4. VIIth nerve nuclei

Fig 3—24. — Supranuclear innervation of facial nerve nuclei.

arterial system occlusion and hemispheric infarction) causes a weakness (not a paralysis) of voluntary left lower facial movement that is especially noticeable while the patient is talking, grimacing (usually elicited by asking the patient to bare his teeth or gums), or resting. In the latter instance, loss of facial tone is evident in the orbicularis oculi muscle by a widening of the palpebral fissure and in the orbicularis oris by a drooping of the corner of the mouth and a flattening of the nasolabial crease (Fig 3 – 25).

The forehead is normally creased when a person raises his eyebrows or looks toward the ceiling; the eyebrows are equally elevated by the bilaterally innervated frontalis muscles. On occasion, there is some minimal weakness in the contralateral frontalis muscle with a unilateral supranuclear lesion, presumably because some contralateral supranuclear innervation is predominant in a few individuals. In these situations, however, the weakness is almost always greater in the lower face, thus distinguishing the involvement from the total face weakness, which is

uniform in intensity and secondary to nuclear or nerve dysfunction.

On recovering from the dysfunction of unilateral motor cortex destruction (this recovery presumably from the remaining functional motor cortex in the same and particularly the opposite hemisphere), a striking phenomenon can frequently be observed. The patient may still have mild weakness of grimacing on the affected side, but on spontaneously smiling the affected side of the mouth may actually turn up more than the normal side. The patient has unilateral hypermimia attributed by many to limbic-basal ganglia release from cortical inhibition, essentially a focal hyperemotionality. In contradistinction, a patient with advanced parkinsonism, which afflicts mainly basal ganglia structures and not the pyramidal system, can grimace without much difficulty but rarely smiles (hypomimia).

Uniform weakness of the face follows destruction of the facial motor nucleus in the brain stem. This is almost always associated with various combinations of involvement of

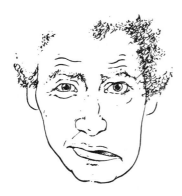
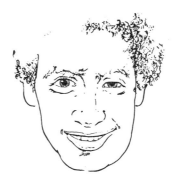

Lower face weakness at rest and on voluntary grimace

Left hypermimia with spontaneous emotion

Fig 3–25.—Left facial weakness following lesion of the right motor cortex. After a delay of weeks to months, hypermimia may appear on the left side of the face, which remains weak to voluntary grimacing and with speech.

proximate cranial nerves such as the vestibular nuclei, nerve VI, spinal nucleus of nerve V, and long tracts such as the pyramidal tract, lemniscal and spinothalamic tracts, the medial longitudinal fasciculus and descending sympathetic pathway, and the close-by cerebellum and cerebellar-connected structures. A uniform weakness also occurs following destruction of the facial nerve proper in its course from the nucleus through the brain stem (review the extraordinary looping course of the facial nerve in the brain stem), the subarachnoid space, the auditory canal, the facial canal above and bordering the middle ear, and after it exits through the stylomastoid foramen to pass through the parotid gland before extending over the face.

The most common cause of involvement of the facial nerve nucleus is infarction of the brain stem, but this is far less common than involvement of the facial nerve in its peripheral course. Bell's palsy, possibly a viral or vascular affliction of the facial nerve and its peripheral pathways, is a common disorder. Its effects would be less marked were it not for the narrowness of the facial canal (the nerve fills almost three quarters of the diameter of the canal). Swelling of the inflamed nerve causes compression against the bony walls, which leads to compression of the blood supply, ischemia, and further swelling. In its most severe form, infarction of the nerve may occur with a prolonged and not infrequently incomplete process of regeneration.

Observation of the patient's face during conversation and at rest almost always reveals facial weakness and differentiates nuclear from supranuclear involvement. Further testing includes having the patient close his eyes and lips tightly and the examiner attempting to open them, having the patient grimace (show his teeth), and also having the patient fill his cheeks with air with his lips tightly pursed. If one or both sides of the face are weak, he will have difficulty holding the air in. Tapping each cheek accentuates the difficulty on the appropriate side. The frontalis muscles are tested by having the patient look up, elevating eyebrows and furrowing the forehead.

TASTE

The course of the facial taste fibers is from the taste buds of the anterior two thirds of the tongue, joining the lingual branch of cranial nerve V and then separating away as the chorda tympani (which travels through the temporal bone via its own canal) to emerge into the middle ear. The chorda tympani travels just medial to the tympanic membrane and then joins the facial nerve to travel inward to its cell body origin, the geniculate ganglion, at the junction of the facial and internal auditory canals. The fibers continue inward with the facial nerve and on reaching the brain stem separate to pass to the nucleus solitarius in its rostral extent. The thalamic and cortical localization of taste has not been clearly delineated in humans. The parietal opercular region and the insula seem important, and proximate seizure foci, particularly in the inferomesial temporal lobe, sometimes give rise to hallucinations of taste. Unilateral cortical lesions have rarely been described as causing changes in the threshold for taste because taste, like olfaction, is presumably bilaterally represented.

It is particularly useful to evaluate taste in a person who has Bell's palsy and by this means determine the localization of involvement, which may vary. If the face is paralyzed and taste is intact, the site of the lesion is probably in the facial canal distal to the takeoff of the chorda tympani. If taste is involved, the locus of difficulty is proximal to the separation of the chorda tympani at the middle ear.

Bell's palsy is the most common cause of loss of taste. Another potential but surprisingly unusual source of decreased taste (hypoageusia) is suppurative otitis media. Recently hypoageusia and dysageusia (unpleasant taste) have been associated with zinc deficiency and also with diabetes mellitus.

To test taste, the examiner holds the patient's tongue out with a piece of gauze and paints the anterior portion of each side of the tongue separately with a well saturated solution of sugar. The patient is then asked to report his taste perception on each side and whether or not there is a noticeable difference. Between testings the patient should wash his mouth out with tap water. In most cases it is not necessary to test the other three basic taste percepts (salt, sour, and bitter) because if there is loss of taste in the anterior tongue, it is almost always reflected in depressed perception of sweet substances.

SOMATIC SENSATION

The major somatic sensory distribution of the facial nerve is in the skin of the external auditory canal and over the tympanic membrane where it overlaps with the small somatic branches of cranial nerves IX, X, and possibly V. Additionally, nerve VII variably supplies small branches to the earlobe and over the mastoid, which overlap with cranial nerve V and the dermatomes of cervical nerves II and III. The geniculate ganglion houses the cell body of the seventh-nerve fibers, and the central distribution is the spinal tract and nucleus of nerve V. It is not surprising with the considerable overlap of dermatomes that sensory testing seldom reveals hypoesthesia over the distribution of an involved seventh-nerve. However, the positive or irritative signs of nerve involvement are frequently present in persons with Bell's palsy who complain of pain in the external canal and over the mastoid region. Herpes zoster, a viral affliction of dorsal root ganglia (usually only a single ganglion is affected, most commonly thoracic and other spinal segments, but also trigeminal, particularly the ophthalmic division) occasionally affects the geniculate ganglion and manifests itself as pain over the preceding distribution. Additionally, the viral vesicular eruption is seen over the peripheral distribution of the nerves, particularly in the external auditory canal and over the tympanic membrane. Facial weakness or paralysis is frequently but not always associated and is presumably secondary to concomitant viral involvement of the motor fibers or compression of the motor root by the swollen geniculate ganglion.

STAPEDIUS MUSCLE

edius muscle, when contracted,
ossicular system of the middle
hought thereby to dampen loud,
injurious, low-frequency noises
tympani supplied by the trigeminal mandibular branch has a similar function). When the seventh nerve is afflicted proximal to the middle ear, its stapedius function is lost, and persons frequently complain of an irritating quality of loud noises (hyperacusis) as perceived by the involved ear. In New York City a frequent complaint from persons who have Bell's palsy is that the noise of the subway is so intolerable that they must cover the involved ear.

One of the more common types of old-age hearing loss (presbycusis) involves predominantly the high-frequency range. A speculative hypothesis suggests that the stapedius and tensor tympani muscles, which protect against low frequencies, allow the loud, high frequencies that are so common in our mechanized society through to the hair cells. Indeed, these sounds may get through a tightened system more efficiently. As a result, chronic hair cell damage would occur in greater amounts in the high-frequency receptors.

VIII. Auditory Vestibular Function

AUDITORY FUNCTION

Hearing acuity is depressed with unilateral lesions of the peripheral neural apparatus (the inner ear and nerve VIII) or with processes that occlude the sound conduction pathways (the external auditory canal and middle ear and the ossicles). The cochlear nuclei, dorsal and ventral, which are on the lateral aspect of the pontomedullary junction, are the site of the second-order neuron, the first central synapse, in the ascending auditory system. Destruction at this level also causes ipsilateral hearing loss. Beyond the cochlear nucleus level the auditory system makes multiple decussations up to the medial geniculate, and therefore each auditory apparatus is bilaterally represented from above the cochlear nucleus to the auditory cortices in Heschl's gyri of the posterior-superior temporal lobes. Significant loss of hearing therefore does not occur following unilateral lesions of the auditory system above the cochlear nuclei. Bilateral lesions are necessary to cause major hearing loss and rarely occur in isolation in the brain stem or hemispheres; the destruction of other major functional structures in the brain stem or hemispheres usually precludes meaningful testing of auditory function.

Large unilateral cerebral cortical lesions cause deficit in auditory localization that is most marked when the primary auditory cortex is involved but also with large lesions of the frontal and/or parietal cortex. Such a person is unable, with eyes closed, to localize an auditory stimulus with his hand in the auditory field opposite the lesioned hemisphere. This can be tested at the bedside using snapping fingers or other stimuli. Double simultaneous stimulation can also be useful, with the patient extinguishing the stimulus opposite the lesioned hemisphere. Acuity testing is usually normal. Frontal and especially parietal lesions also result in this phenomenon, so it is assumed that the extinction represents a stimulus neglect or inattention phenomenon.

Rare irritative lesions of the auditory cortex (e.g., neoplasm, scarring, occasionally ischemia) cause hallucinations of sound (tinnitus) and frequently also of movement (vertigo), which are essentially focal epileptiform seizures (see chap. 9). They can be differentiated from eighth-nerve dysfunction by auditory acuity and vestibular testing (see below), which are abnormal with peripheral disease but not with hemispheric disease. The full neurologic examination may bring out associated defects such as visual-field abnormality or language dysfunction, which also help make the distinction.

The vast majority of hearing problems result from peripheral disease, i.e., involvement of the eighth nerve or inner ear. Testing of the peripheral system at the bedside is simple and rewarding. More detailed clinical evaluation including special audiometric testing is carried out in otolaryngological laboratories and can be very useful in differentiating cochlear (inner ear) disease from direct eighth-nerve involvement. At the bedside the examiner can differentiate between hearing loss caused by defects in the conduction system (conduction deafness) and that caused by the inner ear–auditory nerve system as a unit (nerve deafness).

Two basic instruments are necessary for this test: a C512 tuning fork (C256 is adequate but not as sensitive; C128 is inadequate except for testing for hyperacusis and, most important, cutaneous and bony vibratory perception) and a nonelectric watch (watch-ticking is in the 1,500-cps range). The watch is placed next to the patient's ear and gradually moved away. The distance at which the patient ceases to hear the tick is noted and compared with the distance from the opposite side. If the examiner has normal hearing, a useful comparison can be made. High-tone deafness is measured by this test. The C512 (or C256) fork is then used to test for lower tone falloff and, more important, to determine whether hearing loss is of the conduction or the neural type.

The stem of the tuning fork is placed gently against the maxillary incisor teeth or vertex of the cranium or forehead (Weber's test) and the patient is asked where he hears the buzz. This is a test of bone conduction; sound is transmitted to both sides equally if the conduction and neural apparatus is intact. With neural deafness, the sound transmits best to the normal side. With conduction deafness, the sound transmits best to the side of deafness. This has been thought to occur because ambient sound is prevented from getting to the cochlea on the blocked side, and receptors previously taken up by ambient noises are free to accept the vibrations conducted from the tuning fork through the skull. This would create a greater reception and, therefore, a louder sound in the occluded system. The patient claims to hear the sound best on that side because the normal side is relatively depressed and extinguished. You can check the validity of the Weber test by plugging an ear with your finger, causing conduction deafness, and then doing the test on yourself; even your own voice will be heard better on the occluded side.

You notice the effects of ambient sound competition for receptors when you must talk to a friend at the top of your voice in a noisy, crowded room and then continue talking and walk into a silent room where you find yourselves shouting at each other. Although the explanation given here is probably not entirely correct and much more complex sound biophysics are involved in the Weber test, it is useful for remembering the appropriate responses of conduction and neural deafness.

The Rinné test is next carried out with the tuning fork. This tests both bone and air conduction. The examiner places the butt of the vibrating fork on the mastoid region, and when the patient ceases to hear the vibration, the examiner places the tines close to the external auditory meatus to check air conduction. Vibrations perceived through air are heard twice as long as those perceived through bone, so the normal individual reports, for example, hearing the bone vibration for 30 seconds and then continues to hear the vibration through air for another 30 seconds—60 seconds altogether. If there is conduction deafness, bony conduction is either normal or slightly enhanced, whereas air conduction is decreased. If there is neural deafness, both bone and air conduction are equally suppressed. As with the watch tick, the examiner should compare the ability of both sides to perceive the fork. A comparison of the patient's ability to perceive the fork, as well as the watch tick, with the examiner's ability is also useful (Schwabach test).

For screening persons who do not complain of hearing loss, the Weber test and watch tick are adequate. To this might be added the use of rubbed-finger noise or whispered voice, which represent mid-range frequencies that frequently are involved in neural deafness.

VESTIBULAR FUNCTION

The objective evaluation of vestibular function is actually an evaluation of the vestibular portion of the eighth nerve as seen through its effects on the oculomotor system. In reviewing the anatomy of these interconnections (Fig 3–26), it can be seen that vestibular testing creates an opportunity to evaluate not only the peripheral vestibular apparatus but also an expanse of the brain stem extending from the vestibular nuclear complex in the upper medulla through the third-nerve nuclei in the mesencephalon. Lesions anywhere along this tegmental system are associated with characteristic deficits in vestibular-oculomotor function as determined by observation and vestibular testing.

The cristae within the semicircular canals act as mechanical transducers, responding to the flow of endolymph during acceleration or deceleration in rotation of the body. At rest or at a steady state of rotation, the functionally paired semicircular canal cristae discharge tonically to extraocular muscle agonist-antagonist pairs at a low level that is statistically equal and opposing [right horizontal canal + left horizontal canal = 0 electrical activity (EA) and eye movement (EM); right and left anterior + right and left posterior = 0 EA + EM; right anterior + right posterior = 0 EA + EM; left anterior + left posterior = 0 EA + EM]. No net vestibular-oculomotor effect is therefore caused. If, however, disease, which is almost always destructive and is rarely irritative, affects one set of semicircular canals (e.g., the *right* side), the tonic firing level of the opposite canal system is no longer opposed. Spontaneous vestibular-oculomotor abnormality (nystagmus) is the result of excessive activity in the normal system on the *left* (left horizontal activity + diminished opposing right horizontal activity > 0 EA + EM).

The tonic firing of the anterior and posterior vertical canals on each side, which innervates the vertical and rotational vector eye muscles, has no net effect, so it is not surprising that no significant net dysfunction results from destruction of the opposing vertical canals of either side. The major dysfunction is therefore the result of horizontal canal imbalance, and this is reflected in horizontal nystagmus because the horizontal canals innervate the horizontal directional eye muscles (see Fig 3–26). If only partial labyrin-

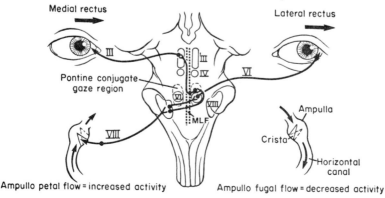

Fig 3–26. — Distribution of horizontal semicircular canal cristae to oculomotor system.

thine destruction occurs and one vertical canal is affected more than another, however, vestibular dysfunction is the result of the sum of both horizontal and vertical vectors. Rotary nystagmus is seen.

Following sudden loss of the right labyrinthine system, for example, as in vestibular neuronitis (a common affliction presumably viral in origin), characteristic vestibular-oculomotor changes are noted. The normal response of the now-unopposed opposite horizontal canal system is to drive the eyes conjugately to the right tonically (Fig 3–27). In an alert individual, there is a reflex attempt to contain the abnormal tonic drive. This checking attempt is called the fast component and, in combination with the tonic or slow component, forms the rhythmic to-and-fro movement—nystagmus. The tonic component encompasses the vestibular-oculomotor brain stem systems, whereas the fast component depends on the integrity of the cerebral hemispheres. The right hemisphere, including cortex, basal ganglia, and diencephalon, is responsible for the fast compo-

nent to the left and the left hemisphere for the fast component to the right, just as for voluntary and visual tracking horizontal gaze (see Figs 3–15 and 3–16). With loss of hemispheric function and preservation of basic brain stem functions (e.g., in a coma from sedative overdose), the fast component becomes weak, irregular, and finally disappears, leaving only tonic deviation of the eyes following vestibular-oculomotor activation. With acute unilateral hemispheric depression, such as caused by a middle cerebral artery occlusion, the fast component to the opposite side is depressed. The tonic component is predominant during vestibular-oculomotor activation and drives the eyes toward the side of the abnormal hemisphere, which is capable of little, if any, checking.

On examining a patient with suspected vestibular dysfunction, observation for nystagmus is of primary importance prior to formal testing. A person with, for example, acute right vestibular apparatus destructive disease has horizontal nystagmus with the

Fig 3–27.—Dorsal view of brain stem and cerebral hemispheres. Eyes are also seen from behind, as if reader is looking through eyes from the intracranial position. Loss of right vestibular influence releases the left vestibular apparatus to unopposed tonic driving of eyes to the right through neuronal apparatus illustrated by solid lines. Opposing phasic impulses that constitute the fast or checking component of nystagmus and arise from the right hemisphere are illustrated by broken lines.

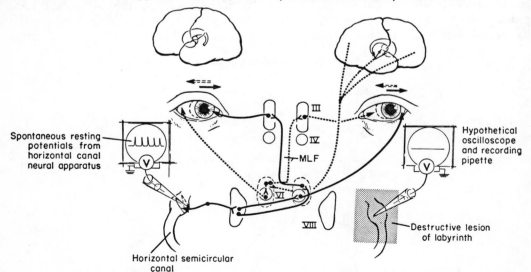

tonic component toward the diseased right side (release of the normal left) and the fast component toward the left (see Fig 3–27). Usually he complains of vertigo (illusion of movement of self or environment), saying that the room is spinning in the direction of the fast component, to the left—an illusion caused by the forced tonic movement of the eyes and retinae. This is called *object* (or objective) vertigo as opposed to *subject* (or subjective) vertigo, which is the sensation that the subject is spinning and which occurs almost exclusively with the eyes closed. Subject vertigo is true vestibular illusion, unsuppressed by the retinal image. The patient usually complains that he feels he is rotating in the direction of the clinically observed fast component of the nystagmus.

With chronic, slowly progressive disease such as acoustic neurilemoma (a tumor arising from the neurilemmal sheaths of the eighth nerve at the internal auditory meatus), a person is much less likely to complain of vertigo or to have significant nystagmus. This is true also in persons following recovery from an acute destructive process despite the lack of effective function in the destroyed system. The lack of symptoms and signs is due to central compensation and in large part, though not entirely, depends on visual fixation. If a patient with chronic disease or compensated acute disease closes his

eyes, the examiner can usually note the reappearance of the nystagmus by using a polygraph-recorded electro-oculogram or simply by feeling the elevated corneas move through the closed lids. Vertigo usually does not reappear, which suggests that there are means other than visual for suppressing the illusion of movement. An excellent example of the suppression of nystagmus and vertigo is seen in the figure skater who subjects himself to marked acceleration and deceleration of the horizontal endolymph-cristae systems every time he spins. Using visual fixation (a fix on one object as long as possible while spinning), skaters learn to suppress afterspin nystagmus and vertigo almost entirely. Imagine what figure skating would look like if this were not possible!

The position of the horizontal semicircular canal is diagrammed in Figure 3–28. The canal lies in the petrous portion of the temporal bone at an angle of approximately 20 degrees from the anatomical horizontal (a line drawn between the inferior orbital margin and the center of the external auditory meatus). The ampullary portion that is anterior lies above the horizontal.

The Barany rotation test as carried out in the laboratory in a spinning chair was once standard for evaluating vestibular function. It is very awkward for use in the clinic and creates considerable discomfort for the sub-

Fig 3–28.—The horizontal canals lie in the petrous portion of the temporal bone at an angle of approximately 20 degrees from Reid's anatomical horizontal baseline.

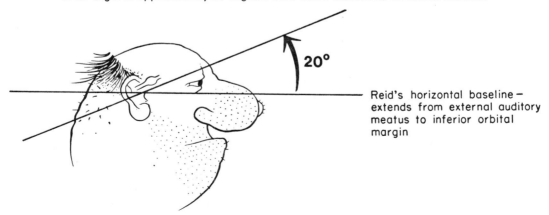

20°

Reid's horizontal baseline—extends from external auditory meatus to inferior orbital margin

ject, particularly nausea, so it has been replaced by caloric testing, which is easier to carry out and tends to be less noxious. In addition, only one horizontal canal is involved and therefore evaluated in routine caloric testing, whereas both are involved in Barany rotation. Barany rotation is more useful for testing the vertical canals; this can also be done with bilateral simultaneous caloric testing with, however, some inconsistency in the results. Vertical canal testing is rarely necessary, so a rotating barber's chair need not be part of a physician's clinical armamentarium.

Caloric testing is carried out most simply by irrigating the external auditory canal (observed by otoscope to be wax-free, not infected, and with no tympanic perforation) with water warmer or colder than body temperature, the presumed resting temperature of the labyrinths. The differential warming or cooling of the horizontal semicircular canal where it lies closest to the external auditory canal causes a decrease or increase, respectively, in the specific gravity of the endolymph at that point. If the head is positioned so that the horizontal canal is vertical, significant convection currents are caused in the canal by the induced changes in specific gravity (Figs 3–29 and 3–30). Vertical

upward currents are caused by warming because of the decreased specific gravity, and if the face is up (face down makes observation difficult), the current is ampullopetal—toward the ampulla and crista (see Fig 3–30). In the horizontal canal, this direction of flow is excitatory to the crista (the opposite is true for the vertical canals), causing increased firing over the pathways diagrammed in Figures 3–26, 3–27, and 3–30 and tonic deviation of the eyes to the contralateral side. The reflex checking or fast component appears and nystagmus is the result. In many texts, nystagmus is described with reference to the fast component. Nystagmus "to the right" means nystagmus with the fast component to the right. Clarity is best maintained by describing what is seen. It is well to understand this terminology, but the directions of the fast and slow components should both be described so there will be no confusion. Cold-water irrigation with the horizontal canal in the vertical position and face upward increases the specific gravity of the endolymph closest to the external auditory canal and therefore flows downward and away from the crista—ampullofugal (see Fig 3–30). This decreases the spontaneous firing of the ipsilateral horizontal canal vestibular system and therefore causes an imbalance;

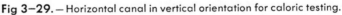

Fig 3–29.—Horizontal canal in vertical orientation for caloric testing.

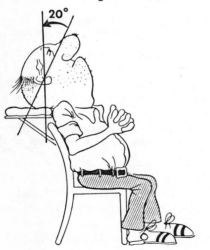
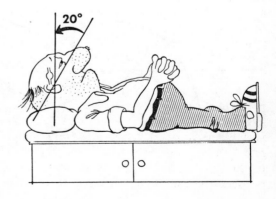

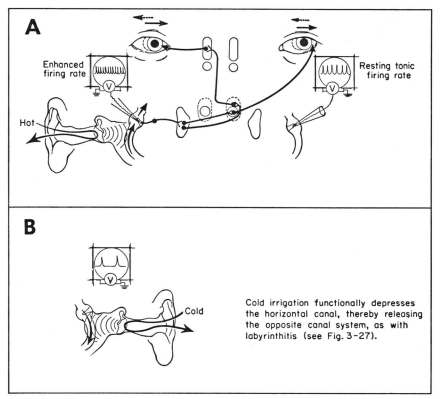

Fig 3–30.—A, mechanism for contralateral tonic deviation of eyes on irrigation of external auditory canal with hot water (horizontal canal in vertical position, see Fig 3–29). B, ipsilateral tonic deviation of eyes on irrigation of external auditory canal with cold water. Increased temperature decreases endolymph specific gravity in the horizontal semicircular canal, and endolymph flows ampullopetally—toward the crista—increasing its rate. Cold water causes the opposite effect, essentially a temporary ablation of the irrigated apparatus.

the resting tone of the opposite horizontal canal system becomes dominant. The eyes are thus driven tonically toward the irrigated side and the checking or fast component is opposite in direction. The same nystagmus and concomitant vertigo are seen in persons with ablative disease of the vestibular apparatus (see Fig 3–27).

As a routine, the alert person who complains or has a history of vertigo, nausea, imbalance, and/or signs of vestibular involvement (nystagmus, past pointing, imbalance) should have warm (approximately 48 C) irrigation of the canals. Warm irrigation is particularly useful in the person who has

compensated for his imbalance, when the acute episode (e.g., acute vestibular neuronitis or labyrinthitis) is past, or when the process is *slowly progressive* (e.g., acoustic neurilemoma) with compensation occurring simultaneously with progression of the disease process. Cold caloric irrigation on occasion gives hypoactive responses with irrigation of either side in these circumstances.

At the bedside, 20 cc of approximately 48 C water is irrigated into the external auditory canal, which should be clear of wax, uninfected, and with no tympanic membrane perforation (Fig 3–31).

Each auditory canal should be irrigated

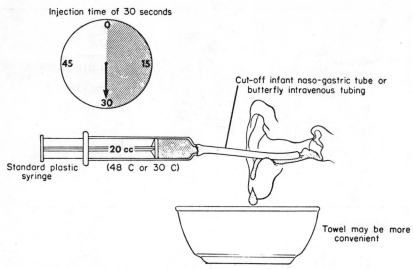

Fig 3–31.— Simple apparatus and technique for irrigating auditory canal.

separately for the same duration (30 seconds is convenient), and the time of onset of nystagmus from the beginning of irrigation and its duration and direction should be recorded. The findings from the two sides should be compared; a difference of approximately 20% is considered significantly abnormal. The patient should be asked whether he is experiencing spinning sensations or nausea and whether there is a difference between the two sides; a lesser experience suggests hypofunction. At least five minutes should elapse between irrigations to allow the stimulated canal to return to body temperature.

You may have surmised that vestibular-oculomotor testing has considerable diagnostic usefulness in the unconscious patient. This is because the vestibular-oculomotor system encompasses an expanse of the brain stem (upper medulla through mesencephalon) that contains a large portion of the reticular formation necessary for the maintenance of consciousness. Vestibular-oculomotor testing is particularly useful when the cause of the unconsciousness is not clear at the time of examination (see chap. 19).

The pathophysiologic basis of depressed consciousness can be diffuse bilateral hemi-spheric disease, bilateral suppression of the brain stem reticular formation, or both. The checking or fast component of nystagmus also depends on the integrity of the brain stem reticular formation and cerebral hemispheres. Loss of either causes depression or loss of this component. In the unconscious patient, therefore, the fast component disappears, leaving the more primitive and resistant brain stem vestibular-oculomotor apparatus intact. Caloric irrigation thus elicits only tonic deviation of the eyes. If the disease process lies above the midbrain, warm caloric irrigation causes tonic conjugate deviation of the eyes to the side opposite the irrigation, and cold irrigation elicits deviation of the eyes toward the irrigated ear (Fig 3–32, A). A destructive process (e.g., infarction, hemorrhage, or tumor) at the midbrain level involves the oculomotor complex with subsequent loss of the medial rectus portion of conjugate horizontal deviation, and only the lateral rectus deviation is seen on irrigation (Fig 3–32, B). A bilateral lesion of the pons, involving the abducens nuclei and the proximate medial longitudinal fasciculi, destroys the vestibular-oculomotor reflexes entirely (Fig 3–32, C). What effect would be

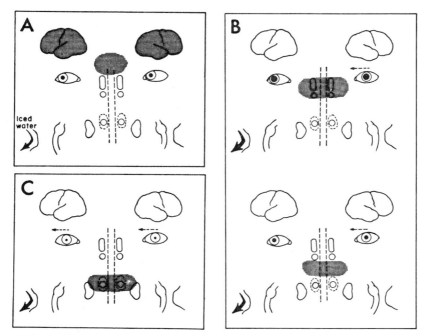

Fig 3–32.—Lesions causing pathologic depression of consciousness and associated vestibular-oculomotor changes elicited by caloric irrigation or the oculocephalic maneuver.

seen after complete transection of the basis pontis sparing the tegmentum (see Figs 3–15 and 3–26)?

Ice-water irrigation is routinely used in the comatose patient because it creates maximal suppression. Water hot enough to be as far above body temperature as ice water is below body temperature would damage the tympanic membranes, so it is less practical.

The poorly named "doll's eye" maneuver is a simple mechanical test that is particularly useful in the patient with suppressed consciousness. More appropriately called the oculocephalic maneuver, it is composed of a rapid passive rotation of the head laterally, which causes an inertial flow of the horizontal-canal endolymph in the opposite direction of the head rotation. As seen in Figure 3–33, the eyes are driven in a direction opposite the head rotation.

If the patient is awake, the hemispheric checking component (this has the same substrate as the fast component of the nystag-mus) keeps the eyes from deviating from midposition and actually may drive the eyes beyond the midposition toward the direction of turning. If the patient is in a coma from bilateral hemispheric disease or combined hemispheric and brain stem reticular formation suppression, as with metabolic disease (e.g., sedative overdose or uremia), which spares the oculomotor-vestibular pathways until very late, the checking component (also the fast component of nystagmus) is lost. The eyes then deviate away from the direction of rotation unchecked, and the reflex response is therefore considered disinhibited or hyperactive. In the patient who is comatose from bilateral midbrain disease, there is full deviation of the appropriate lateral rectus but loss of medial rectus function. With loss of the lower pons, including the medial longitudinal fasciculus and abducens nuclei, the eyes remain fixed on rotation of the head, as in the alert patient. In the alert patient, however, there are always some erratic compen-

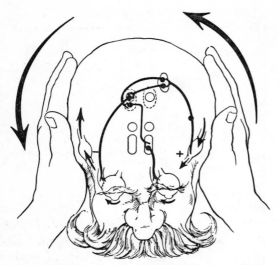

Fig 3–33.—Mechanism for reflex vestibular-oculomotor response to oculocephalic maneuver. Checking component from the right hemisphere as seen in alert patient with intact pathways is not illustrated.

satory eye movements including active movement beyond the midposition in the direction of head movement during oculocephalic testing.

Caloric testing by eliciting full nystagmus differentiates more clearly the alert patient with hysterical coma from the patient with alterations of consciousness whose response is pathologically modified. The patient who is alert and quadriplegic following lower pontine transection (usually infarction or hemorrhage) manifests intact voluntary convergence and vertical gaze but has no responses to vestibular-oculomotor testing unless the pontine tegmentum is spared, thereby preserving the reflex pathway (see chap. 20).

Metabolic suppression of the hemispheres and brain stem spares the oculomotor-vestibular pathways until quite late and also respiratory and cardiovascular control and pupillary function. The response to oculocephalic maneuvers and caloric irrigation finally becomes sluggish and disappears; respirations become depressed at about the same level of toxicity. The pupils continue to respond until much later as long as respira-

tions are supported and hypoxia does not complicate the metabolic suppression (see chap. 20).

Two other types of vestibular-oculomotor dysfunction must be considered: (1) vertical nystagmus and (2) positional nystagmus and vertigo. Vertical upward or downward nystagmus, unless elicited from the vertical labyrinthine canals by double simultaneous caloric irrigations or appropriate Barany rotation, is pathognomonic of dysfunction in the brain stem vestibular apparatus and its connections. The rare, bilateral, perfectly symmetric peripheral disease is associated with vertical nystagmus. Horizontal and rotary nystagmus occur with both peripheral and central disease and are therefore not of value in differentiation. If not present on forward gaze, vertical nystagmus is best observed by having the patient look directly up or down (Fig 3–34).

In addition to the presence of vertical nystagmus, acute central vestibular involvement as contrasted with acute peripheral disease is associated with less vertiginous symptoms. Very marked nystagmus may be seen, for example, in persons with demyelinating disease of the brain stem (multiple sclerosis) and may be associated with very little, if any, vertigo or autonomic symptoms. With peripheral vestibular involvement (e.g., labyrinthitis), nystagmus, vertigo, and autonomic symptoms are almost directly proportional in severity (Table 3–1). Presumably this is

Fig 3–34.—Vertical nystagmus with slow component downward.

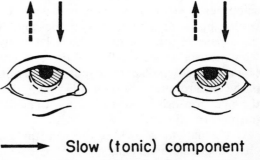

→ Slow (tonic) component

---→ Fast (checking) component

TABLE 3-1.—PERIPHERAL VS. CENTRAL VESTIBULAR DYSFUNCTION

DISEASE	NYSTAGMUS		ASSOCIATED PHENOMENA		CALORIC IRRIGATION
	TYPE	VERTIGO			
Peripheral	Horizontal or rotary; unidirectional	As severe as nystagmus	Hearing and tinnitus frequent	Long-tract sensory, motor involvement unusual	Depressed response
Central	Horizontal, rotary, or vertical; multidirectional	Relatively mild or absent	Tinnitus and hearing loss rare	Associated sensory, motor, cerebellar, other cranial nerve involvement more common	Variably affected and unreliable

because labyrinthine disease, by suppressing the major portion if not all of one input, causes a much greater proprioceptive imbalance than involvement of only a small portion of the widespread brain stem vestibular system by brain stem disease processes. Additionally, brain stem involvement is frequently bilateral and more balanced. Vertical nystagmus may well represent a vectoral sum of this bilateral involvement.

Positional nystagmus and vertigo are rela-

tively common disorders associated with both peripheral and central vestibular disease states. The patient complains of vertigo only when the head is in certain positions, commonly looking up. The vertigo may persist if the head is kept in the same position (this is particularly true with central disease) or it may rapidly fade (typical of the more common peripheral disease). A characteristic complaint is of vertigo after turning in bed, which makes frequently suspected

Fig 3-35.—Technique for testing macula-otolith apparatus and rotary nystagmus elicited in patient with abnormal apparatus. The patient should be dropped from the sitting position to his head hanging in each of three positions: head to right, to left, and without turning, i.e., head facing forward. As a rule, nystagmus is best elicited when the head is turned toward the abnormal side and less intensively in the head-forward position.

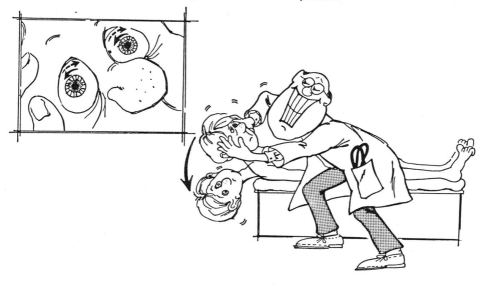

orthostatic vascular insufficiency an unlikely diagnosis. Some examples of etiologic significance are head trauma, frequently of only minor severity, vertebrobasilar distribution ischemia, and acoustic neurilemoma, the latter involving both the nerve directly and the brain stem by compression. The most commonly affected individual is the elderly patient with no predisposing factors and no threatening pathology. Presumably the dysfunction, which is called *benign positional vertigo*, is caused by aging and minor degenerative changes in the macula-otolith apparatus.

Testing for positional nystagmus and vertigo is done by rapidly dropping the patient backward as in Figure 3–35. The patient's head is held right side down, left side down, and in the midline on each of three manipulations.

Nystagmus, if unilaterally caused, normally appears when the diseased side is down, and with peripheral disease typically has an onset latency of 5–10 seconds, is rotary in nature (see Fig 3–35), terminates within one minute, and is associated with marked vertigo. With central disease the nystagmus tends to start with longer latency, up to 20–30 seconds, is variable in type, persists for longer periods, and is associated with only mild vertigo.

Macula-otolith system dysfunction in the utriculus and possibly also in the sacculus and their central connections is thought to be the basis for positional nystagmus, both central and peripheral. The mode of elicitation certainly suggests this, particularly when one notes that position not necessarily associated with significant accelerating or decelerating movement is all that is necessary to bring on the dysfunction.

With aging, cervical osteoarthritis becomes common, and occasionally the bony overgrowth impinges on the transverse foramina through which the vertebral arteries course. Turning the head increases the foraminal narrowing and may compress the vertebral arteries to such a degree that brain stem ischemia occurs. Vertigo on head turning may be the presenting symptom, but usually other evidences of brain stem involvement clarify the picture. The vertigo and other symptoms and signs should be reproducible by turning the head; full head dropping (see Fig 3–35) is unnecessary.

It has been shown that the dorsal root fibers coming from the cervical musculature have connections with the vestibular nuclei. These connections probably communicate head-neck-trunk axis orientation information, and at least part of the reflex response system is channeled through the vestibular-oculomotor and vestibulo-spinal motor systems. Upper cervical dorsal root impingement in osteoarthritic-narrowed cervical foramina may therefore be an alternative explanation for positional vertigo in some individuals.

IX, X. Glossopharyngeal and Vagus Nerves

These two nerves are considered together because they arise from or distribute to many of the same brain stem columns of nuclei (dorsal motor nucleus of the vagus, nucleus ambiguous, nucleus solitarius, spinal nucleus of the trigeminal), exit from the brain stem side by side, and have similar and frequently side-by-side and overlapping functional and anatomical distributions in the periphery.

PHARYNX

The pharynx is innervated by nerves IX and X with motor and sensory contributions from both. There is a great deal of overlap in distribution, but some segregation persists in that the oral pharynx and soft palate are mainly innervated by nerve IX, whereas the more caudal pharyngeal structures lying behind the tonsilar pillars are predominantly innervated by nerve X.

Contraction of the paired and fused muscles of both sides of the soft palate causes upward and outward movement vectors (Fig

3–36). The sum vector is an upward, midline movement of the palate. If the innervation of one side is interrupted (e.g., by a tumor at the jugular foramen, compressing nerve IX and likely also nerve X), the palate elevates asymmetrically, being pulled up toward the strong side and away from the weak half of the palate (Fig 3–37).

If both sides of the palate are weak, as occurs in persons with bilateral supranuclear lesions or focal bilateral invasion by tumor (most commonly this is a retropharyngeal carcinoma that spreads along the base of the skull, involving cranial nerves at their foraminal exits), the palate does not elevate normally during phonation and a nasal quality is imparted to the voice. This is because the voice is more deflected into and damped by the nasal passages.

The gag reflex is mainly a IX + X/IX + X sensory/motor arc confined to the oral and pharyngeal region. In very sensitive individuals, much more of the neuraxis may be involved; a simple gag may enlarge to retching and vomiting in some. A greater extent of visceral musculature (esophageal, gastric, and small bowel) and somatic musculature (abdominal and thoracic) then comes into play. The gag response varies greatly from individual to individual but is relatively constant in any one person. It is fortunate for the patient-physician relationship that in most subjects it is confined to the oral and pharyngeal region. Otherwise, the examiner might avoid routinely testing the reflex!

Palate function is tested by having the patient say "aah," a maneuver that normally elevates the palate in the midline (see Fig 3–36). The pillars and the posterior pharyngeal wall of each side are then gingerly probed with a tongue blade. The normal gag response is a mass contraction of both sides of the posterior oral and pharyngeal musculature and an indication by the patient of an unpleasant experience. In peripheral nerve involvement, most commonly noted with tumor compression of the nerves at or external to the jugular foramen, the gag response and experience are absent or depressed on the affected side. Stimulation of the normal side elicits only a unilateral response; no consensual response is seen. This is because both the motor and sensory nerves are involved on the affected side. With a lesion (most commonly ischemic) of the nucleus ambiguous, which is the motor nucleus to the pharynx and larynx, the same hyporesponsivity ipsilateral to the lesion occurs with stimulation of either side. Because the sensory limb is intact on the weak side, however, a

Fig 3–36. — Elevation of soft palate.

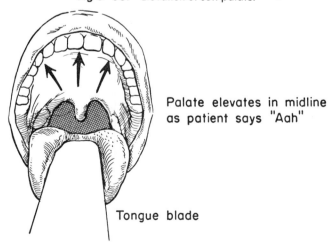

Palate elevates in midline as patient says "Aah"

Tongue blade

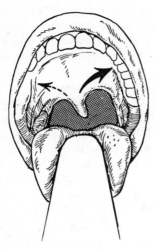

Fig 3–37. — Elevation of palate away from weakened right side (Rideau or curtain sign).

contralateral consensual response occurs when the weak side is probed.

The gag reflex is frequently under such strong voluntary control that probing causes very little or no response. This could make differentiation of normal suppression of the gag from symmetric pathologic depression of motor and/or sensory function difficult. However, by having the subject swallow some water, the examiner should be able to make this differentiation. Swallowing is unimpeded if the gag is normally suppressed, but if there is bilateral sensory and/or motor deficit, escape of fluid into the unprotected larynx and subsequent choking and coughing are likely (which the patient may well confirm in the history). This is because closure of the epiglottis, a normal concomitant of swallowing and also gagging, is deficient. The water-swallowing test is also useful in helping to determine how a patient with significant neurologic deficit eats. Being told of a recently admitted patient's choking and possibly asphyxiation on food is a poor way to discover that he has a deficit in swallowing.

To differentiate between involvement of the peripheral and nuclear portions of any cranial nerve, the examiner looks in the latter instance for the associated involvement of other cranial nerves, cerebellar functions, and, most particularly, long-tract involvement in the brain stem (corticospinal and autonomic motor, and lemniscal and spinothalamic sensory path). It is unusual for brain stem lesions to involve one or several cranial nerves in isolation from the contiguous long-tract and cerebellar system structures. Poliomyelitis with isolated viral involvement of the cranial motor nuclei, though rare today, is an exception to this rule as is motor neuron disease, a degenerative disease involving upper and lower motor neurons exclusively.

Laryngeal control is primarily a function of the vagus nerves. It is worth reviewing the anatomy of the principal vagal innervation of the vocal cords, the recurrent laryngeal nerves. These nerves take a long, circuitous route before reaching the larynx. The left nerve passes all the way to the aortic arch, which it encircles before turning back up through the mediastinum and the root of the neck to reach the left larynx. Mediastinal lesions (e.g., carcinoma of the esophagus and aortic aneurysms) not uncommonly are first evidenced by hoarseness, the manifestation of paralysis of the left vocal cord. The same is true for malignancies in the neck, where both the right and left recurrent nerves can be affected. The right recurrent nerve does not enter the thorax; it reaches only as far as the right subclavian artery, which it encircles before turning back to reach the larynx.

Loss of the function of one or both recurrent laryngeal nerves causes dysphonia, as manifested by hoarseness. Beyond the usual maximum three-week duration of a laryngitic inflammatory process, hoarseness, a persistent difficulty in producing intonated sounds and decreased intensity of vigor of the voice, should alert the examiner to the possibility of unilateral or bilateral vocal cord weakness or paralysis and warrants examination of laryngeal appearance and function. Indirect laryngoscopy is the most convenient technique for bedside examination; it requires a simple curved dental mirror and a light source (a bedside lamp shining over the physician's shoulder or a flashlight held by an assistant) (Fig 3–38). The tongue is held protruded with cotton gauze or is depressed gingerly with a tongue blade, and the mirror, previously warmed with tap water to avoid fogging by the patient's breath, is then placed face down just posterior to the soft palate, not touching the pharyngeal walls to avoid gagging. If the patient cannot avoid gagging, it is sometimes useful to spray the nasopharynx with a small amount of a weak topical anesthetic such as 1% Xylocaine. With the light showing into the pharynx, the mirror allows a view of the superior aspect of the larynx covered by the epiglottis. The patient is asked to say "aah." The epiglottis then uncovers the vocal cords, which should be in a relatively unopposed position. If the patient then attempts to say "eee," a high-pitched sound, the cords should closely oppose unless they are paralyzed on one side or both (see Fig 3–38). Though difficult to master at first, this technique is well worth learning. It is not part of a routine bedside examination, however; it should be done only when phonation changes are persistent.

Supranuclear motor pathways to the palate, pharyngeal, and laryngeal musculature are bilateral, with the motor systems of each cerebral hemisphere innervating equally the nucleus ambiguous of both sides. Lesions of the supranuclear connections therefore must as a rule be bilateral to cause difficulties with palate, pharyngeal, and laryngeal function; as an empirical rule, 50% supranuclear innervation of a muscle group is adequate for normal function. Bilateral acute or subacute loss of hemispheric connections to the nucleus ambiguous causes difficulty with swallowing, phonating, and, initially, a depressed gag reflex. In time, the gag reflex becomes uncontrollably hyperactive as do many other skeletal and autonomic reflexes that are separated from supranuclear modulation. The initially hypoactive gag is comparable to the hypoactive deep-tendon reflexes seen in patients with spinal shock and for this same reason is even seen on occasion with large and acute unilateral hemispheric lesions. It is usually bilaterally depressed but occasionally with a contralateral predominance, presumably in individuals with some predominance of contralateral supranuclear innervation.

Both nerves IX and X have taste and somatic sensory functions that are not routinely tested when the cranial nerves are evaluated. However, if on routine examina-

Fig 3–38. — Indirect (through mirror) laryngoscopy. Mirror warmed to avoid fogging by patient's breath.

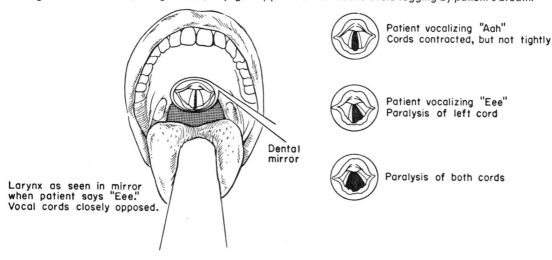

Patient vocalizing "Aah"
Cords contracted, but not tightly

Patient vocalizing "Eee"
Paralysis of left cord

Paralysis of both cords

Dental mirror

Larynx as seen in mirror when patient says "Eee." Vocal cords closely opposed.

tion, palate, pharyngeal, or laryngeal involvement is suggested, testing of these functions is indicated.

The ninth nerve carries the fibers for taste from the posterior third of the tongue; the tenth carries a few fibers from the base of the tongue and upper surface of the epiglottis. The vagal contribution to taste cannot be practically tested, but the contribution of the glossopharyngeal nerve can. A saturated solution of salt, a substance normally tasted best by the posterior and lateral tastebuds (sweet is tasted best by the anterior and midline tastebuds), is used in the testing with the same technique described for cranial nerve VII.

In addition to the palate, pharynx, and larynx, nerves IX and X supply sensory nerves to the external auditory canal. They share this supply with the seventh nerve and, possibly to some extent, with the fifth nerve and cervical roots II and III. This extensive overlap precludes loss of sensation caused by lesions of any one component. Pain in the ear, however, may be a prominent early complaint associated with a lesion that is irritating any one of these cranial nerves. If nerve IX and/or X is involved, pain in the pharyngeal region frequently is also present, helping to differentiate from the pain of seventh-nerve irritation, which would be confined to the ear and mastoid region. If facial weakness is present, it is also a clue, as well as depression of the gag reflex. Fifth-nerve involvement is differentiated by the observation of deficits in sensation and discomfort over the face; involvement of the upper cervical nerves is indicated by hypoesthesia or pain in the scalp and back of the neck.

The carotid sinus reflex is a IX sensory/X motor arc, normally functioning as a baroreceptor feedback control apparatus for the cardiovascular system. Increased intravascular pressure causes increased firing within the carotid sinus, which lies at the carotid bifurcation. The major observable response is slowing of the heart rate and lowering of the blood pressure. Because the receptor

works as a mechanical transducer, any kind of manipulation with subsequent distortion of the sinus can cause slowing of the pulse and hypotension. Firm massaging of the carotid bifurcation while monitoring pulse and blood pressure is the bedside technique for testing the reflex. The occasional and potentially dangerous cardiac arrhythmias caused by this procedure in elderly and middle-aged patients who are predisposed to atherosclerotic cardiac ischemic disease precludes its use as a routine bedside examination. Also in elderly patients the carotid bifurcation is a common site of friable atherosclerotic intimal lesions, which may be broken loose by coarse mechanical manipulations and embolize the cerebral circulation. Reflex IX/X cardiac slowing and the resulting increase in diastolic perfusion of the coronary arteries may alleviate angina pectoris temporarily, and therefore carotid massage is considered by some a useful test for differentiating angina from other types of chest pain. Sublingual administration of nitroglycerin is a proved method for doing the same thing and is recommended as a considerably safer diagnostic technique. The increase in vagal tone elicited by this carotid massage is frequently useful in terminating attacks of paroxysmal atrial tachycardia. It is therefore of both therapeutic and diagnostic use in younger individuals with this not unusual disorder.

XI. Spinal Accessory Nerve

Nerve XI has two major components: (1) a central branch arising from the caudal end of the nucleus ambiguous and probably also the dorsal motor nucleus of the vagus and (2) a spinal accessory branch arising in the first five to six cervical spinal segments from the lateral portion of the ventral horn. The central branch of nerve XI, derived from both the nucleus ambiguous and the dorsal motor nucleus of nerve X, joins the vagus on leaving the brain stem, and with nerve X, innervates pharyngeal and laryngeal musculature and sends autonomic fibers along with the vagus to thoracic and probably also abdominal viscera. Because of the structural contiguity and functional overlap of these two nerves, it is practical to consider them together and many do not even consider nerve XI to contain a central branch of its own. Testing of these components would be the same as for cranial nerve X.

The spinal accessory branch has an unusual derivation. It arises from anterior horn cells in cervical spinal segments 1 through 6, sending its fibers laterally (not with the ventral root system) where they join to form a main trunk, lying just dorsal to the denticulate ligaments, which ascends to pass through the foramen magnum. The trunk then turns laterally to pass to the jugular foramen along with cranial nerves IX, X, and central XI. Passing back down into the neck, the accessory nerve innervates the upper half of the trapezius and most of the sternomastoid muscle. The remainder of each of these muscles is supplied by segmental cervical and thoracic ventral roots.

The sternomastoid muscle rotates the head toward the opposite side. The two sternomastoids contracting together flex the head toward the chest.

The bulk in outline of the sternomastoids should be observed. Sternomastoid weakness, like facial weakness, is frequently evi-

dent before testing is carried out. Atrophy and fasciculations may be obvious with a nuclear or peripheral nerve lesion, and weakness may be indicated by the patient holding his head slightly toward the weak side. With bilateral weakness, the head may be inclined posteriorly for lack of flexor tone; however, the remaining cervical musculature usually compensates adequately and there is no postural head change. Spasmodic torticollis, an excessive activity of unknown etiology, in one (rarely both) of the sternomastoids is very obvious from observation. The subject's head is spasmodically turned away from the involved muscle, which is usually obviously hypertrophied. A striking phenomenon is the frequent ability of a patient to terminate the spasm by simply touching the opposite side of the chin, a reason given by some, surely faulty, for attributing the whole problem to psychiatric disability. Testing entails having the subject turn his head against the examiner's hand, which is pressed against the patient's chin (Fig 3–39). The bulk of the muscle is then easily seen and palpated, and its strength can be determined. Both muscles are tested by having the patient press his restrained chin toward his chest.

Complete paralysis of the sternomastoid (e.g., by a tumor in the jugular foramen or

Fig 3–39. — A, testing of right sternomastoid muscle. B, testing upper portion of trapezius muscles.

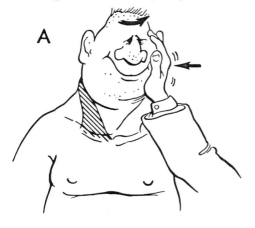

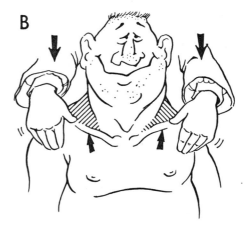

along the base of the skull) does not cause complete loss of head-turning toward the opposite side. Cervical paraspinal and strap muscles are capable of carrying out adequate though weak versions.

The corticobulbar (supranuclear) supply to the accessory motor neurons of either side in the cervical spinal cord is derived from both cerebral hemispheres in approximately equal proportions. Therefore, unilateral lesions of the supranuclear, corticospinal motor system do not cause significant weakness of the sternomastoid muscles. Nevertheless, on occasion an interesting instructive disability occurs with unilateral supranuclear lesions at the telencephalic level. There is a weakness of *voluntary* turning of the head and also the eyes (review cranial nerves III, IV, and VI) toward the opposite side. But the muscle involved is the ipsilateral sternomastoid. The right hemisphere causes the right sternomastoid to turn the head to the contralateral side; the left hemisphere the reverse. We frequently lose sight of the fact that the cortical motor system causes *movement* in or toward the opposite side and that this may entail ipsilateral musculature, particularly when axial turning (eyes, head, trunk) is carried out. This turning function, however, is usually depressed only transiently by unilateral hemispheric lesions. Presumably this is due to the bilaterality of innervation of each muscle group, allowing either hemisphere, if isolated by loss of its partner, to produce turning to either side. Recent experimental evidence suggests that careful testing, particularly of the vestibular-oculomotor system, reveals residual minor turning deficits not seen on ordinary testing (i.e., depression of the checking component of nystagmus). Bilateral supranuclear denervation causes weakness of voluntary turning of the head to either side and weakness of voluntary depression of the head on chest. No atrophy is present in the sternomastoid muscles. Other brain stem-innervated musculature is affected similarly.

The spinal accessory nerve innervates the upper half of the trapezius muscles, which elevate the shoulders. Denervation is evidenced by atrophy and often fasciculations. The shoulder droops on the side of the weak muscle and there is downward displacement of the scapula posteriorly. Shrugging the shoulders against resistance is the standard way of testing the upper trapezius (Fig 3–39).

The trapezius anterior horn cell pools are also bilaterally innervated from the hemispheres as are all axial muscles, but a contralateral predominance is usually present. For this reason, supranuclear lesions usually cause mild to moderate contralateral weakness of the shoulder elevation, rarely as severe as weakness associated with peripheral lesions of the nerve.

XII. Hypoglossal Nerve

Nerve XII is entirely motor in function, innervating the muscles of the tongue. It originates from the columns of motor neurons lying on the surface of the fourth ventricle along the midline of the medullary tegmentum. From the nucleus the nerve descends and exits as a row of small radicals between the olive and the pyramid of the medulla. After a short course through the subarachnoid space, it condenses into a single nerve root and passes through the hypoglossal foramen and canal to emerge at the base of the skull, passing through the posterolateral buccopharyngeal wall to reach the tongue.

The supranuclear innervation of the hypoglossal nerve follows the rule of all axial musculature. It is bilateral; however, there is some contralateral predominance of innervation in most individuals. For this reason, unilateral supranuclear lesions involving the major pathways from the motor cortex cause a contralateral weakness of mild to moderate degree with some variation among individuals.

The tongue muscles are arranged as paired

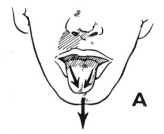
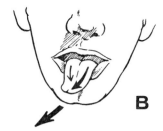
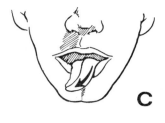

Vectors of normal tongue protrusion

Left corticobulbar system loss

Right hypoglossal nucleus or nerve destruction

Fig 3–40.—A, normal vectors of tongue protrusion. **B,** weakness without atrophy of right side of tongue with left corticobulbar lesion. **C,** weakness and atrophy (and fasciculations) with lesion of right hypoglossal nucleus or nerve. The tongue always deviates toward the weak side whether the lesion is nuclear or supranuclear.

groups, fused in the midline and oriented in multiple planes and attitudes that allow the extremely varied and complex movement capability of the tongue in speaking, chewing, swallowing, and buccal cleaning processes.

Weakness of the tongue manifests itself as a slurring of speech. The patient complains that his tongue feels "thick," "heavy," or "clumsy." Lingual sounds (i.e., l's, t's, d's, n's, r's, etc.) are slurred and this is obvious in conversation even before direct examination.

Observation of the tongue for atrophy and fasciculations is the first step of the examination. With supranuclear lesions, weakness, frequently mild, is not accompanied by loss of muscle mass or fasciculations. With nuclear lesions (e.g., paramedian vertebrobasilar vascular distribution ischemia, bulbar poliomyelitis, motor neuron disease) or nerve damage (e.g., hypoglossal neurilemoma, nasopharyngeal tumor along the base of the skull, basal skull fracture), the tongue displays weakness, atrophy, and fasciculations on the side of the involvement (Fig 3–40). Atrophy and fasciculations in combination are almost exclusively the signs of nuclear-peripheral denervation. Fasciculations are fine, multifocal twitches, evaluated in this instance by having the patient keep his tongue at rest on the floor of his mouth. They

are best seen along the lateral aspect of the tongue. Protrusion frequently causes a fine tremor in the normal tongue, which can obscure or mimic fasciculations. Strength is tested simply by having the patient protrude his tongue in the midline. The normal vectors of protrusion are illustrated in Figure 3–40, A. As with the jaw in opening the mouth, the tongue protrudes toward the weakened side (Fig 3–40, B). A repetitive or complex lingual sound (e.g., "la la la la" or "Methodist artillery") adequately tests fine coordination and usually signals difficulties secondary to lesions in the speech executive area (e.g., Broca's region), motor cortex, basal ganglia, cerebellum, brain stem, nucleus, and nerve.

The most common process causing major involvement of the twelfth nerve is probably motor neuron disease (amyotrophic lateral sclerosis), a degenerative disease of the supranuclear and nuclear motor systems that may have a predilection for early and severe involvement of the hypoglossal nucleus and later the nucleus ambiguous. This is almost always bilaterally symmetric involvement. Tumors or trauma involving the base of the skull are the most common causes of unilateral involvement of the peripheral apparatus, whereas stroke involving the upper brain stem, or more commonly the cerebral hemisphere, is the usual cause of unilateral supranuclear dysfunction.

REFERENCES

Brodal, A.: *Neurological Anatomy in Relation to Clinical Medicine*, ed. 2. New York, Oxford University Press, 1969.

Cogan, D. G.: *Neurology of the Ocular Muscles*, ed. 2. Springfield, Ill., Charles C Thomas, Publisher, 1956.

Monrad-Krohn, G. H., Refsum, S.: *The Clinical Examination of the Nervous System*, ed. 12. London, H. K. Lewis & Co., 1964.

Spillane, J. D.: *Atlas of Clinical Neurology*, ed. 2. New York, Oxford University Press, 1975.

Walsh, F. B., Hoyt, W. F.: *Clinical Neuro-ophthalmology*, ed. 3. Baltimore, Williams & Wilkins Co., 1969.

4

Motor System Evaluation

IN THIS CHAPTER we discuss in general terms the system that is responsible for voluntary and reflex somatic behavior. The motor system can be divided into (1) the peripheral apparatus, which consists of the anterior horn cell and its peripheral axon, the neuromuscular junction, and muscle, and (2) the more complex central apparatus, which includes the pyramidal and extrapyramidal systems, which initiate and modulate motor activity through the peripheral apparatus.

Dysfunction in individual components of the peripheral and central systems results in fairly specific abnormalities that can be observed or elicited at the bedside. Although multiple components may be involved, particularly with diseases of the central nervous system, isolated involvement of the various components commonly occurs and examples of these should help you establish an orderly approach to motor system evaluation (Table 4–1).

Examination for motor dysfunction should consist of a fairly rigid routine. Table 4–2 lists the components of a comprehensive and efficient screening examination that will elicit and localize most motor system dysfunctions. Table 4–3 lists the findings expected with diseases listed in Table 4–1.

Peripheral Apparatus (see chap. 8)

Weakness is the major complaint of a person who has a problem in any part of the motor unit (anterior horn cell-peripheral axon, neuromuscular junction, and muscle). The characteristics of the weakness in most instances decide which part of the system is involved.

Typically, muscle disease (myopathy) has its earliest and greatest effects on proximal musculature. There is no definitive explanation of this phenomenon. Certain rare myopathies involve primarily the distal muscles; however, as a rule neuronal disease is present when weakness is mainly distal. The best explanation for the distal weakness in neuronal disease is that motor (also sensory) neurons die back first at their most distant and therefore most tenuous reaches of supply. This is supported by the observation that in most diffuse peripheral neuropathies, the feet, which are most distant from the anterior horn cell, weaken earlier as a rule than do the hands, which are less distant. In the diffuse polyneuropathy of Guillain-Barré syndrome (presumed to be an autoimmune process), weakness may begin in the proximal muscles. There is no explanation for this exception; however, it suggests that the involvement is separated from the trophic effects of the anterior horn cell.

Almost all excitable membranes in the body (neurons and smooth, cardiac, and skeletal muscle) transform mechanical energy into electric energy, and, in the case of muscle, a local contraction can be elicited by this transduction. Normal skeletal muscle contracts locally when percussed. Primary disorders of muscle decrease the excitability to percussion, and the localized muscle con-

TABLE 4–1.— MOTOR SYSTEM COMPONENTS
WITH EXAMPLES OF ISOLATED INVOLVEMENT

COMPONENTS OF MOTOR SYSTEM	EXAMPLE OF ISOLATED INVOLVEMENT
Muscle	Myopathy
Neuromuscular junction	Myasthenia gravis
Peripheral and cranial nerve	Neuropathy
Ventral root	Polyradiculopathy, motor type
Anterior horn cell and cranial nerve motor neuron	Poliomyelitis, amyotrophic lateral sclerosis
Pyramidal system	Primary lateral sclerosis
Extrapyramidal	
Cerebellum	Alcoholic degeneration
Basal ganglia	Parkinsonism, Huntington's chorea, ballism
Reticular	Decerebrate rigidity

tractions are depressed or absent even when the deep-tendon reflex involving the same muscle remains intact. In disorders of the peripheral nerves, muscle excitability to percussion remains normal or may be hyperresponsive, and this frequently contrasts with depression or loss of the deep-tendon reflex involving the same muscle. Therefore, preservation of deep-tendon reflexes in weak muscles that have a depressed response to percussion indicates primary muscle disease, whereas loss of deep-tendon reflexes in weak muscles that have preserved or hyperactive response to percussion indicates neuronal disease.

In persons with myopathy, the deep-tendon reflexes are decreased in proportion to the weakness. In neuropathic conditions, because afferent fibers are frequently involved at the same time and often earlier and more severely than motor fibers, the deep-tendon reflexes are depressed out of proportion to the weakness. In typical symmetric peripheral neuropathy, the Achilles tendon reflex (ankle jerk) is depressed or absent long before significant weakness of the calf muscles can be elicited.

Muscles weakened by any peripheral process atrophy. An apparent exception to this is in some dystrophies where certain muscles (e.g., the calf muscles) appear greatly enlarged because of overgrowth of fibrous and fatty tissue. However, the muscle fibers

themselves are dropping out, so the term *pseudohypertrophy* is appropriate.

In myopathy the proximal muscles show the earliest and greatest loss of substance, whereas in most neuropathic processes the distal muscles atrophy earliest. There are exceptions in both myopathy and neuropathy. Nevertheless, the atrophy is almost invariably in the distribution of the weakness.

Any muscle without activity for a prolonged time atrophies. Muscles inactivated by a fracture cast or by pain begin to lose bulk and strength within two weeks. Recovery of this loss may require prolonged, vigorous exercise. The quadriceps muscles are for some reason particularly susceptible to this change. If a muscle is temporarily weakened and inactivated by a reversible neuropathic or myopathic process, disuse atrophy compounds the losses caused by the primary process. Although some controversy exists on this point, many recommend continued active use of weakened muscles to avoid what sometimes may be a significant disuse component of the disability.

Disuse atrophy and weakness may be of great significance in the person who has suffered a past neuromuscular insult such as poliomyelitis and who has, through vigorous physical therapy, made maximal and effective use of residual motor units. A short period of inactivity caused by hospitalization for another illness or simply from "taking it

TABLE 4-2.—MOTOR SYSTEM EXAMINATION AND ANCILLARY STUDIES

1. Observation.
   a. Muscle group size, symmetry; limb and trunk posture (e.g., contractures).
   b. Involuntary movements.
      i. Adventitious movement disorder (e.g., chorea, dystonic posture, tremor, myoclonus, seizures).
      ii. Fasciculations.
      iii. Myotonia on attempted active movement.
2. Palpation and percussion.
   a. Tenderness, consistency (less reliable in differential).
   b. Response of muscle to direct percussion.
3. Passive resistance to manipulation.
   a. Spasticity, rigidity (plastic/cogwheel or perseverative/paratonic).
   b. Hypotonia.
4. Strength.
   a. Sampling of distal and proximal musculature of extremities in addition to cranial, neck, and trunk muscles (e.g., cranial nerve exam, trapezius and sternomastoids, neck extensors, deltoids, biceps, triceps, wrist dorsiflexion, grip, interosseus fingerspread, abdominals, psoas, quadriceps, hamstrings, gastrocnemius-soleus, anterior tibialis, dorsiflexion of foot and large toe). If weakness or other indication of motor involvement is observed, more detailed exam is necessary.
   b. Grading of strength:
      0 No evidence of movement
      1 Trace muscle movement
      2 Complete range with gravity eliminated
      3 Complete range against gravity
      4 Complete range against gravity with some resistance
      5 Normal
5. Coordination.
   a. Rapid rhythmic alternating movements (RRAM) of upper and lower extremities (e.g., tapping thumb against index finger, tapping heel on opposite knee).
   b. Finger-to-nose, eyes open and eyes closed; heel-to-shin.

6. Gait.
   a. Basic form observation—ataxia, spasticity, weakness, apraxia, rigidity in extension or flexion; turning behavior—en bloc, ataxic, apraxic.
   b. To test anterior tibialis and coordination: walk on heels. To test gastrocnemius and coordination: walk on toes.
   c. Coordination: tandem heel-toe, walk backward, hop on one foot at a time.
7. Deep-tendon, superficial, and pathologic reflexes.
   Ancillary Studies As Indicated (see chaps. 8 and 18)
1. Electromyography and nerve conduction studies (EMG and NCV).
   a. To differentiate neuronal disease from muscle disease, to differentiate axonal from demyelinating neuropathy.
   b. To substantiate or rule out neuromuscular junction disorders.
2. Neostigmine or edrophonium tests in myasthenia gravis suspect (e.g., a patient with nontender muscle disease, particularly if he has increasing weakness on exercise or unexplained extraocular muscle or bulbar weakness even if only one or a few muscles are involved).
3. Neostigmine IM to enhance fasciculations in anterior horn, ventral root, and peripheral nerve disease.
4. Muscle—nerve biopsy.
5. Enzyme studies: creatine phosphokinase (CPK) elevated in acute and subacute disease of muscle; minimally or not elevated with slowly progressive muscle disease, and peripheral or central nervous system disease.
6. Vitamin B_{12}, folate levels; thyroxine—T3, T4 tests; glucose tolerance, K+; urine porphobilinogen.
7. Lumbar puncture.
8. Electroencephalogram.
9. Neuroradiologic studies: skull and spine x-rays, brain scan, angiography, pneumoencephalogram, myelography, cisternography, computerized axial tomography.

easy" can result in major disuse disability. We recently were called to see a patient who had residual severe weakness from old poliomyelitis. She had been hospitalized for many weeks following an emergency abdominal operation. Prior to hospitalization she was able to transfer from bed to wheelchair and from wheelchair to toilet and had been relatively independent. She could now no longer do either and it was suspected that she had late-onset, postpolio progressive

motor neuron disorder. In fact, she had received no physical therapy in the hospital and had rapidly lost her marginal compensation. It took three months of active physical therapy for her to regain her former independence.

Atrophy is observed with involvement of the central motor apparatus, although it is not so great as that seen with neuromuscular disease. It is most likely also caused by decreased use of the involved limbs.

TABLE 4-3.—ISOLATED MOTOR SYSTEMS INVOLVEMENT: GENERAL CHARACTERISTICS ON EXAMINATION

EXAMINATION KEY: 1. Observation. 2. Palpation and percussion. 3. Passive resistance. 4. Strength. 5. Coordination: a. RRAM; b. Finger to nose, etc. 6. Gait. 7. Deep-tendon reflexes.

MUSCLE: MYOSITIS AND DYSTROPHY

Examination
1. Proximal wasting prominent.
2. Myositic muscle may be tender to palpation.
3. Decreased resistance.
4. Proximal weakness predominant with late distal involvement.
5. a. Slow and irregularly clumsy.
   b. Slow, but accurate if strong enough.
6. Difficulty climbing and descending stairs, running, rising from chair or floor, or crossing obstacles; waddling gait.
7. Tendon reflexes usually present, but depressed in parallel to weakness.

Special Studies
1. EMG and NCV: Decreased units diffusely with small, fast, myopathic potentials; normal conduction time.
2. Normal edrophonium or neostigmine test (i.e., no increased strength).
3. No fasciculations with neostigmine.
4. Biopsy: diffuse muscle degeneration, inflammatory infiltrate in myositis, noninflammatory degeneration if dystrophy.
5. Elevated level of serum muscle enzymes (creatine phosphokinase most sensitive); may not be elevated in late or chronic myositis and dystrophy. A useful measurement in evaluating course of disease and results of therapy.
6. Thyroid deficiency or excess may be present.

NEUROMUSCULAR JUNCTION: MYASTHENIA GRAVIS

Examination
1. Extraocular muscle system most frequently involved early. Other bulbar muscles frequently involved. Distal and proximal muscles of extremities affected less and later as a rule. Atrophic changes occur from disuse; dystrophic features in *long-standing* disease, possibly related in part to chronic anticholinesterase effect.
2. Nontender.
3. Decreasing tone with increasing weakness.
4. Characteristic increasing weakness with exercise with usually prompt recovery to *almost* normal strength on resting early; increasingly irreversible weakness with progression of disease.
5. Slow but usually accurate.
6. As with diffuse weakness, but frequently not severely involved because extremity muscles are less affected.
7. Progressive decrease in DTR response with repeated tendon tapping.

Special Tests
1. EMG and NCV: Progressively decreasing muscle potentials with exercise or repeated motor nerve stimulation.
2. Neostigmine and edrophonium cause prompt strengthening and resistance to fatigue in affected

muscles (less reliable with extraocular myasthenia).
3. Biopsy nonspecific.

Special Study
Neuromuscular postsynaptic membrane antibodies detectable in serum.

PERIPHERAL NERVE: NEUROPATHY

Examination
1. Distal atrophy prominent, occasional fasciculations.
2. *Sensory abnormalities* usually associated, and therefore patients have concomitant sensory symptoms (hypoesthesia, paresthesia, etc.)
3. Decreased tone.
4. Distal weakness predominates.
5. Where proprioception is lost, closure of eyes results in misplacements (if in lower extremities, positive Romberg sign).
6. As with distal weakness and proprioceptive loss.
7. Depressed to absent DTRs.

Special Studies
1. Decreased conduction time with demyelinating neuropathies, occasional fasciculations and giant summation potentials on EMG.
2. Neostigmine may bring out fasciculations.
3. Biopsy reveals motor unit dropout and neuronal damage.
4. Evidence for malnutrition (folic acid level decreased), diabetes mellitus, thyroid deficiency, vitamin B_{12} deficiency, uremia, porphyria, heavy metal poisoning to be sought among others by appropriate blood, urine, and stool studies.

VENTRAL ROOT: ACUTE AND SUBACUTE POLYNEUROPATHY

Examination
1. Nonspecific, occasional fasciculations.
2. Nonspecific, nontender.
3. Decreased tone.
4. Ascending weakness frequent (Landry, Guillain-Barré, and carcinomatous radiculopathy) with distal prominence though occasional major proximal prominence early.
5. Slow, but accurate if able.
6. Nonspecific.
7. Usually absent DTRs.

Special Tests
1. Nerve conduction slowed; EMG with occasional fasciculations and decreased mass response (interference pattern).
2. Neostigmine may increase fasciculations.
3. Level of protein in cerebrospinal fluid up; cells normal (if cells are increased or not, cytologic tests should be done for malignant cells).

ANTERIOR HORN CELL: POLIOMYELITIS, AMYOTROPHIC LATERAL SCLEROSIS

Examination
1. Patchy *atrophy* from single muscles to large masses; fasciculations not prominent. (In amyotrophic lateral sclerosis, there tends to be

TABLE 4-3.—(Cont.)

EXAMINATION KEY: 1. Observation. 2. Palpation and percussion. 3. Passive resistance. 4. Strength. 5. Coordination: a. RRAM; b. Finger to nose, etc. 6. Gait. 7. Deep-tendon reflexes.

symmetric involvement with prominent fasciculations.)
2. Tender early in polio.
3. Decreased tone, unless contractures. (In ALS, tone may be increased, decreased, or normal depending on balance of anterior horn/long-tract involvement.)
4. Weakness appropriate to distribution and severity of atrophy.
5. Nonspecific.
6. Depends on muscle groups involved.
7. Depressed to absent DTRs in proportion to weakness. (In ALS, increased, decreased, or normal depending on balance of anterior horn/long-tract involvement.)

Special Studies
1. EMG: fasciculations, fibrillations, and giant summation potentials in involved muscles.
2. Neostigmine may cause marked increase in fasciculations.
3. Throat, stool virus cultures for polio suspect. Most recent cases of polio are related to live virus vaccine complications.

PYRAMIDAL SYSTEM: PRIMARY LATERAL SCLEROSIS*
Examination:
1. Minimal atrophy; prominent flexor hypertonus; flexor spasms occur with severe involvement.
2. Nonspecific.
3. Clasp-knife rigidity.
4. Distal muscles tend to be predominantly involved with unilateral involvement.
5. Slow, irregularly clumsy.
6. Spastic—scissors and stiff leg gait; decreased arm swing.
7. DTRs hyperactive with clonus; abdominals depressed; Babinski response present.

Special Studies
To determine site of lesion, neuroradiologic studies such as myelogram, angiography, CT scan, brain scan may be needed to supplement more routine tests (i.e., lumbar puncture, EEG, skull and spine x-rays) when diagnosis is not secure.

CEREBELLUM
Examination
1. Intention tremor (rhythmic oscillatory tremor—three to eight per second, absent at rest) on side of lesion.
2. Nonspecific.
3. Decreased tone.
4. May see *mild* weakness of diffuse nature in involved extremities.
5. Past and under pointing, severe dyscoordination on RRAM.
6. Wide-based ataxic (drunk) gait with falling to side

of lesion; may see narrow or normally based gait with severe retropulsion when lesion is in midline vermis region.
7. DTRs usually normal but may be pendular.

Special Tests
CT scan, brain scan, angiography of vertebrobasilar system, pneumoencephalogram (PEG).

BASAL GANGLIA: PARKINSONISM
Examination
1. a. Three to eight per second tremor, present with tonic posturing and at rest. (Muscle must, however, have resting *tonus* to see tremor.)
   b. Bradykinesia (e.g., difficulty initiating movement, masked facies).
2. Nonspecific.
3. Cogwheel—plastic rigidity.
4. May have some weakness of disuse.
5. Bradykinesia; may be quite coordinated after movement is initiated.
6. Flexed trunk, small steps; retropulsion if pushed backward or walks backward.
7. Normal reflexes, occasionally depressed.

BASAL GANGLIA: HUNTINGTON'S CHOREA
Examination
1. Irregular, jerky, involuntary movements associated with progressive dementia; autosomal dominant so family history is the rule.

Special Test
PEG reveals loss of caudate nucleus outline in lateral ventricles.

BASAL GANGLIA: HEMIBALLISM
Examination
1. Gross flailing to mild choreic movements (contralateral to subthalamic nucleus lesion) make diagnosis obvious. Patient may die of exhaustion; however, movements are normally self-limited if caused, as is frequently the case, by ischemia-infarction.

BASAL GANGLIA: ATHETOSIS
Examination
1. Slow, writhing movements, particularly involving proximal muscles and trunk, associated with progressive dementia. (Huntington's chorea frequently has athetoid components.)

RETICULAR SYSTEMS
Examination
1. Lesions characterized by decerebrate or decorticate rigidity if between low pons and low diencephalon (see text).

*A form of motor neuron disease presumed to be part of the spectrum of amyotrophic lateral sclerosis with little detectable anterior horn cell involvement.

GENERAL DIFFERENTIATING CHARACTERISTICS OF NEURONAL AND MUSCLE DISEASES

Examination

NEURONAL	MUSCLE
Distal weakness and atrophy predominate	Proximal weakness and atrophy predominate
Sensory abnormalities common	No sensory abnormalities
Fasciculations prominent with anterior horn cell degeneration, less often present with radiculopathy and peripheral nerve involvement	No fasciculations
Response of muscle to direct percussion hyperactive	Response to percussion decreased, myotonic response to percussion in myotonias and hypothyroidism

Special Studies

NEURONAL	MUSCLE
EMG: fasciculations, fibrillations, giant potentials; slowed nerve conduction with demyelinating peripheral nerve involvement	EMG: myopathic potentials (high-frequency, low-amplitude); decreased motor units in general; normal conduction velocities
Neostigmine: increased fasciculations	No response to neostigmine
Muscle enzymes usually not increased in blood	Muscle enzymes (CPK most sensitive) increased in active disease
Biopsy: atrophy and degeneration of groups of muscle fibers (motor units); degeneration of nerve fibers may be seen	Biopsy: diffuse, patchy atrophy and degeneration of muscle fibers; inflammatory infiltrates seen in active myositis
Sedimentation rate normal in most	Sedimentation rate elevated in some myositis

Parietal lobe involvement is also associated with atrophy of the contralateral limbs, and this is presumed by some to be a function of inactivity of the limb.

As mentioned, neuropathic processes frequently also involve the sensory systems, resulting in loss of sensation or symptoms of sensory nerve hyperactivity (e.g., pins-and-needles paresthesias, burning, aching, hypersensitivity to stimuli). Pure anterior horn cell disease (e.g., motor neuron disease) is an exception, with no observable sensory system involvement. Because of this, the deep-tendon reflexes are depressed in proportion to weakness as in myopathy. In myopathies, sensory symptoms and signs are unusual with the exception of some inflammatory processes (e.g., polymyositis) in which pain and tenderness may be present.

During normal motor activity, motor units contract in a synchronous and graded fashion. On occasion, single normal motor units may fire spontaneously and independent of any purposeful or reflex movement. This causes a visible twitch called a *fasciculation*. Most individuals experience occasional isolated fasciculations. These are more likely to follow exercise. If the exercise is particularly strenuous and prolonged, the fasciculations may occur in great numbers in the most exercised muscles, for example, the gastrocnemius in long-distance runners. As a rule, however, multiple fasciculations represent a pathologic hyperexcitability of the anterior horn cell or its axon. Direct degenerative involvement of the anterior horn cell is the most common cause of multiple fasciculations. The pathophysiology is presumed to be a hyperexcitability of the degenerating (or regenerating) motor neuron dendritic membrane to random excitatory synaptic inputs or simply an autoexcitability of a defective, leaky neuronal membrane. Peripheral axon degeneration is also associated with fasciculations but to a lesser degree than anterior horn cell involvement. These fasciculations may represent retrograde changes in the anterior horn cell membrane or possibly a denervation hypersensitivity of the neuromuscular junction to small amounts of circulating acetylcholine or other cholinergic substances.

Small doses of neostigmine, a cholinesterase inhibitor that increases acetylcholine availability at the end-plate (and does not cross the blood-brain barrier), are effective in enhancing or eliciting fasciculations in peripheral neuropathic conditions. This supports the hypothesis that fasciculations seen in peripheral neuropathy are secondary to a denervation hypersensitivity phenomenon. Increased fasciculations also follow neostigmine injection in anterior horn cell disease presumably for the same reason. Fasciculations are not elicited by cholinesterase inhibitors in patients with myopathic disorders and are elicited only to a small degree in normal persons.

The most common primary disorder of the neuromuscular junction is myasthenia gravis. The best evidence indicates that its pathogenesis is defective or blocked muscle endplate receptivity. Characteristically the weakness is excessive and rapid muscle fatigue, with extraocular and bulbar muscles being earliest involved, followed by limb and trunk muscles. On resting, the fatigued muscles regain some strength, although as the disease progresses this becomes less and less possible. Increasing the available acetylcholine by use of cholinesterase inhibitors such as edrophonium or neostigmine is both diagnostic and therapeutic, though not curative.

Myotonia is a resistance to active movement in muscle caused by a persistent and involuntary contraction of antagonist muscles that normally are inhibited by reciprocal neuromuscular mechanisms. It occurs in several rare conditions, and it appears to be a striated muscle abnormality and not an abnormality of innervation. It can be elicited easily by asking the individual to reverse a muscle action quickly; for example, opening a tightly clenched fist occurs very slowly.

Electric recording shows continued contraction of the hand flexors, which are normally silent when the extensor muscles are activated. The increased resistance to movement caused by cooling of muscle appears similar to myotonia and cooling may in fact exacerbate myotonia but is presumably a passive phenomenon. The response to percussion in myotonic muscle is abnormal and is used as a diagnostic test. Tapping the thenar muscle group of the hand causes depolarization and contraction and the thumb adducts. Normally the contraction is brief and the thumb promptly returns to its neutral resting position. The myotonic thenar muscle group continues to contract and the thumb only sluggishly returns to the resting position.

Central Apparatus

Voluntary motor behavior reaches its phylogenetic peak in humans and is reflected best in the fine movements of the articulatory apparatus that are involved in verbal language and in the highly skilled capabilities of the hands. The greatly enlarged neocortical mantle is presumed to be the substrate for most if not all volitional movement in humans.

Most neural science texts still consider the pyramidal system the executive of purposive or voluntary motor activity. This is not entirely correct. The motor cortex in and around the precentral gyrus, from which arises at least 40% of the pyramidal tract as it passes through the pyramids of the medulla, does not have the capacity for voluntary behavior in the absence of the remaining neocortical mantle. Destruction of the motor cortex alone, however, causes contralateral weakness and loss of skilled movements. One can therefore conclude that the motor cortex and presumably the remainder of neurons in other regions, particularly the postcentral gyrus and premotor cortex, which give rise to the pyramidal tract, represent a major, final station through which motor commands, particularly for skilled distal movements, are relayed to the final efferent circuitry in the brain stem and spinal cord. Purposeful or voluntary motor activity is probably best considered to arise from many areas of the cerebral cortex; it is modified by subcortical systems such as the basal ganglia, reticular formation, thalamus, cerebellum, vestibular network, and major sensory projections.

There are other corticospinal and cortico-bulbar systems including the cortico-rubro-bulbospinal, cortico-reticular-bulbospinal, cortico-striatal-bulbospinal, and cortico-cer-ebellar-bulbospinal pathways. There are no good clinical data to implicate any of these extrapyramidal systems as a major motor executive. However, destruction of the py-ramidal system in isolation at the base of the medulla or in other parts of the cortico-spinal-corticobulbar descending pathway— i.e., precentral gyrus, internal capsule, cere-bral peduncle, basis pontis, lateral spinal col-umn—results in a transient weakness from which considerable recovery can and usually does occur. It must be assumed that, beyond resolution of the pathologic process itself, these other systems are the main basis for recovery. When the destruction extends be-yond the traditional descending motor path-way to include the extrapyramidal projec-tions, it is not surprising that less recovery of purposeful motor activity occurs.

In lower vertebrates, particularly those with no significant cerebral cortex, such as reptiles, amphibians, and fish, purposeful motor activity is simpler. The word *volun-tary* probably has little meaning at this level of phylogeny. It can be more easily catego-rized as a stereotype of behaviors, therefore almost reflex in nature, directed toward pres-ervation of self and species. These animals rely on what appear to be motor patterns laid down at the spinal cord and brain stem level, which are released and modulated by de-scending influences from the basal ganglia, upper brain stem reticular formations, tec-tum, and vestibular system. As the cerebral (and cerebellar) cortex evolved through the

phylogenetic scale, finally mushrooming in size through the mammalian line to reach its peak in humans, these primitive motor sys-tems remained but increased only minimally in size and complexity. Their role in motor function also became less and less important, so that in humans isolated loss of parts of these systems (e.g., the globus pallidus, a very important efferent system in fish and reptiles) is not associated with any significant change in motor activity (see chap. 13). Loss of the vestibular system causes only tran-sient and readily compensated dysfunction in humans (see chap. 3). If much of the cerebral cortex is destroyed in humans, for example by severe hypoxia to which it is exquisitely and preferentially susceptible, the basal gan-glia, reticular formation, vestibular system, and spinal cord can execute very basic vege-tative functions that are, however, inade-quate for independent existence of any kind. We cannot revert to the full capabilities of our distant relative the salamander.

If this is true then what are the functions of the subcortical motor systems in humans? Are these systems, particularly the globus pallidus, simply appendices, vestigial in func-tion but not discarded in evolution? To some degree this is probably so; however, it is quite clear from clinical observations that most subcortical structures subserve some basic motor functions. The basal ganglia and ves-tibular system remain, for example, impor-tant substrates for automatic postural adjust-ment (see chaps. 3 and 13) but have come under cortical control. The reticular forma-tion appears to be one of the major systems through which extrapyramidal cortical influ-ences affect voluntary behavior and may be particularly prominent in the recovery of voluntary motor activity following pyramidal loss. In contrast, the tectal descending sys-tems (particularly from the superior collicu-lus) appear to be almost vestigial in lower primates and probably also in humans, be-cause their removal in apes results in no ob-vious motor dysfunction; in lower mammals removal is associated with major deficits in orientation of the body and eyes toward all modalities of external stimuli. Presumably the visual, somatesthetic, auditory-vestibular, and olfactory primary cortices have taken over these functions in higher primates.

From this short preamble it should be fairly clear that we know only little about the substrates of voluntary motor activity in humans. Nevertheless, although destructive or irritative processes involving the nervous systems are limited in what they can teach us about normal function, the abnormal patterns of function associated with various lesions are well described and fairly specific for involvement of the various parts of the central and peripheral motor systems. Using a standard examination (see Table 4–2) these abnormalities can be readily recognized and aid in localization of the abnormal process or processes.

Disorders of language (dysphasias) and other highly skilled motor functions (dyspraxias) are associated with lesions in various parts of the association cortices and were described in chapter 2. In this section we confine ourselves to a description of abnormalities associated with involvement of the corticospinal and corticobulbar pathways and the major subcortical motor systems.

PYRAMIDAL-EXTRAPYRAMIDAL (CORTICOSPINAL-CORTICOBULBAR) SYSTEM

Lesions involving the corticofugal motor system almost always affect the pyramidal and also the extrapyramidal projections to varying degrees. The pyramidal system can only be involved in isolation at the base of the medulla where it appears to be relatively free from extrapyramidal contamination. This involvement occurs rarely and is usually the result of occlusion of a paramedian penetrating branch of a vertebral artery. Although persons with this lesion are rare, it is worth describing the syndrome because it helps to separate out the basic components of the much more common syndrome that

results from involvement of both pyramidal and extrapyramidal corticofugal influences.

Acutely, contralateral paralysis of distal limb movements is characteristic, while proximal limb movements are severely weakened and trunk movement minimally involved. Muscle tone (measured as passive resistance to manipulation) is depressed and may remain so permanently. The deep-tendon reflexes are initially absent, recovering in time to normal or slightly hyperactive levels. The superficial reflexes (abdominal and cremasteric) opposite the lesion are depressed or absent. A Babinski response (dorsiflexion of the hallux and in its fullest form with flexion at the knee and hip) can be elicited by noxious stimulation of the lateral aspect of the plantar surface in the paralyzed leg. The Babinski response appears to be a disinhibition of a primitive spinal reflex that comes under inhibitory control when the pyramidal system myelinates during infancy. When the reflex disappears, it is replaced by the normal plantar response—flexion of the hallux and toes.

Over weeks to months proximal strength improves to a significant degree, whereas distal movements make only a poor recovery. A rudimentary grasping capability is frequently all that remains in the hand. Extension, opposition, and individual finger movements remain severely depressed or are entirely lost. The little recovery of distal movements that occurs is presumed to be related to preserved extrapyramidal corticofugal systems such as the cortico-rubro-spinal tract and, to a much lesser degree, to ipsilateral projections from the preserved opposite pyramidal system. The pyramidal projection to the spinal cord is approximately 95% crossed for motor neurons that innervate distal movements, and has a contralateral predominance for proximal muscle groups, although to a lesser degree. The motor neuron circuits that innervate axial muscles receive an approximately equal pyramidal supply from each cerebral hemisphere, with variable small contralateral predominance.

The latter is most apparent in several cranial nerves, particularly those that innervate the lower facial muscles and the tongue (see chap. 3).

Neuroanatomy texts and clinical observation are frequently at odds concerning the proximal motor innervation of limbs by the corticofugal motor systems. Traditionally we are taught that approximately 90% of the corticospinal pathway crosses in the pyramidal decussation and that approximately 70% of the remaining uncrossed fibers ultimately cross to the opposite anterior horn at segmental spinal levels. This means that 97% of the descending corticospinal pathway ultimately innervates contralateral anterior horn cell systems. If only 3% of the descending fibers remain ipsilateral, one is left with a major contradiction to the preceding statements concerning the bilaterality of proximal control. Recent data have clarified and reconciled the issue. Approximately half the descending fibers destined to innervate proximal muscle anterior horn cells *recross* at segmental levels to reach the medial portion of the anterior horn, which contains the proximal musculature anterior horn cells.

It has been shown that the major basal ganglia descending motor systems predominantly innervate proximal musculature, and this may also account for residual proximal capability following corticospinal involvement. However, this residual basal ganglia capability is more likely related to preserved involuntary or automatic postural adjustments and not voluntary activity (see chap. 13).

This gradation in the ratio of contralateral to ipsilateral pyramidal influence on the distal, proximal, and axial muscle groups is probably an adequate explanation for the gradation of weakness (distal > proximal > axial) that follows unilateral pyramidal tract lesions and also for the relatively better recovery of proximal and axial strengths and skills.

Lesions involving the other parts of the pyramidal tract (motor cortex, corona radia-ta, internal capsule, cerebral peduncle, basis pontis, and lateral columns of the spinal cord) invariably also involve other corticofugal pathways that are intermixed with the pyramidal projection. The weakness accompanying these lesions is qualitatively and quantitatively similar to that described for pure pyramidal lesions. Added to the weakness, however, is a release of phasic reflexes and muscle tone from higher inhibitory influences. This release is manifested as hyperactivity of the deep-tendon reflexes (see chap. 6) and what is traditionally called *spasticity*, which is elicited on passive manipulation of the muscles. The muscles at rest do not have excessive tone, and unless a fairly brisk stretch is applied to them, no significant abnormality of tone is noted. With the brisk stretch of a muscle group, particularly the flexors in the upper extremity and the extensors in the lower extremity, there is a short period of normal or reduced resistance followed by a catch at about midlength of the muscle and then a sudden release of the catch and relaxation of the muscle. The last two components, the catch and release, have been likened to a closing pen knife, which is the origin of the term "clasp-knife" spasticity or rigidity. It is difficult to distinguish hyperactive deep-tendon reflexes from spasticity, and many consider them identical. Destruction of the dorsal roots from the extremities involved abolishes both the reflexes and the spasticity. The giving away or release portion of the clasp-knife phenomenon is presumed to be caused by increased firing of the inhibitory golgi tendon organs of the stretched muscles, and is possibly a defense against potential damage caused by excessive muscle tension.

If the lesion extends beyond the confines of the traditional corticospinal-corticobulbar path, more descending pathways are involved and a greater degree of spasticity is noted; also there is a poorer recovery from weakness. This is presumably because of loss of more inhibitory influences on the segmental reflex arc and loss of more facilitatory influences on the motor neuron effector systems.

Lesions like those caused by severe hypoxia, which extensively destroy the cerebral cortex and basal ganglia and preserve at least some of the diencephalon, release the lower brain stem and spinal cord motor systems to severe spasticity and hyperreflexia. Recovery of motor function is limited to a stereotyped flexion of the upper extremities and extension of the lower, with some extension of the trunk. Noxious stimulation is necessary to elicit this reflex activity, which has been called *decorticate posturing* (Fig 4–1). It has been thought, on the basis of experimental data, that release of the rubrospinal motor system is, at least in part, responsible for decorticate posturing. This is because

Fig 4–1.—Postures and major motor reflexes associated with lesions at different levels of the central nervous system. A, lesion in motor cortex and internal capsule: unilateral hemiparesis with residual excess flexor tone in upper extremity and extensor tone in lower extremity. B, bilateral midbrain transection above the red nucleus (rn): *decorticate posturing* with bilateral upper-extremity flexion and lower-extremity extension on noxious stimulation. C, bilateral pontine transection above vestibular nuclei (vn): *decerebrate posturing* with upper-extremity extension and pronation and lower-extremity extension on noxious stimulation. D, upper cervical spinal cord or lower medullary transection: lower- and upper-extremity flexion withdrawal from noxious stimulation at somatic levels below the lesion. E, thoracic spinal cord transection: flexion withdrawal of lower extremities from noxious stimulation at somatic levels below the lesion. These postures usually appear with some delay following the lesion and a period of acute shock with lack of response. The lower the lesion in the nervous system, the longer the shock state.

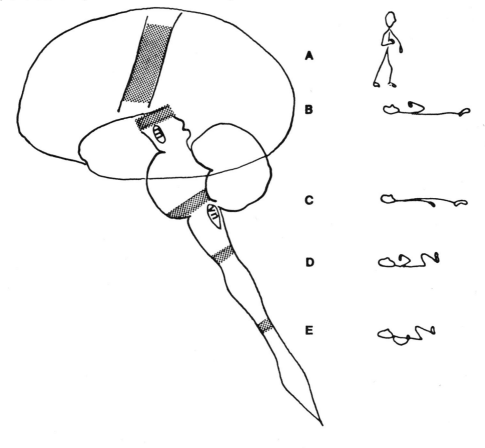

preservation of the red nucleus appears necessary for the posturing and also because the rubrospinal system distributes mainly to the neuron pool of the flexors of the upper extremities and to the extensor pool in the lumbosacral segments.

Transection of the brain stem, for example by stroke, at the level of the midbrain or pons is followed after a period of neuraxis shock by severe spasticity and reflex extension and pronation of the upper extremities with extension of the lower extremities and trunk on noxious stimulation (see Fig 4–1). This response is called *decerebrate posturing* and depends on the release of the vestibulospinal motor system from higher influences.

Lesions transecting the brain stem and also destroying the vestibular nuclei with transection of the medulla below the vestibular nuclei or transection of the spinal cord result in quadriplegia and severe spasticity after a period of shock, but no decerebrate posturing. In time, reflex flexion movements can be elicited with noxious stimulation (see Fig 4–1). These probably represent primitive spinal withdrawal responses.

Acute destructive lesions of the descending motor pathways cause a transient shock state of flaccid, areflexic paralysis. Lesions at the level of the motor cortex produce the least shock, occasionally none. When progressively greater amounts of the descending pathways are involved, a longer period of shock ensues. Acute cortical destruction may result in only hours to days of shock, whereas acute transection of the spinal cord can cause a shock state that persists for many weeks to months before spastic hyperreflexia and rudimentary spinal reflex behavior return.

Chronic or slowly progressive destruction of the descending motor pathways is not associated with a shock state. Presumably this is because compensatory reorganization of motor function occurs in pace with the losses.

The pathophysiology of motor shock is not at all clear. It has been speculated that it simply represents a loss of neuronal membrane excitability occasioned by massive loss of descending synaptic input. Recovery to a hyperactive state has been thought to be the result, at least in part, of replacement of bare synaptic zones, which were formerly occupied by descending inhibitory influences, with sprouts from axons of local and predominantly facilitatory neuronal systems. Arguing against this hypothesis is the clearing of shock and the emergence of spasticity following cortical lesions, which proceed much faster (sometimes hours) than would be anticipated for synaptic loss and reorganization.

As a rule, lesions that involve different levels of the pyramidal corticofugal motor system cannot be differentiated. The abnormalities of motor function—paresis, spasticity, hyperactive deep-tendon reflexes, depressed superficial reflexes, and the Babinski response—are the same and therefore do not help to localize the level of the lesion. The lack of spasticity with the rare medullary pyramidal lesion may be useful. Another exception is the greater likelihood of differential involvement of the limbs with lesions of the motor cortex where there is a wide zone of somatotopic representation of body parts. One of the most common cortical motor syndromes follows occlusion of the middle cerebral artery or its rolandic branches. Reviewing the blood supply to the frontal lobe, you can see that the motor representation for the arm, face, and trunk lie within the supply of the middle cerebral artery, whereas the leg lies within the distribution of the anterior cerebral artery (Fig 4–2). Loss of middle cerebral cortical perfusion therefore causes a greater degree of weakness of the upper extremity than of the lower extremity. Because of bilateral cortical distribution to the axial neuronal segments, including the face, less weakness of these groups ensues (see chap. 3). Occlusion of the anterior cerebral artery, an uncommon event, is associated with

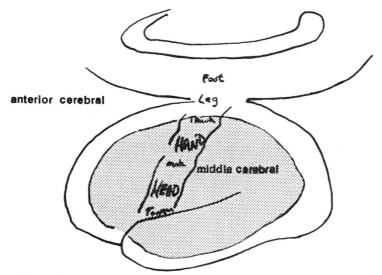

Fig 4–2.—Relationship of motor cortex somatotopic representation to the anterior and middle cerebral arterial supply.

greater weakness in the leg than in the arm.

A pyramidal-extrapyramidal syndrome with no sensory loss, although unusual, usually indicates a lesion in the posterior portion of the posterior limb of the internal capsule where the corticospinal-corticobulbar system courses in isolation from the more anteriorly and medially placed thalamocortical sensory projections. Or it can be the result of a lesion in the corticospinal tract as it runs through the basis pontis or, rarely, a lesion isolated to the pyramids of the medulla.

In most cases, the presence of signs of segmental involvement are necessary to localize definitively lesions at various levels of the corticospinal-corticobulbar system. Language difficulties, visual field abnormalities, dyspraxias, and other disorders of higher integrative function suggest cortical localization. Cranial nerve involvement localizes the lesions to the various segments of the brain stem, whereas spinal cord lesions involving the corticospinal system usually also involve segmental motor and sensory functions and the spinothalamic and/or dorsal column sensory systems that indicate a sensory level on examination (see chap. 5).

BASAL GANGLIA

The abnormalities associated with lesions and degenerative processes in the basal ganglia are discussed in some detail in chapter 13. In this chapter we discuss only the rigidity characteristic of idiopathic and drug-induced parkinsonism so that you can differentiate it from the spastic rigidity associated with corticospinal lesions. As mentioned, spastic rigidity appears to be hyperactivity of the phasic stretch reflex system and can therefore be abolished by sectioning the afferent arc of the reflex. The rigidity of parkinsonism is present in all ranges of passive manipulation and cannot be abolished by sectioning the dorsal roots. Also, as a rule, the stretch reflexes are not abnormal in parkinsonism. Presumably the abnormality is mainly increased tonic firing of the motor neurons. This may well be the result of excessive tonic motor cortex activity driven by a disinhibited globus pallidus (see chap. 13).

CEREBELLUM

Clinical observations confirm that the major function of the cerebellum is inhibitory modulation of motor activity. In humans this function is subserved mainly by the neocerebellum, which has enlarged in parallel with the cerebral cortex. The more primitive archicerebellum, which comprises part of the posterior vermis and the fastigial nuclei, has remained through phylogeny a modulator of vestibular function, and the medulloblastoma, a neoplasm of childhood that originates here, confirms that this continues to be true in humans. The associated syndrome is initially one of ipsilateral vestibular disinhibition as would be predicted from experimental studies. As the neoplasm enlarges, a neocerebellar syndrome and brain stem signs supersede the archicerebellar dysfunction.

The paleocerebellum, also part of the midline cerebellum (the vermis), plays a prominent inhibitory role in lower animals. When the anterior vermis is destroyed in cats, a marked spastic rigidity develops. Animals already rendered decerebrate by brain stem transection have their decerebrate posturing markedly enhanced by paleocerebellar removal. Despite these obvious changes in lower animals, no clear-cut paleocerebellar syndrome has been described in humans. This is presumed to be so because it is very difficult if not impossible for a lesion to involve the paleocerebellum alone without also affecting overlapping neocerebellar elements that share the vermis.

It is necessary for you to learn several clinically important somatotopic relationships of the neocerebellum. Each lateral hemisphere modulates the motor activity of the ipsilateral limbs. This modulation is directed mainly through the efferent projection of the dentate nucleus onto the contralateral motor and premotor region (dentato-rubro-thalamo-cortical pathway). The decussation of the corticospinal pathway redistributes the cerebellar effect to the limbs ipsilateral to the cerebellar hemisphere of origin. Therefore, for example, lesions of the right cerebellum and its pathways cause difficulties in the right limbs.

Because the cerebellar outflow tract (brachium conjunctivum or superior cerebellar peduncle) crosses in the midbrain, lesions of the red nucleus in the midbrain and ventrolateral thalamus create cerebellar system difficulties in the limbs opposite the lesion. In addition lesions in the frontal lobes anterior to the motor cortex (e.g., the so-called premotor cortex), to which the cerebellum also projects, are associated with motor difficulties occasionally indistinguishable from direct cerebellar involvement and they are opposite the lesion. The descending fronto-pontine systems that lie in the anterior limb of the internal capsule project to the pontine nuclei (in the basis pontis), which innervate the opposite cerebellar hemisphere through the brachium pontis (middle cerebellar peduncle). Lesions in this descending system also lead to cerebellar motor dysfunctions either contralateral to the lesions, if in the pathway from the frontal lobe through the pontine nuclei, or ipsilateral to the lesion, if in the brachium pontis or cerebellum itself.

The midline cerebellum (vermis) modulates axial motor activity, contributing to head and trunk stability and the smoothness of articulation and eye movements.

Tremor, ataxia, and hypotonia are the major components of the neocerebellar syndrome. The *tremor* is rhythmic, variably 3–8 per second in oscillation, and occurs predominantly on voluntary activity and reaches its peak of oscillation toward the end of the movement. It disappears with posturing or at rest. Fine limb movements are therefore affected as well as articulatory movements and phonation.

The patient may complain that he no longer is able to write and has difficulty drinking without spilling the contents of the container. Testing the patient by asking him to write, for example to copy a spiral, or drink from a filled cup is a simple way of semiquantitating the difficulty. Rapid rhythmic alternating movements, for example rapidly tapping the thumb and index finger together or rapidly alternating pronation and supination of the hand, are also broken up by the tremor. An increasing distance of oscillation occurs toward the end of a voluntary movement and causes the hand or foot to undershoot or overshoot the mark, for example the nose or shin. This phenomenon has been called *dysmetria* (disordered distance).

Increasing muscle tension of any origin increases the tremor. This is generally true for all tremors and adventitious movement disorders. Simply increasing the patient's anxiety level, for example by talking about his tremor and the difficulties it is causing, may markedly increase muscle tension and the tremor, whereas putting the patient at ease may decrease the severity of the tremor.

Tremor of phonation may be mild and only obvious when the patient is asked to sustain a note, for example "a a a a a h." The tremor modifies the note to a rhythmic "ah-ah-ah-ah-ah." When the tremor is severe, speech may be broken into a rhythmic production with irregularities of tone and volume caused by a combination of the rhythm and voluntary attempts to correct it. Explosive increases in volume may occur and are comparable to the dysmetria of limb tremor. In some persons, speech may be very slow and monotonous (possibly a compensation for the tremor). In lesser degrees this slowing may take on a metered or scanning quality in which inappropriate syllables are stressed.

The dysmetria of conjugate eye movements is probably also tremor. The eyes overshoot a target and then may oscillate several beats before settling on it.

Both speech and ocular abnormalities, as with other axial dysfunctions, have been associated with lesions of the vermis in its middle portion. A tremor of the head has also been associated with lesions in this region.

Cerebellar *ataxia,* an imbalance of walking, standing, and sitting, appears to have at least two origins: (1) intention tremor of the legs giving a dysmetric gait and (2) truncal imbalance, the result of a dysmetric response of the trunk to the stresses of walking or sitting.

Leg ataxia alone may be present with involvement of the lateral hemispheres, for example by neoplasm or stroke, whereas only truncal ataxia may be present with involvement of the vermis, as in early alcoholic cerebellar degeneration where the anterior vermis is involved in isolation. Both may be present in persons with diffuse involvement of the cerebellum as in acute sedative excess or chronic degenerative processes. A third element, vestibular-cerebellar dysequilibrium, may be added particularly with sedative excess, and nystagmus is the best evidence for this. It is not clear, however, whether this represents primary archicerebellar dysfunction (flocculo-nodular lobe or fastigial nucleus) or vestibular apparatus involvement, or both. Medulloblastoma is associated with ataxia and nystagmus and this is usually attributed to archicerebellar involvement. When no other signs are present to implicate brain stem involvement, this is a fair assessment; however, the tumor frequently compresses the proximate vestibular nuclei in the brain stem, giving direct vestibular dysfunction.

Ataxia is fairly easy to elicit. If advanced, the patient has a wide-based compensatory gait, and if there is lateralized limb involvement, he tends to lean and fall toward the affected leg. If the trunk alone is involved, as in early alcoholic degeneration or with a tumor of the vermis, there is a tendency to fall to either side, forward or backward. Some persons with midline involvement have a stronger tendency to fall backward. This is called *retropulsion* and has also been associated with basal ganglia dysfunction, particularly parkinsonism, and frontal lobe disorders. With cerebellar involvement, the retropulsion frequently has an involuntary tonic character. Even at rest, sitting, or standing, there is a tendency to lean or fall backward. With frontal lobe dysfunction and parkinsonism, the retropulsion is usually passive rather than active. The patient has difficulty recovering from being pushed backward or from a backward-leaning position, but he has no active or forced retropulsion at rest.

A sensitive test for ataxia is heel-to-toe tandem walking; this should be part of any neurologic screening examination because it detects early cerebellar dysfunction.

Cerebellar dysfunction may be limited to midline (i.e., axial) difficulties with midline cerebellar lesions. Therefore, it is imperative to examine a patient standing and walking. Examination of the patient in bed limits the testing to limb functions.

Cerebellar *hypotonia,* a decreased resistance to passive manipulation of the limbs frequently accompanied by flabbiness of the muscles to palpation, is considered the result of increased descending inhibition on the segmental reflex system. Presumably the descending inhibitory pathways are released from neocerebellar inhibition. The examiner should check for tone abnormalities by asking the patient to relax and not resist. The limbs are then moved rapidly by the examiner in several ranges. A lack of resistance or a floppiness is noticed with hypotonia. The legs may be tested by having the patient sit with his legs swinging free. The leg is lifted by the examiner and released. Normally the leg swings back and forth several times and then stops, arrested by inertia and the normal resting muscle tone, which is increased by the stretch placed on the muscle by the swinging leg. With the hyperactive stretch reflexes of spasticity, the arresting occurs more rapidly. With cerebellar hypotonia, the leg swings freely, unchecked, like a pendulum, arrested mainly by passive limb inertia.

Examination of the motor system can be relatively objective and Tables 4–2 and 4–3 outline an approach using isolated segments of the motor system as models. Mixed-system involvements do occur with variable symptom and sign predominance, depending on such variables as the dominance of the various motor systems involved and the extent of the lesion(s) in each system.

Lack of cooperation caused by patient fatigue, misunderstanding of the tasks demanded, or lack of physician-patient rapport must always be considered. Feigned weakness or hysterical weakness usually can be distinguished by its bizarre localization, the absence of expected involvement of other systems (i.e., reflex, sensory, cranial), and the irregular ratchet-like giving way of muscles tested.

Detailed segmental examination of muscle function becomes necessary when complaints or findings suggest specific regional difficulties. It is beyond the scope of this book to describe individual muscle testing. We recommend the use of a handbook (e.g., *Aids to the Examination of the Peripheral Nervous System)* for immediate bedside or office reference. This type of examination is learned through practice and not memorization.

REFERENCES

Brodal, A.: *Neurological Anatomy in Relation to Clinical Medicine,* ed. 2. New York, Oxford University Press, 1969.

Medical Council of the U.K.: *Aids to the Examination of the Peripheral Nervous System.* Palo Alto, Calif., Pendragon House, 1978.

Monrad-Krohn, G. H., Refsum, S.: *The Clinical Examination of the Nervous System,* ed. 12. London, H.K. Lewis & Co., 1964.

5

Sensory System Evaluation

EVALUATION OF SENSATION is hindered by several striking problems. Sensation belongs to the patient and the examiner must therefore depend almost entirely on his cooperation and reliability. A demented or psychotic patient is likely to give only the crudest, if any, picture of his perception of sensory stimuli. An intelligent, stable patient may refine asymmetries of stimulus intensity to such a degree that insignificant differences in sensation, usually due to the inconsistency of the examiner, are reported and only confuse the picture. Suggestion can modify a subject's response to a marked degree (e.g., to ask a patient where a stimulus changes suggests that it must change and may therefore create false lines of demarcation in an all too cooperative patient). Obviously the examiner must not waste time and efficiency on detailed sensory testing of the psychotic or demented patient, he must warn the perceptive individual that minute differences taking more than a few moments to decipher are probably of no significance, and he must avoid any hint of predisposition or suggestion. After considered precaution, problems still arise, however. Uniformity in testing is almost impossible and there is considerable variability in response in the same patient.

Factors that may affect the patient's variability and should be controlled are fatigue and mood. Fatigue is particularly likely to be induced by a long, detailed, unnecessary, and tedious sensory examination during which the examiner is frequently exhorting the pa-

tient's undivided attention. A *rapid, efficient* exam is the most practical means of diminishing fatigue. Mood is less subject to modification.

Use of a pressure transducer allows more consistent stimulus intensities and therefore more objectivity in the examination; however, this is impractical at bedside and does not eliminate the patient's variability.

Sensory changes unassociated with any other abnormalities (i.e., motor, reflex, cranial, hemispheric dysfunctions) must be considered weak evidence of disease unless a pattern of loss in classical sensory distribution is elicited (i.e., in a typical peripheral nerve or root-dermatomal distribution). Bizarre patterns of abnormality, loss, or irritation usually indicate hysteria or simulation of disease, but the examiner must beware of personal limitations. Peripheral nerve distributions vary considerably, less so dermatomes, from individual to individual, and even the classic distributions are hard to keep in mind unless one deals with neurologic problems frequently. Therefore it is advisable for the examiner to carry a booklet on peripheral nerve distribution, sensory and motor (e.g., *Aids to the Examination of the Peripheral Nervous System,* published by the Medical Council of the U.K.).

As in the motor system examination, an efficient screening exam must be developed for sensory testing. This should be more detailed when abnormalities are suspected or detected. Basic testing should sample the major functional subdivisions of the sensory systems. The patient's eyes should be closed throughout the examination. The stimuli should routinely be applied lightly and as close to threshold as possible so that minor abnormalities can be detected. Spinothalamic (pain [pin] and light touch), dorsal column (vibration, proprioception, and light touch), and hemispheric (stereognosis, graphesthesia) functions should be sampled.

Pain (pin), vibration (C128), and light touch should be compared at distal and proximal sites on the extremities, and the right side should be compared with the left. Proprioception should be tested in the fingers and toes and then at larger joints if losses are detected. Stereognosis, the ability to distinguish objects by feel alone, and graphesthesia, the ability to decipher letters and numbers written on skin by feel alone, should be tested in the hands if deficits in the simpler modalities are minor or absent. Motor weakness in the hand may, because of defective finger manipulations, cause apparent abnormalities in stereognosis despite normal sensation. Frequently, significant deficits in the basic modalities cause dysgraphesthesia and stereognostic difficulties whether the lesion or lesions are peripheral or central. However, significant defects in graphesthesia and stereognosis occur with contralateral hemispheric disease that is not associated with a major loss of perception of vibration, position, pain, and temperature. This is particularly marked with parietal lobe lesions. A less striking disorder or no defect is found with lesions involving other lobes unless the lesion or lesions are quite extensive.

It may be surprising that the more basic modalities are not greatly affected by hemispheric and particularly cortical lesions. With acute hemispheric insults (e.g., cerebral infarction or hemorrhage), an almost complete contralateral loss of sensation may occur. It is relatively short-lived, however; perception of pin and light touch, as routinely tested, return to almost normal levels, whereas proprioception and vibration may remain deficient though considerably improved in most cases. The initial marked loss of basic sensation has been explained by some to be secondary to hemispheric shock, a little-understood phenomenon most often recognized in the motor system. The lack of a significant long-term deficiency in basic sensation with hemispheric lesions has been variously explained. A popular explanation is that pain and possibly light touch are perceived at the thalamic level. This is unsatisfactory, however, because bilateral cortical devastation sparing the thalamus leaves only a vegetative existence, certainly with no perception of pain and touch consciously as we know them. A better explanation with some experimental and clinical corroboration is that the basic sensations have considerable bilateral projection to the hemispheres.

A productive modification of standard unilateral light-touch testing is the utilization of double simultaneous stimulation (DSS). The value of paired stimuli presented rapidly, simultaneously, and at minimal intensity to homologous areas on the body (distal and proximal samplings on extremities) lies in the ability of this method to pick up very minor threshold differences which, if consistent on repeated testing, are significant; and neglect phenomena identified with association cortex lesions.

Neglect may be hard to distinguish from involvement of the primary sensory systems unless abnormalities are found in multiple sensory systems (i.e., visual, auditory, and somatesthetic), thus making a single primary projection system lesion unlikely because of the disparate anatomical localization of all these systems. Association cortex lesions, particularly involvement of the right posterior parietal cortex, may become apparent only on double simultaneous stimulation.

The face-hand test is a further modification of DSS that takes advantage of the presence of facial perceptual dominance over the rest of the body. This dominance is best illustrated in children and in demented and therefore regressed patients. Before the age of 10, most strikingly earlier than age 5, stimuli presented simultaneously to the face and ipsilateral or contralateral hand are frequently (more than three in ten stimulations) perceived at the face alone. Perception of the hand and, if tested, other parts of the body is extinguished. In an older child or adult, several initial extinctions of the hand may occur, but very quickly both stimuli are correctly perceived. In the patient with diffuse hemispheric dysfunction, dementia, a regression is frequently seen to consistent extinction of the hand stimuli.

This test therefore can be doubly useful, first as an indication of diffuse hemispheric function and second by stimulating the face and *opposite* hand, a means of detecting minor hemisensory defects (e.g., if the patient consistently extinguishes only the right hand and not the left, a sensory threshold elevation due to primary sensory system or association cortex involvement on the left is suspect).

It is worthwhile now to review some profiles of sensory system involvement. You should be able to understand each of the elicited patterns of abnormality utilizing your knowledge of the functional anatomy of the various sensory systems.

1. *Peripheral neuropathy* is most frequently seen in this country associated with diabetes mellitus and the malnutrition of alcoholism. A symmetric stocking-glove loss of sensation is characteristic. The periphery is most affected because it is the farthest removed from the neuron cell bodies in the dorsal root ganglia. The feet are usually involved before the hands. The cell body in the normal state has a trophic effect on the remainder of the neuron, and with disease the most distant portions of the "supply line" are the least supportable and therefore the first to drop out. The receptors of the feet are considerably farther removed from the dorsal root ganglia than are the receptors of the hands, which accounts for the usual first appearance of lower-extremity loss. Over

the trunk, peripheral loss is noted first along the anterior midline (Fig 5 – 1).

Vibration perception is often the earliest affected modality followed by loss of pin, temperature, and light-touch perception and, variably, proprioception. Metabolic involvement of the peripheral nerves first affects the wide-diameter, thickly myelinated, fast-conducting fibers that carry vibration and position sense information and later affects the smaller, less myelinated, slower conducting fibers that carry pain, temperature, and light touch. Proprioception is usually not involved early because the testing procedure, moving the toes or fingers up or down, is quite crude and is not likely to pick up early loss.

Fig 5–1. — Distribution of typical sensory loss with diffuse symmetric peripheral neuropathy. Darker stippling represents greatest deficit.

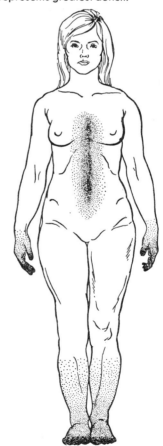

The peripheral deep-tendon reflexes are depressed early, particularly the Achilles reflex. Information is relayed from the stretch receptors over large myelinated fibers.

As a rule, symptomatic motor involvement is late, and when it occurs, it affects the intrinsic muscles of the feet first.

2. *Radiculopathy* (dorsal root involvement) is characterized by a pattern of loss characteristic of the dermatomes represented (Fig 5–2). Single-root involvement may be reflected only by positive (irritative) phenomena, pain, and paresthesias, because of the striking overlap of dermatomal sensory distribution (Fig 5–3). Herpes zoster, which affects individual dorsal roots, nicely demonstrates dermatomal distribution because, despite the lack of sensory loss (attributable to overlap), vesicles ("shingles") appear at the nerve endings in the skin (see Fig 5–3).

Pain referable to root irritation is more often referred to the muscle (myotomal) and bone (sclerotomal) distributions of the root than to the dermatomes. The person usually complains of a deep aching sensation. Myotomes should not be memorized but can be looked up easily by referring to the motor root innervations of muscles which are essentially the same as their sensory innervations.

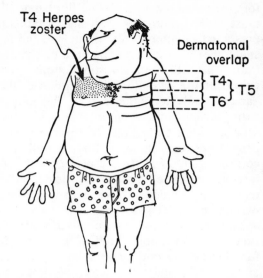

Fig 5–3.—Dermatomal distribution pattern on trunk showing overlap. Herpetic lesions on the right demarcate the major distribution of the single dorsal root involved (T4 in this instance).

Sclerotomal overlap is so great that localization on their basis proves impractical.

3. *Spinal cord involvement* is characterized by both sensory and motor segmental and long-tract system abnormalities. Segmental changes in the distribution of dermatomes and myotomes are used by the examiner for narrow localization of the lesion or lesions. Long-tract sensory involvement is less localizing because of considerable overlap of segmental input (review particularly the spinothalamic system and its input from Lissauer's tract); long-tract (corticospinal) motor involvement is even less so. (Why?)

Compression of the spinal cord from without, if the mass is lateral or ventrolateral, first involves the spinothalamic paths representing the sacral region, and a "saddle" loss of pin and temperature perception is therefore present in isolation even though the lesion is high in the cord as determined by the segmental or root involvement (Fig 5–4). With progression, involvement includes the remaining portions of the body below the segment (see Fig 5–4).

Fig 5–2.—Approximate dermatomal separation lines.

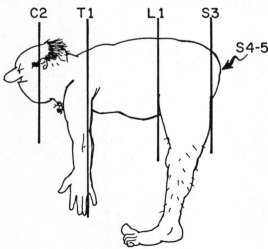

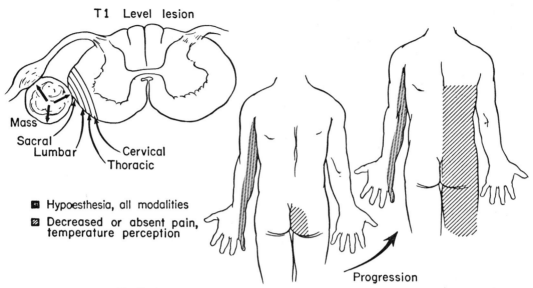

T1 Level lesion

Mass
Sacral
Lumbar
Cervical
Thoracic

■ Hypoesthesia, all modalities
▨ Decreased or absent pain, temperature perception

Progression

Fig 5–4. — Characteristic pattern of sensory loss with extradural lesion compressing the lateral aspect of cord and T1 dorsal root.

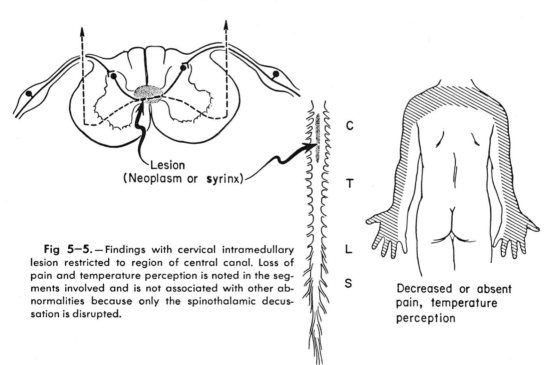

Lesion
(Neoplasm or syrinx)

C
T
L
S

Fig 5–5. — Findings with cervical intramedullary lesion restricted to region of central canal. Loss of pain and temperature perception is noted in the segments involved and is not associated with other abnormalities because only the spinothalamic decussation is disrupted.

Decreased or absent pain, temperature perception

Intramedullary lesions do not present a characteristic early pattern unless the involvement is in or around the central canal as with a syrinx, ependymoma, or central glioma. An isolated segmental loss of pain and temperature perception is characteristic because the crossing spinothalamic systems are interrupted (Fig 5–5). The dorsal column is spared, leaving touch, vibration, and proprioception intact. This dissociated sensory loss is in contrast to the loss in all modalities associated with root lesions. Sacral segment sparing of pain and temperature may occur with progression of an intramedullary neoplasm because the more peripheral sacral spinothalamic fibers may be the last to be involved (see Fig 5–4).

Complete hemisection of the cord results in a characteristic picture of sensorimotor loss (Brown-Séquard syndrome), which is easily recognized (Fig 5–6).

4. *Brain stem involvement*, like involvement of the spinal cord, is characterized by long-tract and segmental (cranial nerve) motor and sensory abnormality and is localized by the segmental signs. The picture of ipsilateral cranial nerve abnormality and contralateral long-tract dysfunction is quite consistent (Fig 5–7). The decussation of the dorsal columns and pyramids at the transition between the medulla and cervical spinal cord and the spinothalamic system in the cord accounts for the typical crossed presentation. Until the midbrain level, the spinothalamic and dorsal column (medial lemniscus) systems remain separate and therefore lesions may involve the pathways separately. For example, an infarction caused by occlusion of the posterior inferior cerebellar artery typically involves only the lateral portion (lateral plate) of the medulla. The ipsilateral trigeminal tract and nucleus and

Fig 5–6.— A, findings following stab wound hemisection of spinal cord at T5 on right (Brown-Séquard syndrome). **B,** segmental overlap of Lissauer's tract allowing pain-temperature bypass of lesion from several segments below the lesion on the left and explaining the lowered demarcation of pain-temperature loss on the left.

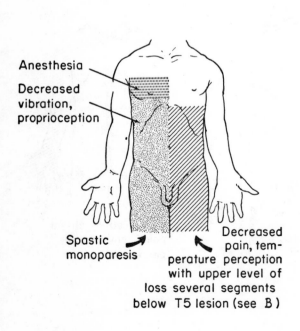

A

Anesthesia

Decreased vibration, proprioception

Spastic monoparesis

Decreased pain, temperature perception with upper level of loss several segments below T5 lesion (see B)

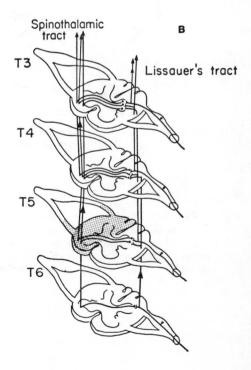

B

Spinothalamic tract

Lissauer's tract

T3

T4

T5

T6

Left Pontine Destructive Lesion

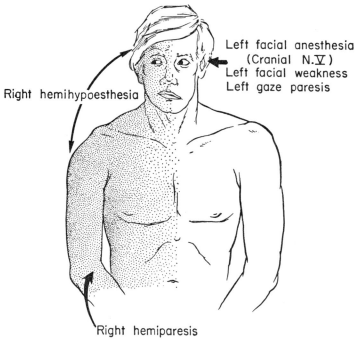

Fig 5—7.—Ipsilateral segmental and crossed long-tract deficits associated with left pontine lesion. Of note and frequently missed is the bilateral decrease in facial perception. There is anesthesia on the left from involvement of the trigeminal complex and hypoesthesia on the right associated with total hemihypoesthesia from involvement of the crossed trigeminal thalamic, spinothalamic, and medial lemniscal systems. Review the section on conjugate gaze in chapter 3 to explain gaze paresis.

the spinothalamic tract are frequently included in the lesion, leaving a loss of pain and temperature perception over the ipsilateral face (see chap. 3) and the contralateral limbs and trunk. The medial lemniscus and its modalities are spared.

5. *Thalamic lesions* are associated with contralateral hemihypoesthesia. Initially, if the lesion is acute, there is considerable loss bordering on anesthesia, but some recovery is expected over time, especially of touch, temperature, and pain perception. Vibration and proprioception remain more severely defective. A striking and not infrequent residual of thalamic destruction is episodic

paroxysms of contralateral pain, probably an irritative phenomenon. These can be controlled only occasionally with anticonvulsants. An additional residual that develops over time is marked contralateral hyperpathia in spite of the presence of a raised threshold for pain perception. Stimulation cf a site with a pin causes a very unpleasant, poorly localized and spreading sensation, which is frequently described as burning.

This is presumably an irritative phenomenon released by the pain system input; although it is most often seen and most marked with thalamic lesions, it can occur as a residual of lesions in any portion of the central sensory systems. A hypersensitivity to cold sensation frequently accompanies the hyperpathia.

6. *Cortical lesions,* as discussed earlier, tend to leave minimal basic sensation deficits but, especially if in the parietal lobe, are associated with striking contralateral deficits in the higher perceptual functions. Stereognosis and graphesthesia are abnormal in spite of minor difficulties with vibration and proprioception and even less, if any, difficulty with pain, temperature, and light-touch perception. Higher perceptual functions are defective with lesions anywhere in the sensory system and, with the exception of cortical and less so thalamic deficits, are marked in proportion to the amount of loss of basic sensory perception.

Higher sensorimotor integration functions such as body-part recognition, musicality, and certain visuospatial capabilities, depend on the integrity of the association cortex, particularly the parietal lobes. The greatest defects occur with right parietal damage (see chap. 2).

REFERENCES

Brodal, A.: *Neurological Anatomy in Relation to Clinical Medicine,* ed. 2. New York, Oxford University Press, 1969.

Medical Council of the U.K.: *Aids to the Examination of the Peripheral Nervous System.* Palo Alto, Calif., Pendragon House, 1978.

Monrad-Krohn, G. H., Refsum, S.: *The Clinical Examination of the Nervous System,* ed. 12. London, H. K. Lewis & Co., 1964.

6

Reflex Evaluation

MOST REFLEXES when reduced to their simplest level are sensorimotor arcs, sometimes represented anatomically with only two neurons: a receptor neuron (e.g., muscle spindle apparatus) and an effector neuron (e.g., alpha motor neuron). Multiple inhibitory and facilitatory influences affect this arc and arise from all levels of the nervous system. Inputs, intrasegmental and intersegmental in the spinal cord, from the brain stem, cerebellum, basal ganglia, and cerebral cortices all influence the motor neurons, both alpha and gamma, directly or indirectly. The sensory or afferent side of the simple reflex is also influenced by centrifugal and centripetal pathways from all levels of the nervous system.

As a general rule the major portion of higher influence on the reflex is inhibitory. For this reason the net result of lesions that isolate the spinal reflex arc but do not directly affect it is facilitation. With few exceptions this means that the reflexes become hyperactive. They usually pass through a stage of hypoactivity if the lesion involving the spinal cord (above the segment of the reflex arc), brain stem, or cerebral hemispheres is acute. This stage has been called a diaschesis or shock state and is more severe and long-lasting in proportion to the amount of higher influence lost. Transection of the spinal cord removes the greatest amount of higher influence and may be associated with weeks of hypoactivity. Small, acute lesions of the cerebral cortex cause very little shock and indeed very little subsequent hyperactivity because very little higher influence is lost.

When reflexes return after spinal transection, they become extremely hyperactive, even massive. Great overflow with the elicitation of many reflexes may occur on examining a single arc such as the patellar reflex.

Lesions that affect the sensory or motor portion of the arc (peripheral nerve and receptors, dorsal root or ganglion, dorsal horn, anterior horn cell [alpha and/or gamma], ventral root, peripheral nerve, neuromuscular junction, and muscle) depress the reflexes.

Lesions of the cerebellum and basal ganglia in humans are not associated with consistent reflex changes. Classically, destruction of the major portion of the cerebellar hemispheres in humans is associated with pendular deep-tendon reflexes. The reflexes are poorly checked so that the leg, for example, in a seated person with foot hanging may swing to and fro like a pendulum on elicitation of the patellar reflex; normally the stretching of the antagonist muscles, in this case the hamstrings, dampens the elicited reflex almost immediately. When this type of reflex is elicited and other signs of cerebellar disease (motor system examination) are present, it is significant. However, as a lone sign it is unusual and not clearly diagnostic. Normal reflexes are compatible with cerebellar disease.

Basal ganglia disease (e.g., parkinsonism) usually is not associated with predictable reflex change; most often the reflexes are normal.

Reflex elicitation and evaluation are the

most objective part of the neurologic examination. In some situations they may be the major part of the examination (e.g., the comatose patient). It depends on a minimal amount of cooperation on the part of the patient. A list of all possible reflexes would be almost endless and a tangle of eponymic jargon for those with an historical bent. It is necessary to know the most commonly elicited reflexes and this knowledge is not terribly difficult to acquire. Table 6–1 is a list of the most commonly tested reflexes. It covers most of the segmental levels of the nervous system from the cerebral hemisphere through the spinal cord.

Reflexes are graded at the bedside in a semiquantitative manner. The response lev-els of deep-tendon reflexes are graded $0-4+$, with 2+ being normal. 0 signifies no response at all, $1+$ means depressed, and the term *trace* means just that. $3+$ means excessive or hyperactive, and $4+$ means hyperactive with clonus. Clonus is a repetitive, usually rhythmic, and variably sustained reflex response elicited by manually sustaining the tendon stretch. Superficial and autonomic reflexes are graded simply as *normal, hyperactive, depressed,* or *absent.* This terminology is modified with some reflexes (e.g., the pupillary light reflexes may be sluggish or slow as with the tonic pupillary response of ciliary ganglion dysfunction [Adie's pupil]; a numerical drop in blood pressure is recorded with carotid sinus or

TABLE 6–1.—THE MOST COMMONLY TESTED REFLEXES

CATEGORY	REFLEX	SEGMENTS
Stretch reflexes (deep tendon reflexes)*	Jaw jerk	V sensory (s) and motor (m)
	Biceps	C5-6 (s, m)
	Triceps	C6-7 (s, m)
	Brachioradialis	C6, 7, 8 (s, m)
	Finger flexor	C6, 7, 8 (s, m)
	Knee	L2, 3, 4 (s, m)
	Ankle	S1, 2 (s, m)
Superficial reflexes	Corneal*	V (s) and VII (m)
	Nose tickle	V (s) and VII + (m)
	Gag*	IX, X (s, m)
	Abdominal	T7–T12 (s, m)
	Cremasteric	S1 (s, m)
	Plantar*	S1, 2 (s, m)
	Anal wink	S4, 5 (s, m)
Visceral (autonomic) reflexes	Pupillary—light accommodation*	II (s) and III (m)
	Oculocardiac	V (s) and X (m)
	Carotid sinus	IX (s) and X (m)
	Bulbocavernosis	S2, 3, 4 (s, m)
	Rectal (internal sphincter)	S2, 3, 4 (s, m)
	Orthostatic blood pressure and pulse change	

Reflexes associated with diffuse bilateral hemispheric dysfunction (see chaps. 2 and 11)
 Glabellar
 Forced grasping (feet and hands)
 Feeding reflexes (sucking, biting, rooting)
 Oculocephalic and nuchocephalic disinhibition
Miscellaneous: Vestibulo-oculomotor responses (see chap. 3)
 Oculocephalic reflex
 Caloric irrigations

*These reflexes are considered part of a routine screening examination for neurologic disease. The other reflexes are examined when suspicion of abnormality exists on the basis of history or screening examination.

oculocardiac reflex elicitation). Reflexes associated with *diffuse* bilateral hemispheric dysfunction are recorded as absent or present (inhibited or disinhibited).

Practice observing normal reflexes in patients and initially among students is the best way to determine the range of normalcy. Asymmetry of reflexes, symmetrically tested, is abnormal, but it must then be decided, when extremes of response do not make designation obvious, which is abnormal: the more active or the less active side. If this is a problem, the remainder of the neurologic examination and findings usually clarifies the issue.

We now list the reflex changes associated with dysfunction at various levels of the nervous system.

1. *Muscle: Stretch reflexes* are depressed in parallel to loss of strength.

2. *Neuromuscular junction: Stretch reflexes* are depressed in parallel to loss of strength.

3. *Peripheral nerve: Stretch reflexes* are depressed, usually out of proportion to weakness, which may be minimal. This is because the afferent arc is involved early in neuropathy. *Orthostatic hypotension* can be seen in persons with advanced and diffuse peripheral nerve involvement.

4. *Root: Stretch reflexes* subserved by root are depressed in proportion to the contribution that root makes to the reflex. *Superficial reflexes* are depressed in proportion to sensory loss in the dermatomes tested.

5. *Spinal cord and brain stem: Stretch reflexes* are hypoactive at the level of the lesion and hyperactive below the level of the lesion. As noted, during the shock state following acute lesions, the sublesion reflexes are also hypoactive to absent.

Superficial reflexes are hypoactive at and below the level of the lesion and normal above. The abdominal superficial reflexes are not reliably present in normal individuals who are excessively obese, who have abdominal scars, or who have had multiple pregnancies, and they are frequently poorly

elicited in otherwise normal but old persons. Therefore, though classically depressed in persons with corticospinal system involvement, one should not place great emphasis on bilaterally depressed abdominal reflexes if they are the only abnormality found in the examination. Guilt by association is necessary. The *plantar* response is exceptional and is abnormal, extensor (Babinski response), when the upper motor neuron system is involved. The Babinski response is most likely a regressive reflex or release phenomenon, a primitive spinal function seen normally in infants during their first year and usually extinguished during the second year.

Autonomic reflexes are depressed according to the segment of cord or stem involvement. For example, sweating is depressed at the level of the lesion and below if the lesion is in the spinal cord. Brain stem lesions cause ipsilateral depression of sweating over the whole body.

6. *Cerebellum:* Classically the *stretch reflexes* are hypoactive and pendular as mentioned above. When this is so, the test is reliable; however, more often the reflexes are not visibly abnormal as tested at the bedside.

7. *Basal ganglia:* There are no consistent deep-tendon or superficial reflex changes. There is frequently some diffuse cerebral dysfunction (dementia) associated with basal ganglia dysfunctions (e.g., parkinsonism, Huntington's chorea), and this is reflected in a release (disinhibition) of some of the primitive reflexes — e.g., the glabellar, oculocephalic, grasp, and feeding reflexes.

8. *Cerebral cortex: Unilateral* disease releases stretch reflexes to hyperactivity, for unknown reasons depresses abdominal and cremasteric reflexes, and releases a Babinski response, all on the contralateral side, when the motor cortex or proximate areas are involved.

Bilateral disease is associated with the same abnormalities bilaterally and, in addition, the regressive feeding reflexes, forced grasping, and glabellar reflexes are released from inhibition. The vestibulo-oculomotor reflexes become disinhibited (see chap. 3). The gag reflex is also excessive, particularly if bilateral motor cortex involvement is striking. Why is the gag reflex not hyperactive with unilateral disease?

When bilateral neocortical motor control is depressed, particularly when corticobulbar system involvement is prominent, inhibitory control of the complex emotional expression reflexes becomes defective. These individuals cry or laugh with minimal emotional provocation. If the disease is isolated to the motor system, the patient says he does not understand why he is crying or laughing,

agreeing that he has not really been provoked to feel nearly so strongly as he is acting. These complex emotional reflexes are subserved by the limbic cortex, basal ganglia, and brain stem, presumably under inhibitory modulation by the neocortex.

REFERENCES

DeJong, R. N.: *The Neurologic Examination*, ed. 4. New York, Paul B. Hoeber, Inc., 1958.

Monrad-Krohn, G. H., Refsum, S.: *The Clinical Examination of the Nervous System*, ed. 12. London, H. K. Lewis & Co., 1964.

Wartenberg, R.: *The Examination of Reflexes: A Simplification.* Chicago, Year Book Medical Publishers, 1945.

Part II

Symptoms, Systems, and Diseases

7

Basic Principles in Neurologic Disease

DISTURBANCES OF THE NERVOUS SYSTEM, both peripheral and central, are manifested in four basic ways:

1. *Ablative or deficiency phenomena* associated with destructive (e.g., infarction, tumor, trauma) and depressing processes (e.g., anesthesia).

2. *Irritative phenomena* as typified by seizures and the pins-and-needles or burning paresthesias of peripheral neuropathy, both of which represent excessive neuronal firing secondary to pathologic depolarization.

3. *Release phenomena* as typified by the hyperactive reflexes and spasticity of corticospinal system involvement, the tremor of Parkinson's disease, the excessive emotional behavior following bilateral corticobulbar system loss, and sedative withdrawal hyperactivity.

4. *Compensation phenomena,* either appropriate, as typified by visual-motor compensation for the nystagmus and vertigo of vestibular disease, circumduction of the paretic leg on walking to avoid tripping, a high-stepping gait to avoid tripping when a foot drops, or inappropriate, as typified by tendon contractures.

Combinations of these disturbances are the rule. The person who has cerebral infarction is hemiparetic, develops spasticity, may develop seizures early or late, and com-

pensates for hemiparesis appropriately with a circumducting gait. If physical rehabilitation is not carried out, he can develop a functionally inappropriate flexion contracture of his arm.

Momentum of disease is another phenomenon that should be considered. This refers essentially to the rate of involvement of the nervous system. An acute destructive lesion (e.g., infarction) causes an early maximal deficit, whereas a chronic, slowly progressive lesion (e.g., tumor) usually produces considerably less deficit because compensating mechanisms (e.g., mechanical adjustment, redundancy of function in other regions) parallel the destructive forces. We have seen a slow-growing meningioma compressing the frontal lobes reach the size of a lemon over at least 25 years and cause no clear-cut neurologic deficit; the patient was admitted to the hospital for onset of seizures. Malignant glial tumors (glioblastoma) frequently infiltrate neuronal tissue and many neurons lying within the tumor continue to function; this is a reason for the surprisingly small deficit occasionally associated with very large tumors, which as a rule grow rapidly. It is not surprising, therefore, that removal of these tumors almost invariably leaves the patient with greater neurologic deficits because many functioning neurons are lost.

Recuperation of function following the

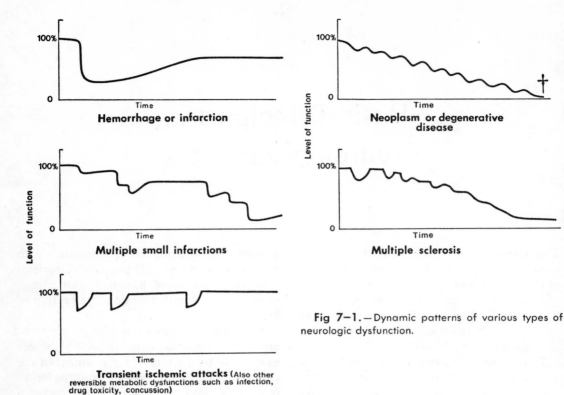

Fig 7-1.—Dynamic patterns of various types of neurologic dysfunction.

removal of lesions of the nervous system takes two basic forms: resolution and recuperation.

Resolution of the lesion (as seen by the clearing of edema, ischemia, hemorrhagic or tumor compression of tissue, and metabolic suppression of neurons, for example, drugs, uremia, hypoxia, etc.) is the main mechanism of recovery in adults and older children with major dysfunctions.

Reorganization as derived from redundancy and/or multipotentiality of function in the remaining normal neurons is an important mode of recuperation following minor destructive lesions. In young children (5 years or younger) this can be the major mode of recuperation following destructive lesions. In adults and older children plasticity or multipotentiality of neuronal function is minor, whereas in young children it can be very marked for certain major functions (e.g., speech—left-hemisphere lesions that leave an adult with permanent and severe dysphasia can be well compensated by development of speech in the right hemisphere in young children; residual hemiparesis in children following large hemispheric lesions is less than that seen in adults). Redundancy assumes multifocal localization of function. Although it is not the major source of recuperation following large lesions, it is the reason for the lack of dysfunction in some capabilities. For example, memories of past events, well imprinted, are very resistant to hemispheric lesions because they are diffusely represented in both cerebral cortices.

REFERENCE

Monrad-Krohn, G. H., and Refsum, S.: *The Clinical Examination of the Nervous System*, ed. 12. London, H. K. Lewis & Co., 1964.

8

Neuromuscular System Disorders

JOSÉ OCHOA

IF ONE DEFINES the nervous system as a reflex arc designed for analyzing the environment through sensation and ultimately for modifying the environment through movement, then the neuromuscular component of the nervous system is made up of the first and the last links in that intricate chain. It consists of the first sensory element (the sensory unit) and the last motor element (the motor unit). These two extremities communicate through short circuits in the cord and brain stem (the spinal reflexes). Table 8–1 lists the parts of this peripheral machine.

The neuromuscular machine has a simple design and a simple physiology, and therefore its clinical expression is very limited. However, from the *quality* and the *distribution* of those simple manifestations, it is possible to achieve a good deal of diagnostic resolution and to do the following:

1. Confirm that such manifestations arise in the sensory unit or the motor unit as opposed to in the CNS.
2. Determine which part of the system is affected (e.g., weakness caused by defect of nerve fiber versus end-plate versus muscle).
3. In the case of nerve fiber disease, determine the level of the lesion along the nerves or roots.
4. Again, in the case of nerve fiber disease, obtain an idea of the type of pathologic process: Schwann cell disease versus neuronal disease.

Our responsibility goes beyond this; we have to aim at a diagnosis. Here we depend very much on *histology of nerve and muscle* and also on *applied electrophysiology;* these are almost part of the physical examination of the patient.

In the rest of this chapter we attempt to give an integrated picture relating normal and abnormal structure, function, and clinical manifestations.

Motor and Sensory Anatomical Units

The parts of this peripheral machinery are organized in anatomical units, each formed by one neuron with its peripheral neurite (axon) and its terminal branches plugged to a number of sensory receptors, or muscle fibers.

The noble element is the neuron, which carries trophic material to muscle and sensory endings and seemingly also to Schwann cells. Defective synthesis or impaired axoplasmic transport of trophic material results in metabolic derangement and atrophy *(denervation atrophy)* of sensory receptors and atrophy of muscle fibers and also in dystrophic changes in Schwann cells and myelin. The simplest example of this neurotrophic influence follows transection of the axon: *wallerian degeneration.* In the distal stump the axon and myelin start disintegrating in the first couple of days. The peripheral end-organs eventually atrophy also.

A more refined example of neurotrophic

TABLE 8-1.—NEUROMUSCULAR SYSTEM

PARTS	PHYSIOLOGY	DISORDER	CLINICAL
Sensory receptors	Transduction	Elementary sensory defect	Sensory loss (may cause ataxia), paresthesia, pain
Neurites			
Nerve fibers	Conduction		
Schwann cells			
Motor end-plates	Neuromuscular transmission	Simple motor defect	Weakness (wasting), muscle twitching, cramps, myotonia
Striated muscle fibers	Shortening	Reflex loss (and reflex muscle tone)	Weakness, wasting, occasionally pseudohypertrophy

influence follows destruction of axonal microtubules and neurofilaments. These fibrous proteins are probably responsible for axoplasmic transport, at least of particulate material. Substances that destroy microtubules (spindle inhibitors), such as colchicine, cause denervation atrophy of peripheral end-organs. This is eventually also followed by degeneration of the myelin and of the axon itself. An interesting feature of these disorders of synthesis or transport of trophic factors is that they affect first the longest neurons, starting from their distal extremities. This has been called the *dying-back phenomenon.* Such a pattern of degeneration is seen in a variety of toxic and metabolic disorders and also in various degenerative diseases. Dying back explains why the symptoms of disease of the peripheral neurons so often start and predominate distally. There is distal anesthesia and paresthesia (stocking and glove), weakness and atrophy, and loss of ankle jerks.

There are other expressions of neuronal influence on peripheral tissues. Depending on the speed (time to peak) of the mechanical muscle twitch that follows the discharge of a motor neuron, motor units can be classified into fast-twitch and slow-twitch units. It so happens that the structure of the muscle fibers is different for each type. In some mammals with muscles made of one separate fiber type, this structural difference can be guessed with the naked eye; those muscles made exclusively of fast fibers are white (type II with high levels of ATPase on histochemical examination). Those made of slow fibers are red (type I with low ATPase). In humans the majority of muscles contain mixtures of type I and type II fibers.

If the nerve to a white muscle is cross-anastomosed with the nerve to a red muscle and reinnervation is allowed to take place, the twitch properties and the corresponding histochemical features of the muscle fibers are reversed. The neuron has induced a specific adaptation in the periphery.

There is a growing body of evidence indicating that some disorders that we used to regard as primary muscle diseases may in fact be neurogenic in origin. What appeared to be "primary" muscle degeneration with muscle fiber atrophy of random distribution has been shown in several instances to correspond to selective atrophy of a particular histochemical type of fiber and therefore motor unit. Also, some neuropathies we used to regard as primary Schwann cell disease are tentatively explained as secondary to defective neuronal support to Schwann cells.

Functional Units

The motor unit is also a physiologic unit. Normally contraction of striated muscle is not possible except through firing of motor neurons that are activated through descending pathways and also through reflex connections.

The muscle fibers in a motor unit respond

in an *all-or-none* fashion to excitation of the motor neuron (both to natural excitation and artificial stimulation, for example, to electric nerve stimulation). There is little variation in the terminal delays of different terminal branches of any motor neuron. The nervous impulse reaches all the muscle fibers in the unit almost at the same time. The result is a brisk twitch. The electric counterpart of this muscle discharge is a *motor unit potential*. It can be recorded with needle electrodes from muscle. It is the "envelope" of the summated action potentials of many single muscle fibers. Its amplitude roughly expresses the numbers of muscle fibers activated. Its duration represents the range of terminal conduction times to those activated muscle fibers (temporal dispersion). Repeated activation of the same unit results in minimal variation in the shape and size of this envelope because normally the times for terminal nerve conduction and neuromuscular transmission are quite constant for any given nerve branch, and because all muscle fibers in the unit respond every time.

What is the behavior of motor units in effort? The answer is fundamental for understanding types of weakness. At rest there is normally no motor unit activity. With increasing effort, tension increases by (1) increasing the firing rates of units: 5 to 40–50 per second, and (2) recruiting more units into the effort.

It is impossible to achieve high firing rates in disorders of the upper motor neuron (UMN), that is, weakness caused by CNS disease has a low firing rate. Weakness with a high firing rate is not caused by a UMN lesion.

Composition of Nerves and Nerve Action Potentials

Most nerves contain a mixture of myelinated and unmyelinated fibers distributed in three well-defined sizes of populations: large myelinated fibers, small myelinated fibers, and many small unmyelinated fibers. Nor-mally the largest-diameter fibers conduct the fastest, and fibers of similar diameter conduct at similar velocity. Therefore, following simultaneous stimulation of all fibers in a nerve, the action potentials of individual nerve fibers summate in time, giving rise to compound nerve action potentials (NAP). In the clinic, NAPs are recorded routinely, but we can only record the NAP corresponding to large myelinated fibers.

Absence of a NAP indicates either few large-diameter myelinated fibers or asynchronous conduction by those fibers.

In the clinic we can also measure *nerve conduction velocity* (see chap. 18).

Disease

Based on these basic considerations, let us review the manifestations of disorders of *neurons* (and neurites), *Schwann cells, endplates*, and *muscle*.

PERIPHERAL NERVE FIBER DISEASE (PERIPHERAL NEUROPATHY)

This disease may affect one isolated nerve or root (mononeuropathy), several isolated nerves (mononeuropathy multiplex), or peripheral nerves diffusely (polyneuropathy). The primary disorder in each case may involve the neuron (or its neurite) or the Schwann cell.

NEURONAL (OR AXONAL) DISEASE.—Anatomically, at the level of the nerve fiber neuronal disease results in disintegration of myelin and axon; Schwann cells survive, and indeed they multiply.

In dying-back neuropathies, the time sequence of changes is stereotyped and similar to that of wallerian degeneration. However, the changes are displayed as a perfect space sequence by virtue of the smoothly ascending course of the defect.

How does this repair? Although differentiated neurons do not multiply, they are good at regenerating axons. Two basic processes occur: (1) terminal regeneration from the end of the proximal stump, and (2) collateral regeneration from unaffected neurites. Axonal regrowth progresses at about 1 mm/day, or 30–40 cm/year.

What will a *nerve biopsy* show in neuronal disease? Findings depend on the level of the sample (too high gives an intact nerve; too low gives total degeneration), but usually a distal biopsy reveals some intact fibers, some degenerating fibers, some empty Schwann cell columns or "bands," and even some regenerating fibers from neurons that have not been insulted and produce collateral sprouts or from neurons that have overcome the insult and regenerate terminally.

One of the most subtle criteria to assess nerve damage is the identification of denervated Schwann cell bands. This requires electron microscopy. Unfortunately one cannot simply rely on counts of nerve fibers. There is a wide normal variation among individuals, so despite a substantial decrease in the number of fibers, a particular case may still fall within the normal range.

Regenerating myelinated fibers that tend to be arranged in clusters also indicate previous axonal damage. One can only identify regenerating unmyelinated sprouts while they are immature; they distort the axon-diameter histogram, leading to a bimodality of smaller regenerating axons and larger normal axons.

Effect of neuronal disease on nerve conduction. — Nerve action potentials are reduced in amplitude in proportion to the fiber loss. Maximal motor conduction velocity (velocity of the fastest fiber) is normal (50–70 m/second in upper limbs) as long as there are any large-diameter fibers connected to muscle. In general, therefore, neuronal polyneuropathies cause minimal or no slowing of nerve conduction velocity. However, conduction is slowed under two unusual circumstances in neuronal disease: (1) selective degeneration of large fibers, and (2) conduction along a diseased nerve containing exclusively small-diameter axonal sprouts; this slows velocity considerably.

Effects of neuronal disease on muscle. —

The most significant effects are muscle-fiber atrophy and spontaneous fibrillation. Because muscle fibers from different motor units are intermingled in a kind of checkerboard pattern, disconnection of a motor neuron results in scattered atrophy of muscle fibers, all of the same histochemical type (Fig 8–1). At the functional level, disconnection from the neuron involves a progressive change in the properties of the muscle cell membrane: sensitivity to acetylcholine (ACh), which is normally confined to the end-plate region, extends to the whole surface of the muscle fibers because ACh receptors are profusely synthesized. Now muscle fibers discharge spontaneously, presumably in response to circulating ACh, giving rise to abnormal contraction of individual muscle fibers. This is called *spontaneous fibrillation,* a phenomenon characteristic of muscle denervation but not visible through the skin. An intramuscular electrode detects fibrillation potentials, the electric hallmark of muscle denervation. It takes a couple of weeks for fibrillation to develop following denervation.

Fasciculations (see chap. 4) are a visible, spontaneous twitch of a single anterior horn cell muscle fiber pool (motor unit). They may occur in normal persons especially after vigorous and frequently exhausting exercise, in association with generalized fatigue, or as an inherited phenomenon. If persistent and associated with historical physical evidence of weakness and atrophy, they are pathologic and probably represent irritability of degenerating (possibly regenerating) or denervated anterior horn cells. Fasciculations are less often seen in persons with motor axon disease (peripheral neuropathy), and when present or uncovered by the use of anticholinesterase medications (see chap. 4) probably represent synchronous fibrillations of a large population of hypersensitive denervated muscle fibers.

Denervated muscle fibers are promptly reinnervated by collateral sprouts from neighboring (motor) nerve fibers (if there are

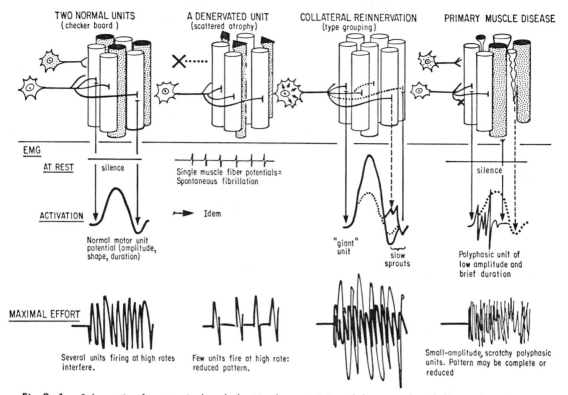

Fig 8–1. — Schematic of anatomical and electric characteristics of the normal and diseased motor unit.

any), and the neuron induces the corresponding histochemical transformation on those reinnervated muscle fibers. This results in (1) motor units with increased numbers of fibers, (2) histochemical type grouping as opposed to a checkerboard pattern, which is normal, (3) giant motor unit potentials, and (4) visible twitchings on mild effort (contraction fasciculation) (see Fig 8–1).

Muscle weakness and wasting are delayed by collateral reinnervation, but eventually even these surviving units denervate; symptoms and signs develop and histochemically there is group atrophy.

SCHWANN CELL AND MYELIN DISEASE.— Schwann cell disease and direct myelin injury may result in *demyelination*. The simplest example is trauma in the form of local nerve compression; this causes what is called *intussusception* at the nodes of Ranvier and eventually leads to paranodal demyelination. Naked axons excite a response in Schwann cells, which multiply and migrate to rewind myelin. Short, intercalated, myelinated segments remain as evidence of repair of previous local demyelination.

Other mechanisms give rise to diffuse demyelination such as direct attack on myelin by chemicals (e.g., lysolecithin) and interference with protein synthesis in the Schwann cell (e.g., diphtheria toxin).

A dramatic form of demyelination became known in the late 1960s as a result of the boom in research on cell-mediated immunity. This is cell-mediated demyelination, in which myelin is eaten away by sensitized lymphocytes. This is definitely the mechanism of demyelination in experimental allergic neuritis and also takes part in natural diseases like acute idiopathic polyneuritis (also called the Guillain-Barré syndrome). The antigen appears to be a basic protein of the myelin.

An important group of demyelinating neuropathies is genetically determined. In some of them, defects of lipid synthesis have been established and some of these have characteristic intracellular inclusions in Schwann cells. Most of these familial demyelinating polyneuropathies cause excessive proliferation of Schwann cells, which become arranged like onion bulbs in cross section. Usually these hypertrophic changes cause visible enlargement of nerves. It must be emphasized that recurrent demyelination, whether genetically determined or not, leads to hypertrophy regardless of its cause.

Demyelination slows conduction. It has been demonstrated that slowing of conduction velocity along a partially demyelinated nerve is not necessarily an artifact due to selective block of fast fibers. It is caused by abnormal conduction in partially blocked fibers that require more time to excite their nodes and, most important, slow conduction in demyelinated fibers remains saltatory. It does not become continuous, as in unmyelinated fibers.

Of course, more severe demyelination may lead to complete block. There may be such a great leak of current along a diseased internode that the following excitable node simply does not receive the density of current necessary for activation.

What are the repercussions of such basic physiologic derangements at a clinical level and in routine diagnostic electrophysiology? Consider first the slowing of conduction. If it affects all fibers equally, then apart from increased nerve conduction time, there is little clinical repercussion. This is an exceptional situation. Second and more common, conduction is slowed to different extents in different fibers. This results in desynchronization; that is, following a single stimulus to a nerve, the action potentials of individual fibers are dispersed in time. They do not summate properly in coherent compound

action potentials and NAPs are small or absent. Clinically, desynchronization upsets those functions that require synchronous nerve volleys: tendon reflexes and vibration sense. The third abnormal level is complete conduction block. Obviously a blocked fiber is no better functionally than an interrupted fiber (except for anatomical continuity, which prevents atrophy of end-organs). Complete block now results in weakness and general sensory loss.

Remyelination of the defects restores conduction and as few as three lamellae may be enough to transform a block into delayed conduction.

So, demyelinating neuropathies lead to diffuse slowing of nerve conduction velocity, whereas axonal or neuronal polyneuropathies as a rule do not.

It is also important to keep in mind that the site of a local nerve lesion giving rise to slowing (or partial) conduction block can often be established by nerve conduction studies, provided one can include the lesion between the stimulating and the recording electrodes (i.e., nerve conduction studies should not be requested for root lesions).

It should be emphasized that there are no pure demyelinating or pure neuronal degenerative conditions. Due to metabolic communication in both directions between neuron and Schwann cell, disease of one may cause secondary involvement of the other.

In general, demyelinating disorders have a better prognosis for recovery than neuronal disorders.

END-PLATE
(NEUROMUSCULAR JUNCTION)

With few exceptions each muscle fiber has one (and only one) end-plate: this is the plug for a nerve terminal branch. It was thought initially that end-plates were electric synapses, that the electric nerve impulse propagated directly from nerve to muscle. There is anatomical discontinuity, however—a neuromuscular (N-M) cleft, which is a chemical synapse. There is also a mediator, acetylcholine. Therefore some time is wasted in N-M transmission (N-M delay).

It was discovered that at rest there are normally intermittent discharges at the end-plate region of fairly constant amplitude and duration (miniature end-plate potentials). These are not capable of triggering propagated muscle action potentials. Subsequently, electron microscopists discovered the synaptic vesicles and that they contain acetylcholine. It was known that ACh is capable of depolarizing the postsynaptic membrane and, in view of the regular size of such synaptic vesicles and the morphologic evidence that vesicles may open to the synaptic cleft, it became obvious that each miniature end-plate potential is the result of spontaneous emptying of a fairly constant number (quantum) of molecules of ACh from a vesicle. Acetylcholinesterase in the end-plates destroys the ACh molecule and the fragments are recycled. Anticholinesterase drugs facilitate the depolarizing effect of ACh, but excess ACh eventually blocks neuromuscular transmission (i.e., cholinergic block).

Arrival of a nervous impulse at the presynaptic terminal causes release of many quanta, and this is normally sufficient to fire an end-plate potential. Then the local end-plate phenomenon spreads at 4 m/second along the whole muscle fiber membrane as the muscle fiber action potential. From here it propagates into the depth of the muscle fiber to trigger myofilaments to slide and shorten the sarcomere.

This refined neuromuscular junction is vulnerable at many points to pharmacologic agents. There are many examples of N-M block caused by toxins but the most common is myasthenia gravis, in many ways still a mysterious disease.

MYASTHENIA GRAVIS.—It is claimed that in myasthenia gravis there is a reduction in the size of the miniature end-plate potentials attributed initially to small quantum size but more recently to a decrease in the number of ACh receptors on the postsynaptic side. Wherever the primary defect may be in myasthenia gravis, its consequence is a reduced safety factor for N-M transmission; successful conduction of a nerve impulse is not followed by efficient transmission to a muscle fiber.

There are degrees of neuromuscular block (as there are of nerve conduction block). The mildest form consists of only increased N-M delay in some junctions of motor units. In severe forms, many end-plates are blocked, but the functional state of a given end-plate varies with time and use. Some end-plates are turned off while others regain function; the cycles repeat randomly during exercise.

So, in myasthenia gravis motor units contract without their full number of muscle fibers; sometimes all contract, sometimes a few, and sometimes none.

A cardinal feature of myasthenia gravis is that repetition makes things worse in the end-plate. This explains why weakness fluctuates in connection with exercise and rest, that is, fatigability. A routine electrophysiologic test that demonstrates this phenomenon is repetitive nerve stimulation and recording of the amplitude of the compound muscle action potential (summation of all muscle fiber potentials from all excitable motor units in the muscle). Normally there is little variation in successive firings. In myasthenia gravis there may be an abnormal decrement due to N-M block (or fatigue). This may be followed by posttetanic facilitation (Fig 8–2).

Acetylcholine or cholinergic substances or anticholinesterases improve this N-M transmission defect (before leading to cholinergic block). However, myasthenia gravis is more than just a functional end-plate disorder. It may lead to muscle fiber atrophy and fixed weakness. Indeed, often there is evidence of neurogenic atrophy of muscle and also selective type II fiber atrophy.

The thymus gland and immune mechanisms (autoimmunity against ACh receptor) have a great deal to do with myasthenia gravis, although their exact roles are not totally

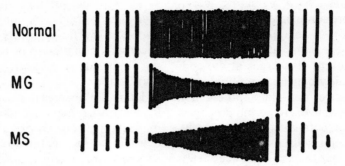

Fig 8–2.—Effect on amplitude of the compound muscle action potential by nerve stimulation at low (2–3 per second) and high (50 per second) frequencies. MG = myasthenia gravis; MS = myasthenic syndrome.

clear. In practice, thymectomy, corticosteroids, and immunosuppressive drugs may be useful in treatment.

MYASTHENIC SYNDROME.—There is another interesting (though rare) disorder of N-M transmission—the myasthenic syndrome associated with carcinoma. It may improve after removal of the tumor (usually bronchogenic small-cell carcinoma). It also causes anatomical distortion of the end-plates (different from myasthenia). The N-M block appears to be caused by reduced numbers of quanta released from nerve terminals in response to a nerve impulse. It causes weakness, which tends to improve with exercise; repetitive stimulation causes facilitation rather than the fatigue seen with myasthenia gravis (see Fig 8–2). The defect can be demonstrated also in vitro in nerve/muscle biopsies from patients. Acetylcholine-releasing agents such a guanidine and 4-aminopyridine may help correct the transmission defect.

Another well-known and, fortunately, rare disorder of transmitter-release blockade is botulism.

MUSCLE

Given the successful transmission of nerve impulse to the postsynaptic element of the end-plate, things can go wrong at various levels on the muscle side: failure to propagate a muscle action potential to invade the T system, failure of electromechanical coupling, and failure in the physical mechanism of sliding filaments.

In recent years we have been overwhelmed by descriptions of "new" muscle diseases based on fancy structural findings in biopsies. Some are rejected as nonspecific.

Electromyography may establish that the disorder lies in muscle as opposed to the neuron or nerve fiber, and muscle biopsy can confirm and classify the myopathy. As you will see, few muscle diseases are treatable.

The following is an oversimplified but practical review. Two major groups can be distinguished. The first group includes disorders of muscle that cause random degeneration of muscle fibers, leading to a reduction in the size of motor units and to muscle weakness and wasting.

1. The main subgroup is the *muscular dystrophies,* which are genetically determined, incurable, and progressive. The types of muscular dystrophy are usually classified according to inheritance and distribution of weakness.

2. Another subgroup of genetically determined myopathies has distinctive structural intracellular abnormalities. They include central core disease, nemaline myopathy, myotubular myopathy, mitochondrial myopathies, and the glycogen storage diseases caused by glyco-

lytic enzyme deficiencies. Some of these are not progressive.

3. Polymyositis is the last subgroup and includes the acquired inflammatory muscle disorders of immune infectious or unknown origin. They are characterized by immunophagocytosis of muscle fibers. Histology may be characteristic and some may be responsive to corticosteroids or immunosuppressants.

Because muscle fibers degenerate randomly in the three groups mentioned, motor units are moth-eaten rather than totally atrophied. The motor unit action potentials are small, brief, and polyphasic (myopathic) (see Fig 8-1). Simple insertion of an electrode into an affected muscle often immediately distinguishes the abnormal motor units and neurogenic versus myogenic muscle weakness. There are, however, limitations due to borderline cases.

The second main group includes diseases that cause more of a functional defect than structural fiber degeneration (little wasting).

1. Here we have *myotonia* and *paramyotonia congenita,* which are disorders of muscle membrane physiology causing improper muscle relaxation. This is equivalent to overexercise and the patients have true muscle hypertrophy.

2. This group includes the *periodic paralyses.* These are thyrotoxic periodic paralysis and familial periodic paralysis (hypo-, hyper-, or normokalemic).

Myotonias and periodic paralyses are rare and present little difficulty in diagnosis. EMG may show typical myotonic discharges. Treatment of symptoms may be rewarding in both groups.

REFERENCES

Brooke, M. H.: *A Clinician's View of Neuromuscular Diseases.* Baltimore, Williams & Wilkins Co., 1977.

Dyck, P. J., Thomas, P. K., Lambert, E. H.: *Peripheral Neuropathy.* Philadelphia, W. B. Saunders Co., 1975.

Walton, J. N.: *Disorders of Voluntary Muscle.* New York, Longman, Inc., 1974.

9

Epilepsy

EPILEPSY is "an occasional, an excessive and a disorderly discharge of nervous tissue" (John Hughlings Jackson, 1889) induced by any process involving the cerebral cortex, and perhaps also the brain stem reticular formation, that pathologically decreases the threshold for depolarization and synchronized firing in neurons. Metabolic intoxication or deficit and mechanical distortion by glial scarring or by the compression of neurons by tumor are considered basic pathophysiologies. Residual glial scarring and other less well-defined changes following trauma, ischemia, anoxia, infection, and possibly also hyperthermia are probably the most common substrates.

Experimentally it is quite easy to demonstrate the mechanical induction of seizures at the single-neuron level. When an electrode approaches a cortical neuron and begins to indent the cell membrane, a marked and excessive burst of firing occurs. If other neurons in the neighborhood are recruited, which is more likely to occur in the cerebral cortex and especially the limbic cortex, a clinical seizure may occur.

All neurons in the nervous system are capable of excessive firing; however, the threshold for this abnormality varies considerably in different areas. The cerebral cortex and, to a lesser degree, the upper brain stem (midbrain and diencephalon) are the only areas from which epileptiform activity arises with any frequency. These areas have the lowest threshold for seizures. The cortex itself can be subdivided into a relatively non-resistant neocortex and a highly susceptible limbic (paleo and archi) cortex. It is very possible though unproved that the majority of clinical seizures arise from the limbic cortex.

The electric activity of a seizure frequently can be recorded from scalp electrodes led into a highly sensitive amplifier system, an electroencephalographic unit. The excessive electroencephalographic discharge recorded can be useful in localizing the source of the seizure activity and occasionally by its pattern can delineate the type of seizure disorder. It is unusual to record an electroencephalogram (EEG) during a clinical seizure, but subclinical electric discharges are frequently recorded and are diagnostic of seizure disorder. A normal EEG in a person suspected of having epilepsy does not rule out the possibility because seizures occur episodically at variable and usually long intervals and interseizure electric activity is frequently normal.

Seizures can and usually do present clinically as excitation phenomena. On occasion and as a rule with certain types of epilepsy, inhibitory phenomena make up the behavioral result of excess neuronal activity. The blank, staring episodes of petit mal, the common childhood seizure disorder, are a good example. Presumably in these cases the excess neuronal activity is manifested by massive pre- and/or postsynaptic inhibition above and beyond any simultaneously occurring depolarization.

The clinical presentation of seizure types depends on the localization of the abnormal neurons and the spread of the abnormal discharges. We present a simplified functional-anatomical categorization of seizure types. It is not exhaustive but it does give the spectrum of major seizure categories (Table 9–1).

Seizures of Generalized Onset

GRAND MAL

These seizures, on presumptive evidence, are thought to arise from the reticular formation of the upper brain stem. A diffuse synchronous depolarization of the reticular formation recruits the cerebral cortex bilaterally and diffusely; the former causes loss of consciousness and the latter causes massive synchronous motor activity. This is manifested by tonic contraction of all muscles of the body. The individual assumes a rigid extended posture because the extensor muscles are more powerful than the flexors, followed in seconds (up to one minute) by synchronous phasic flexion-extension alternation contraction (clonic activity) of the limbs and trunk, and then complete relaxation as the electric seizure dies (Fig 9–1). Usually the

TABLE 9–1.—MAJOR SEIZURE CATEGORIES

I. Seizures of generalized onset
   A. Grand mal (major motor)
   B. Petit mal (absence)

II. Seizures of focal (partial) onset with or without generalization to major motor manifestations
   A. Elementary focal (partial) seizures (elementary cortex involvement)
      1. Motor cortex (jacksonian)
      2. Sensory cortex
         Somatosensory
         Auditory-vestibular
         Visual
         Olfactory-gustatory (uncinate)
   B. Complex focal (partial) seizures (limbic seizures)

III. Continuous seizures
   A. Generalized (status epilepticus)
   B. Focal (epilepsia partialis continua)

seizure is exhausted within several minutes but rarely may continue for hours or days as "status epilepticus." Autonomic motor overflow frequently occurs simultaneously, manifested clinically by emptying of the bladder and less often the bowel. A variable postseizure (postictal) period of depressed consciousness and confusion ensues. The length of this period probably depends on the length of the seizure and to some degree the amount of hypoxia that occurred during the seizure.

Grand mal seizures were considered the most prevalent type of adult seizure until recently when it was realized that limbic cortex foci, which spread excessive activity centrally to recruit the reticular formation and to both cerebral hemispheres through the forebrain commissures, were being overlooked. On questioning patients thought to have grand mal seizures, many claim to have visceral and emotional symptoms immediately prior to losing consciousness. These symptoms are probably the manifestation of limbic foci most often in the mesial temporal region involving the hippocampus or amygdala and neighboring structures, or in the orbitofrontal region.

A smaller group of persons is now considered to have classic grand mal epilepsy arising from a congenital or hereditary low threshold for excessive depolarization and synchronization in the reticular formation. In fact, there is some evidence that all seizures are of cortical origin with secondary involvement of the more resistant reticular formation. Some metabolically induced seizures may well fit the grand mal category. Ionic abnormalities (Na, K, Ca, Mg, BUN, pH, etc.), analeptic toxins (picrotoxin, Metrazol, Megimide, etc.), sedative withdrawal in addicts (alcohol, barbiturates, other sedatives and tranquilizers), hypoglycemia, hypoxia, occasionally hypercarbia (excess CO_2), and hyperthermia, especially in children, are the major metabolic categories. Strychnine and tetanus toxin are usually manifested as spinal cord or peripheral neuromuscular hyperactivity in addition to grand mal seizures.

Grand mal seizure pattern

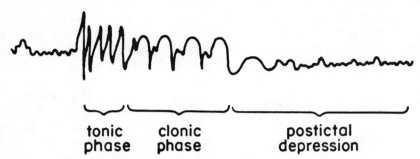

tonic phase clonic phase postictal depression

Fig 9–1.—Electroencephalogram pattern of grand mal seizure.

PETIT MAL

These are generally seizures of childhood that are thought also to originate in the reticular formation. They are manifested in negative fashion by short episodes (seconds) of blank staring for which the patient has no memory. The electroencephalogram is specific and therefore can be diagnostic for this disorder as opposed to the nonspecific excitatory EEG seen with grand mal seizures. The pattern is usually a paroxysm of three spikes and waves per second (Fig 9–2).

This pattern of spike and wave activity may well be a frequent response of the immature cortex to a seizure focus in any cortical or reticular location. Some evidence for this is observed in long-term follow-up of children with petit mal seizures. A significant proportion go on to develop focal seizures, particularly those of limbic origin. Presumably the limbic cortical focus, in many cases mesial temporal or orbitofrontal scarring incurred in or around birth, spreads its abnormal and excessive discharges centrally to the reticular formation, where they are generalized to the remainder of the hemispheres as recorded on EEG. The focal discharge might not be seen on the electroencephalogram because it lies at the depths of the temporal or frontal lobes and possibly, because of immaturity of the cortex, would be impeded in its attempts to spread over the limbic cortex and neocortex. Some reflection

of this suspected focal onset in many cases of petit mal epilepsy is the presence of eye movements, eyelid flickering, chewing movements, and salivation—positive phenomena in an otherwise negative or inhibitory seizure. These are probably behavioral manifestations of limbic or other focal cortical discharge.

You might ask why the petit mal seizure is predominantly a negative phenomenon when there appears to be diffuse hemispheric synchronization. During the grand mal seizure a similar degree of hemispheric synchronization is associated with massive clinical motor activity. Several reasons for this are suggested, and one of these is reflected in the spike-wave electroencephalographic pattern. The spike represents diffuse hemispheric depolarization excitation, whereas the wave is considered to represent diffuse hemispheric hyperpolarization inhibition. This postexcitatory inhibition, possibly initiated by collateral feedback inhibitory systems from the excitable neurons, is presumably adequate to prevent positive behavioral manifestations from being initiated by the massive depolarization. Another reason for lack of positive manifestations is that the immature motor cortex of children may be more resistant to excitatory recruitment. A reflection of this immaturity and relative resistance to excitation may lie in the incompleteness of the long-tract motor system

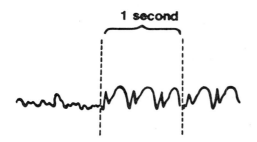

Petit mal spike wave pattern

Fig 9–2.—Electroencephalogram pattern (spike-wave) of petit mal seizure.

myelination in children. This would result in a decreased ability of cortical motor neurons to show excess activity. Additionally, cortical dendritic arborization is less well developed in children, thus allowing less excitable membrane surface for the spread of seizure activity. Children with petit mal usually maintain their posture during the short (seconds) absence attacks. This is presumed to be because the seizure activity does not spread to involve more resistant brain stem postural mechanisms. Incomplete myelination of long tracts may also be of importance here.

Spike-wave electric activity is also seen during the clonic phase of grand mal and major motor seizures; the latter is differentiated from the former only in that they are of focal cortical onset. The spike, which again represents massive and synchronous depolarization, manifests itself clinically as the clonic, flexion motor jerk followed by a phase of relaxation, which electrically is seen as the wave, massive inhibition. The spike is clinically manifest in this circumstance because the motor cortex is more reactive and less resistant to excitatory synchronization, because the synchronization can spread over more completely myelinated pathways, or for reasons inadequately explained on the basis of present data.

Approximately one third to one half of children with petit mal epilepsy are spontaneously clear of their seizures later in child-hood or during adolescence. Neuronal maturation (e.g., dendritic elaboration and spread with increased capacity for receiving inhibitory and excitatory synaptic communication, increasing myelination, etc.) presumably increases the capability of the hemisphere for spontaneously inhibiting excessive synchronous activity. Of the remaining children who continue to have seizures, one group has grand mal seizures with no evidence of focal onset. They presumably can express their diffuse, central (reticular) onset seizures through a mature neocortex capable, when synchronized, of exciting lower motor centers. The remainder of epileptics have their seizures as focal epilepsy, more often limbic, with or without spread to diffuse hemispheric synchronization and major motor clinical manifestation.

Seizures of Focal Nature With or Without Generalization to Major Motor Manifestation

Focal seizures are categorized by their anatomical-functional localization. They are manifested, at least initially, depending on the proximity of the pathologic process (glial scarring, tumor, etc.) to the cortex, by clinically recognizable sensory or motor functions of an either elementary or complex nature. If the seizure is not contained, it may spread to involve both hemispheres via the corpus callosum and/or the reticular formation of the mesodiencephalon and a major motor clinical seizure results, either tonic-clonic or just clonic in nature.

Major motor seizures are differentiated from grand mal seizures mainly on the basis of their focal onset.

ELEMENTARY SEIZURES
(ELEMENTARY OR PRIMARY
CORTEX INVOLVEMENT)

MOTOR CORTEX.—Seizures arising from the motor cortex (or nearby with spread to the motor cortex) appear simply as clonic jerking of the motor structures (muscle groups) innervated by the cortex involved. A focus of excitatory excess in or near the upper extremity of the homunculus is manifested as clonic twitching of part or all of the contralateral extremity. If the focus is not contained, a centrifugal progression to involve other parts of the motor cortex occurs (Fig 9–3), which appears clinically as a march of activity (jacksonian march) from the upper extremity to the face, trunk, and lower limb. Generalization via the corpus callosum or reticular formation frequently culminates in a seizure with bilateral motor excess, a major motor seizure.

SENSORY CORTEX.—The differentiation among transient ischemic attacks, migraine transient dysfunction, and sensory cortex seizures may occasionally be difficult. Age, clinically evident cervical vessel stenotic disease, lack of march, previous history of cerebrovascular disease, fundal changes (e.g., residual cholesterol emboli), involvement of multiple functional systems, motor and sensory, and a normal EEG suggest cerebrovascular insufficiency episodes (see chap. 14). Sensory symptoms followed by headache, usually unilateral, markedly favor migraine (see chap. 16). Headache as a manifestation of seizure is very unusual, although it can occur with transient ischemic attacks on occasion, normally during and not following the attack. The sensory symptoms of migraine march over minutes, those of seizure march over seconds, whereas the symptoms of transient ischemia appear suddenly. If there is generalization to focal or major motor seizure activity, the diagnosis of seizure disorder is almost assured. Rarely transient ischemia initiates a focal seizure.

Somatosensory cortex involvement is manifested by focal or progressive numbness and tingling, which on generalization involve the motor systems and culminate in a major motor seizure.

Auditory-vestibular cortex involvement appears as a hallucination of sound (tinnitus) and vertigo with or without generalization. If generalization does not occur, which is unusual, inner-ear disease (most often Ménière's vestibular-cochlear hydrops) must be differentiated. In the latter condition, standard audiometry results are almost invariably abnormal. (Why not abnormal with a cortical lesion?) An abnormal EEG with a focus of spiking emanating from the posterior temporal region is diagnostic, but the EEG with all seizure forms is frequently normal between seizures.

Fig 9–3.—Diagram of supposed mode of unilateral cortical spread (march) of seizure focus in the motor cortex prior to bilateral generalization via the corpus callosum and/or brain stem reticular formation.

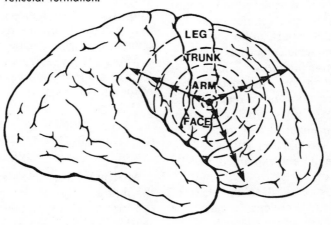

Visual cortex involvement is manifested as hallucinations in the contralateral visual field. Foci in the primary visual cortex (calcarine cortex) appear as unformed flashes, spots, and zig-zags of light, colored or white, whereas foci in association cortex cause more formed hallucinations such as floating balloons, stars, and polygons. Foci intermediary between the visual and the auditory cortex, usually in the temporal neocortex, may be associated with complex sensory hallucinations (e.g., people talking, occasionally described as something like a flashback).

Olfactory-gustatory cortex foci are manifested as hallucinations of smell and taste most often described as acrid and unpleasant. Generalization from the anterior mesial temporal (olfactory) cortex or the region of the insula and its posterior parietal operculum (gustatory) is usually, at least initially, via the contiguous limbic system; as a result the seizure takes the form of the more complex limbic epilepsy. Further spread to involve the reticular formation or neocortex results in a major motor seizure.

COMPLEX FOCAL SEIZURES

Complex focal seizures are almost invariably the result of limbic cortical involvement and appear behaviorally and experientially as visceral and affective (emotional) phenomena. The limbic cortex has the lowest cortical threshold for initiating and sustaining seizure activity. Additionally, the limbic cortex, which includes the hippocampus, parahippocampal temporal cortex, retrosplenial-cingulate-subcallosal cortex, orbitofrontal cortex, and insula—is the cortex most susceptible to metabolic injury. This is particularly true of the hippocampus. It is not surprising then that limbic epilepsy is quite common—probably the most common form of seizure disorder. Grand mal epilepsy was considered the most common form of epilepsy in the past. When it became known that the aura of many grand mal seizures (fre-

quently a peculiar abdominal sensation or detached feeling) represented the limbic focus of seizure onset followed by rapid secondary generalization via the corpus callosum or reticular formation, the category of grand mal epilepsy began to shrink in size. The person with true grand mal epilepsy loses consciousness immediately on initiation of seizure activity because his seizure presumably begins in or near the reticular formation.

If the limbic seizure does not generalize immediately, if it remains confined to the limbic system and its circuits, the visceral and affective psychomotor seizure in its many possible forms results. Simple and/or complex visceral and affective sensory phenomena such as peculiar and unpleasant smells and tastes, bizarre abdominal sensations, fear, anxiety, rarely rage, and excessive sexual appetite are mixed with simple and/or complex visceral and affective behavioral phenomena such as sniffing, chewing, lip smacking, salivation, excessive bowel sounds, belching, penile erection, feeding, running, rarely rage, and sexual behavior. Rarely, a seizure completely isolates the limbic system from the neocortex and reticular formation, which continue to function normally. The patient may carry out complex functions (e.g., drive a car), and because his limbic cortex is electrically synchronized and not functioning normally, on cessation of the seizures he has no idea what transpired. We assume this is because the limbic system is necessary for the imprinting part of learning, and therefore during the seizure inadequate imprinting occurs. This type of behavior, associated with amnesia, is more often caused by transient ischemia of the hippocampal regions than by seizure activity.

You may wonder why focal cortical seizures do not all generalize, why they remain localized clinically and electrically, and indeed why focal excitatory activity seen on the EEG is not always manifested as a clinical seizure. If glial scars underlie many seizure foci, why do we not all have epilepsy? Undoubtedly most, if not all, of us fell on our heads repeatedly as infants and small children and likely sustained a number of microscopic foci of glial scarring. No clear-cut answers to these questions are available; however, some recent experimental evidence is of considerable interest and at least heuristic value.

When a cortical seizure focus is created experimentally (e.g., by placing penicillin, a highly eleptogenic substance, on the cortex) in lower primates or cats, one can measure by intracellular recording a marked excess of depolarization and spiking in the application zone; at a unicellular level, this represents the seizure. From the proximate surrounding neurons one can measure repetitive hyperpolarization waves, which presumably represent collateral inhibition from the excited focus and very possibly block spreading depolarization from the seizure focus. Other evidence suggests that if the exciting focus is large enough and continues to fire, hyperpolarization gradually reverses and becomes depolarization with spiking, essentially an overrunning of the inhibitory surround by the seizure with resulting continued propagation of the seizure. This inhibitory surround may well be the safety factor or one of the safety factors that prevents focal seizures from spreading or indeed keeps excitatory foci small enough never to be clinically manifested as a seizure.

Continuous Seizures (Status Epilepticus and Epilepsia Partialis Continua)

Generalized and focal seizures may on occasion become continuous with very little or no interictal period. Presumably hyperpolarization inhibition, if it is truly a mechanism for the termination of seizures, is overrun by the repetitive depolarization excess emanating from the seizure focus or foci. This does not, however, completely explain the unchecked self-regenerating character of the seizure, which is necessary to maintain continuous activity.

Circumstances that seem to predispose to status epilepticus are similar to those that result in recurrence of single or multiple seizures in individuals who are otherwise medically or physiologically well controlled. An example is acute termination of anticonvulsant medication, which does more than return the patient to his premedication seizure susceptibility. A rebound central nervous system hyperexcitability state occurs, as it does in most individuals with physiologic dependence on sedative medications. However, only about 10%–15% of sedative-dependent (usually alcoholic) subjects develop rebound or withdrawal hyperexcitability great enough to cause seizures. The epileptic is much more susceptible to repeated or recurrent seizures on medication withdrawal because he already has an abnormally low threshold for seizure activity. Although withdrawal of medication is the most common cause, any circumstance that increases central nervous system excitability may lead to seizure recurrence or less commonly status epilepticus. Emotional excess (e.g., fright or anger), fever and other hypermetabolic states, hypocalcemia, hypomagnesemia, hypoxemia, and toxic states (e.g., tetanus, uremia, portacaval shunt encephalopathy) are a few examples.

Continuous major motor seizures (status epilepticus) are a medical emergency. If they are not terminated, the mortality is very high and many survivors are left with brain damage. The massive muscle activity leads to hyperthermia with temperatures as high as 106 F or more, which, if sustained, cause irreversible neuron damage. Hypoxia from inadequate pulmonary ventilation also causes brain damage. Severe lactic acidosis from shock and tissue hypoxia, amplified by excessive muscle activity, probably contributes to neuron damage. Death usually is not from brain dysfunction directly but from overtaxation of cardiopulmonary reserve by the combination of massive continuous exercise, hypoxia, lactic acidosis, shock, and possibly also hyperthermia. Though somewhat controversial, it is possible that brain damage can also be caused by continued seizure activity alone. Therefore, even the person who is paralyzed by a neuromuscular blocking agent (curariform drug), intubated and mechanically respired, and whose blood pressure and temperature are controlled within normal range may need to have his seizure activity terminated as soon as possible.

Continuous focal seizure activity (epilepsia partialis continua) is less threatening. Its tendency to generalize into major motor status epilepticus makes it important to terminate the seizures or, if this is not possible, to contain them as focal seizures with medication until they terminate spontaneously. The etiologic factors are similar to those initiating seizure recurrence and status epilepticus. Occasionally epilepsia partialis continua is the presenting manifestation of a seizure focus. This is most common in adults, and neoplasm or ischemia-infarction of the brain is the most frequent cause.

Therapy

Treatment of epilepsy is based on medical suppression of the excitable focus or surgical removal or isolation of the focus if optimal medical therapy is unsuccessful or if the focus is a tumor and surgery is feasible. Much has been learned about the pharmacologic effects of antiepileptic drugs, but their exact modes of action remain unclear. Seizures that are symptomatic of systemic or localized central nervous system metabolic disorders, such as infection, disorders of fluid and electrolyte balance, exogenous and endogenous toxicities, and renal failure, are best treated by ameliorating the underlying condition, if possible, and the concomitant use of anticonvulsant medications where indicated.

Some anticonvulsant drugs suppress neuronal membrane excitability, probably by hyperpolarization, which possibly reflects a decreased intracellular sodium concentration. Some appear to depress synaptic transmission. Increased inhibitory neurotransmis-

sion may be the mode of action of some others. All these mechanisms could increase neuronal resistance to excessive discharge or protect normal neurons from recruitment by neighboring excessive discharge.

An ideal anticonvulsant decreases abnormal excitability, has a minimal sedating effect, and is free of other significant and deleterious side effects. No medication achieves these goals. Fortunately, diphenylhydantoin and phenobarbital, the mainstays of epilepsy therapy, approach these criteria. Other than these two drugs, primidone, ethosuximide, and diazepam are the major first-line anticonvulsant drugs. Many congeners of these drugs are on the market but because they have less therapeutic effect, more side effects, or both, they are considered second-line medications. Diphenylhydantoin and phenobarbital are the primary medications for most seizure disorders. Primidone, which is metabolized into barbiturate radicals, on occasion is more successful for treating resistant limbic epilepsy. Ethosuximide is the first-line medication for treating children with petit mal epilepsy. Intravenous diphenylhydantoin and diazepam are the drugs of choice for treating continuous seizures, status epilepticus. Carbamazepine, mesantoin, and, more recently, sodium valproate are effective antiseizure medications to be used for the most part if the preceding medications fail.

Medical therapy is successful in decreasing seizures in almost 80% of epileptics. Approximately 30% gain complete arrest of their seizures.

If medical therapy does not adequately control the seizures, surgical removal or isolation of the electric seizure focus can be considered. The focus must be localized by radiodiagnostic and/or electrodiagnostic study and, if localized, must be surgically approachable. The most common operations carried out today are temporal lobectomy and, less often, local corticectomy. Surgical isolation of seizure foci in one hemisphere by corpus callosum section is successful in some cases; the major aim of this type of surgery is to decrease or arrest major motor generalization. Seizures that spread via the brain stem would be unlikely to be affected by corpus callosum section.

As a mode of therapy, removal of neoplasm or other tumor (e. g., abscess, granuloma, clot) causing seizures needs no elaboration. Surgery if possible and radiation and chemotherapy if indicated are the primary therapies. Medical antiseizure treatment serves as pre- and postoperative prophylaxis. Approximately 10% of persons with focal epilepsy have a tumor. The older the patient, the more likely he is to have a tumor as a cause of focal seizures. This agrees with the age-incidence spectrum of neoplasm. Therefore, patients with clearly focal seizures merit more extensive neurologic evaluation, frequently including invasive neuroradiologic procedures (see chap. 18).

REFERENCES

Gastaut, H., Broughton, R.: *Epileptic Seizures.* Springfield, Ill., Charles C Thomas, Publisher, 1972.

Laidlaw, J., Richens, A.: *A Textbook of Epilepsy.* Edinburgh, Churchill and Livingston, 1976.

Schmidt, R. P., Wilder, B. J.: *Epilepsy.* Philadelphia, F. A. Davis Co., 1968.

10

Degenerative and Demyelinating Diseases of the Nervous System

EDWARD VALENSTEIN

Introduction

MANY DISEASES previously classified as degenerative or demyelinating are now associated with specific metabolic deficiencies (Table 10–1). Others are transmitted by viruses (see chap. 12). However, we are still left with a large number of progressive diseases of unknown etiology, and their classification is based on pathologic findings. In this chapter we discuss the more common of these conditions (designated by asterisks in Tables 10–2 and 10–3).

Demyelinating Diseases

In this group of diseases (see Table 10–2) lesions are characterized by loss of myelin with relative sparing of axons. Furthermore, the myelin degradation appears chemically similar to that seen in wallerian degeneration. Thus, demyelinating disorders are distinguished on the one hand from nonspecific demyelination (as seen with ischemia, inflammation, for example) in which axons and myelin are affected together and, on the other hand, from metabolic disorders of myelination characterized by the accumulation of abnormal breakdown products (the "dysmyelinative" disorders, or leukodystrophies—metachromatic leukodystrophy, Krabbe's disease).

DEMYELINATION ON AN ALLERGIC BASIS

Experimental allergic encephalomyelitis is the model for this group of demyelinative disorders. This disease develops several days after central nervous system (CNS) myelin basic protein is injected subcutaneously with Freund's adjuvant. The CNS is peppered with lesions consisting of perivenous lymphocytic infiltration and demyelination. These lesions are similar pathologically to those seen in a naturally occurring human disease, acute disseminated encephalomyelitis (ADEM). This condition may occur

TABLE 10–1.—SOME INBORN ERRORS OF METABOLISM

A. Aminoacidurias (phenylketonurias, etc.)
B. Disorders of lipid metabolism
   1. Sphingolipidoses (Tay-Sachs, etc.)
   2. Leukodystrophies (metachromatic leukodystrophy, Krabbe's disease, etc.)
C. Lipoprotein disorders
   1. Tangier disease
   2. Abetalipoproteinemia (Bassen-Kornzweig disease)
D. Disorders of glucose and glycogen metabolism
   1. Mucopolysaccharidoses
   2. Glycogenoses
   3. Galactosemia
E. Miscellaneous disorders
   1. Wilson's disease
   2. Porphyria
   3. Refsum's disease

121

TABLE 10-2.—DEMYELINATING DISORDERS

A. Allergic
   1. Experimental allergic encephalomyelitis
   2. Acute disseminated encephalomyelopathy (?)
   3. Acute hemorrhagic encephalomyelopathy (?)
   4. Experimental allergic neuritis
  *5. Guillain-Barré syndrome (probable)
B. Unknown etiology
  *1. Multiple sclerosis
   2. Devic's disease
C. Infectious etiology (slow virus infections)
   1. Progressive multifocal leukoencephalopathy
   2. Visna (in sheep)

*These are the more common conditions.

following various viral infections or following vaccinations (and hence is also called postinfectious or postvaccinal encephalomyelitis). In some instances, this disease is shown to be associated with hypersensitivity to CNS myelin. Acute hemorrhagic encephalomyelitis is currently thought to be merely a more fulminant variety of ADEM, in which necrosis of vessels leads to superimposed hemorrhage.

There is evidence that Guillain-Barré syndrome (in which the major pathologic changes are diffuse peripheral nervous system demyelination and perivascular inflammation) is similarly mediated by hypersensitivity to peripheral nerve myelin. There is also an experimental model for this condition (experimental allergic neuritis).

MULTIPLE SCLEROSIS

In multiple sclerosis (MS) the lesions are variable-sized, well-circumscribed plaques of demyclination. They may occur anywhere within the white matter of the central nervous system. Peripheral nerves are not affected, although occasionally the lower motor neurons are demyelinated before they leave the CNS. Lesions of the optic nerves are common; remember that the optic "nerve" is really an extension of the CNS and not a peripheral nerve. The demyelinative lesions may be associated with perivascular cellular infiltration, but the pathologic

picture, as well as the time course of the illness, differs from that seen in experimental allergic encephalomyelitis.

CLINICAL FINDINGS.—The disease is quite common in temperate climates (Japan is the major exception) and appears to be less prevalent among lower socioeconomic groups. It is uncommon in children under the age of 10, and very rarely does it begin after the age of 55.

The typical demyelinative plaque causes a deficit that progresses over hours or days, stabilizes for one to three weeks, and then remits slowly over one to six weeks. Remission probably results from subsidence of the inflammation and edema (short zones, up to 3 mm, of demyelination that do not conduct

TABLE 10-3.—DEGENERATIVE DISEASES

A. Causing dementia primarily
  *1. Alzheimer's disease
   2. Pick's disease
   3. Marchiafava-Bignami disease
B. Causing basal ganglia degeneration primarily
  †1. Parkinsonism
  †2. Huntington's chorea
   3. Progressive supranuclear palsy (Steele-Richardson-Olchewsky)
   4. Hallervorden-Spatz disease
   5. Others
C. Causing visual deficit
   1. Leber's optic atrophy
   2. Retinitis pigmentosa
D. Spinocerebellar degenerations
  *1. Friedreich's ataxia
   2. Olivopontocerebellar degeneration
   3. Familial spastic paraparesis
   4. Others
E. Motor neuron diseases
  *1. Amyotrophic lateral sclerosis (ALS)
   2. Werdnig-Hoffmann disease
   3. Kugelberg-Welander disease
F. Causing peripheral neuropathy
   1. Charcot-Marie-Tooth disease (peroneal atrophy)
   2. Dejerine-Sottas disease
G. Causing myopathy
  *1. Duchenne's muscular dystrophy
   2. Fascio-scapulo-humeral
   3. Limb-girdle
   4. Myotonic dystrophy
   5. Others

*You should know about these conditions.
†Covered in chapter 13 on diseases of the basal ganglia.

impulses during the acute phase may again transmit on clearing of the acute process) and the use of alternate pathways, and not by remyelination. As lesions accumulate, remissions are less complete. Eventually there are so many lesions that new ones are not apparent clinically as discrete events. The disease's course is then steadily progressive. Occasionally, the disease progresses slowly from the start. In either case, the course varies from a few months ("acute MS") to more than 50 years, with the average survival after diagnosis being 15 to 20 years. Death is usually from superimposed infection.

The nature of the deficit depends on the location and size of the demyelinating plaque. Certain locations are especially common. Lesions in the optic nerve produce *optic neuritis*. If the plaque involves the optic disk, edema is seen on funduscopic examination (optic papillitis); if it involves the nerve behind the disk, there are no acute changes on funduscopic examination (retrobulbar neuritis). In either case, optic atrophy supervenes. Acutely, the patient may complain of pain on eye movements (possibly secondary to swelling of the optic nerve), and there is a visual field defect (usually central). Although 40% of persons with MS have optic neuritis, many patients with optic neuritis do not go on to develop MS. Some of these have ischemic optic nerve disorders.

Plaques involving the medial longitudinal fasciculus produce unilateral or bilateral *internuclear ophthalmoplegia* (see chap. 3). On lateral gaze there is paresis of the medial rectus function and nystagmus of the abducted eye. However, convergence movement of the medial rectus is usually spared. Internuclear ophthalmoplegia can be seen in persons with vascular disease, but usually these patients are older. In the younger age group, it is highly suggestive of MS, but occasionally results from tumor, vasculitis, or other inflammatory conditions.

Cerebellar signs, hemiparesis, and evidence of spinal cord involvement (paraparesis, Brown-Séquard syndrome) all occur commonly. Hemispheric lesions may result in dementia, although it usually appears late. Aphasia is uncommon. Sensory loss (especially of vibratory sensation) may occur, but often paresthesias are more distressing. Tic douloureux (trigeminal neuralgia) is sometimes seen. Lhermitte's symptoms, an electric or tingling sensation referred to the trunk and limbs on neck flexion (chin on chest), was first described in association with multiple sclerosis. It is presumed to be caused by distortion of the spinal cord (stretch) with secondary depolarizations of the affected dorsal columns (see chap. 1). Although it is associated with other intrinsic and occasionally extrinsic spinal cord lesions, it is most commonly seen with multiple sclerosis. In some patients, lesions may be predominantly in one portion of the nervous system (most often the spinal cord).

DIAGNOSIS.—The diagnosis of MS is strongly suggested when a person in the appropriate age range has evidence of lesions separated in space and time. The differential diagnosis should include a consideration of multiple emboli and vasculitis. Sarcoid meningitis can produce reversible optic neuritis and other CNS signs. Dementia, spasticity, and posterior column findings suggest vitamin B_{12} deficiency. The examiner should be wary not to miss a single lesion that may affect several different systems. For example, a patient may have cerebellar ataxia and spastic paraparesis that could both result from a lesion compressing the spinal cord and cerebellum at the level of the foramen magnum. Such a lesion would have to be excluded by myelography and/or computerized axial tomography (CT scan). On the other hand, if that person also had optic neuritis or hemiparesis involving the face, one lesion could no longer explain the findings. A history of remissions and exacerbations also helps in the diagnosis of MS, but it must be remembered that the symptoms of neoplasms commonly fluctuate to some degree.

Diagnostic tests should include complete blood count (CBC), antinuclear antibodies

(ANA), serum test for syphilis (STS, VDRL, Kolmer test, etc.), fluorescent treponemal antibody test (FTA), and complete urinalysis. If indicated, appropriate contrast studies (myelography or angiography, CT scan, etc.) should be performed to rule out alternative diagnoses. Spinal fluid examination may show evidence of immunologic activity in the CNS: Cerebrospinal fluid (CSF), pleocytosis, and elevation of gamma globulin can be found in two thirds of the cases. CSF oligoclonal IgG bands and increased globulin to albumin ratio can be found in 90% of cases. There may also be an increase in CSF myelin basic protein levels. Evidence of subclinical demyelinated lesions can be provided by CT scan, visual, somatosensory, or brain stem auditory evoked responses, or the hot bath test (raising body temperature slows conduction in demyelinated plaques—patients with MS may feel worse in hot weather). As yet, there is no pathognomonic test for MS.

ETIOLOGY.—Both autoimmune and infectious mechanisms have received attention recently. Genetic susceptibility to MS is suggested by finding certain histocompatibility antigens overrepresented in patients with MS. The spinal fluid changes noted above indicate production of immunoglobulins in the CNS. A recent study demonstrated reduction in the number of suppressor cells (that normally inhibit immune responses) immediately prior to exacerbations of MS.

An infectious etiology has been suggested by the following evidence:

1. The distribution of MS is very nonuniform. Temperate climates have a higher incidence than warm climates, but the disease is uncommon in Japan. In the Orkney and Shetland islands, north of Scotland, the incidence is extremely high: 1 in 300 persons are affected. Not far away, however, in the Faroe Islands, the disease was unknown until British troops arrived during World War II.
2. Epidemiologic studies suggest that MS is often acquired in childhood or adolescence. Moving from a high-risk to a low-risk area after the age of 15 may not reduce one's chances of developing MS.
3. There is an increased incidence of measles antibody titers in persons with MS.

These findings strongly implicate an environmental factor, probably infectious; however, the identity of the factor is presently unknown. Occasional reports of electron-microscopic or culture evidence of virus in brains of MS patients have so far remained unconfirmed. Epidemiologic evidence implicating distemper virus (closely related to the measles virus) is presently being pursued.

It is thus likely that those infectious and immune mechanisms contribute to the pathogenesis of MS. Possibly a viral infection triggers an inappropriate immune response.

Degenerative Diseases

In the degenerative diseases the major pathologic features are loss of neurons and secondary gliosis (scarring). Demyelination may occur secondary to neuronal death (see Table 10−3).

AMYOTROPHIC LATERAL SCLEROSIS

Amyotrophic lateral sclerosis (ALS) is one of a number of degenerative conditions that selectively involve the motor system. Two inherited conditions (Werdnig-Hoffmann disease in infants and Kugelberg-Welander disease in children and young adults) are characterized by anterior horn cell degeneration only. In ALS, which affects mainly adults 40−60 years of age, there is degeneration not only of the anterior horn cells and cranial nerve motor nuclei but also of the corticobulbar and corticospinal tracts. Clinically, therefore, one sees a combination of atrophy, fasciculations, and hyperactive reflexes. Weakness results from both upper and lower motor neuron lesions. Combined bulbar and pseudobulbar palsies are commonly seen. The disease may start asymmetrically, but usually within months it involves many muscle groups. The average patient survives three years. Death results from weakness of the bulbar and respiratory musculature and resultant superimposed infection.

In primary lateral sclerosis, the upper motor neuron signs predominate, but eventually there is some evidence of lower motor neuron involvement, so that this entity is no longer felt to be distinct from ALS. The course tends to be longer than in the usual variety of ALS, with some persons surviving five to ten years or longer.

SPINOCEREBELLAR DEGENERATIONS

This complex group of diseases defies rational classification. Friedreich's ataxia is by far the most common of these conditions. This disease has its onset in childhood or adolescence, with ataxia that is due to proprioceptive loss and cerebellar ataxia. There is atrophy of the small muscles of the feet, indicating a peripheral neuropathy. Mild spastic weakness and upgoing toes may be seen later. Severe disability and death usually occur by the third or fourth decades; however, mild forms, or *formes frustes,* of the disease are not infrequent. Extraneurologic signs include pes cavus, kyphoscoliosis, and cardiomyopathy, which may result in terminal failure.

The lesions in Friedreich's ataxia involve the dorsal root ganglia, with secondary lesions in the peripheral nerves and dorsal columns. In addition, lesions are present in Clarke's column and in the lateral columns. Sometimes there are lesions in the cerebellum. Other diseases in the group of spinocerebellar degenerations emphasize different aspects of the Friedreich syndrome. In one condition, the lesions are predominantly in the peripheral nerves (the neuronal form of Charcot-Marie-Tooth disease). In another, the lateral columns are primarily affected (familial spastic paraplegia). In others, the brunt of the disease is in the cere-

bellum and brain stem (primary cerebellar atrophy, olivopontocerebellar atrophy). In some persons with the latter disease, extrapyramidal signs and dementia may be prominent. In any of these diseases, optic atrophy or pigmentary degeneration of the retina may be seen. In all variants, symmetric neurologic deficit and slow progression are the rule. Some rare metabolic diseases have many features of spinocerebellar degenerations (Bassen-Kornzweig disease—abetalipoproteinemia—and Refsum's disease). Sorting out this bewildering array of diseases must await a better understanding of their pathogenesis.

ALZHEIMER'S DISEASE

Alzheimer described a presenile dementing illness characterized pathologically by neurofibrillary degeneration and senile plaques. Since the pathologic changes are identical in many cases of senile dementia (occurring over the age of 65), we use the term *Alzheimer's disease* to include this common form of senile dementia. Choline acetyl transferase, an enzyme needed for producing acetyl choline, is diminished in brains of patients with Alzheimer's disease. The disease has a familial tendency.

The pathologic changes in persons with Alzheimer's disease are most severe in the hippocampi and in the phylogenetically newer regions of the cortex. Loss of recent memory is an early clinical feature. Mild anomia and constructional apraxia are also common early signs. More severe cognitive loss and eventually frontal lobe disturbances become prominent as the illness progresses, but paresis, sensory loss, or visual field defects are not seen. Myoclonic seizures may occur. Attempts to improve memory in Alzheimer's disease by increasing dietary choline or its precursors have not been of definite help.

Senile persons with dementia are often diagnosed as having "cerebral arteriosclerosis" when in fact they have Alzheimer's disease. Arteriosclerotic dementia does occur (more rarely than Alzheimer's disease) but is almost always associated with elementary neurologic findings (spasticity, pseudobulbar palsies) and a history of stroke.

PICK'S DISEASE

Pick's disease, rare in this country, is not clinically distinguishable from Alzheimer's disease. The diagnosis must rest on pathologic findings. As for Alzheimer's disease, there is no effective therapy.

MUSCULAR DYSTROPHIES

DUCHENNE'S MUSCULAR DYSTROPHY.— This is the most common type and is a sex-linked recessive trait. It affects young boys, in whom pseudohypertrophy of the calves and weakness of the hip and shoulder girdles progress from early childhood. Levels of serum muscle enzymes (CPK and aldolase) are extremely high, especially early in the course, implying an abnormality in muscle membrane. The children are usually confined to a wheelchair by the age of 10, and they usually die in the second to third decade. No effective therapy is known.

LIMB-GIRDLE MUSCULAR DYSTROPHY.— This probably represents a group of conditions that usually appear in adolescence or adult life with proximal limb weakness. The weakness may progress slowly and may arrest spontaneously. It must be differentiated from the neurogenic and metabolic conditions that cause similar muscle weakness.

MYOTONIC DYSTROPHY.— In this disease myotonia (delayed relaxation of muscles) is combined with dystrophy (muscle atrophy not secondary to peripheral nerve or anterior horn cell involvement). The disease begins in childhood or young adult life. The dystro-

phy, as opposed to most forms of myopathy, is distal, affecting the muscles of the hands before more proximal musculature. In addition, facial and neck musculature are involved early. Evidence points to an abnormality of membranes that is not restricted to muscle. Numerous nonneurologic problems are found: frontal balding, testicular atrophy, diabetes, cardiac arrhythmias, and others. The disease is inherited as an autosomal dominant. It progresses slowly. Many victims succumb to respiratory failure and superimposed infection by the fifth decade.

Other forms of muscular dystrophy are described but fall outside the scope of this book.

Slow Virus Infections of the Nervous System

These conditions are discussed in chapter 12 on infectious diseases. The group of diseases caused by atypical viruses (scrapie, kuru, Jakob-Creutzfeldt disease) provides a possible model for other diseases in which the primary pathologic change is neuronal degeneration and reactive gliosis. Inheritable disorders may not be exempt because Jakob-Creutzfeldt disease has been transmitted to experimental animals from persons who have a familial history of the disease. Transfer of other degenerative diseases has been attempted (ALS, MS, parkinsonism), so far without success.

REFERENCES
McAlpine, D., Lamsden, C. E., Acheson, E. D.: *Multiple Sclerosis—A Reappraisal,* ed. 2. Edinburgh, Churchill and Livingstone, 1972.

Walton, J. N.: *Disorders of Voluntary Muscle,* ed. 3. Edinburgh, Churchill and Livingstone, 1974.

Wells, C. E.: *Dementia,* ed. 2. Philadelphia, F. A. Davis Co., 1977.

11

Dementia

EDWARD VALENSTEIN

DEMENTIA REFERS TO a *loss* of higher intellectual and emotional function. Studies indicate that at least 10% of persons who have symptoms suggestive of dementia turn out to have treatable illness. About half of them will have psychiatric problems, but the remainder will have treatable organic disease. The proportion of treatable cases is less the older the population and the more chronic the dementia; however, even in this group a small number of persons may be helped. Dementia is a very common problem and becomes even more common when looked for, so the clinical importance of this subject can hardly be exaggerated.

Is the Patient Demented?

Several problems often arise in trying to decide whether or not a patient is actually demented.

1. *Senescence:* Mild defects in memory and other higher cortical functions occur normally with age. One may complain of these, but may be able to perform normally on clinical mental status testing and on formal psychological tests that take this normal deterioration into account.

2. *Mental retardation:* Because dementia is defined as a *loss* of function, the history should be adequate to document that the person was once capable of better performance. Educational and occupational histories are valuable in this regard. The person

should be asked at what age he achieved his highest educational grade, to ascertain whether he failed to progress normally.

3. *Psychiatric illness:* Mistakes can be made in both directions. Organic illness can mimic many symptoms of psychiatric disease, especially the psychoses; and some psychiatric illnesses may prevent adequate evaluation of a patient's intellectual functioning. A few rules are useful: (a) With the exception of depression, the functional psychoses rarely arise after the age of 40. A 50-year-old person with his first "schizophrenic break" should therefore be suspected of having organic disease. (b) Depression may accompany mild dementia, but, contrary to what is commonly stated, depression is not the first sign of the usual form of dementia of old age. In fact, depressed elderly persons with normal mental status do not have an increased incidence of subsequent organic dementia. Furthermore, when dementia is moderately severe, a person cannot sustain a deep depression although he may be querulous and at times sad. Severe depression, therefore, is rarely a symptom of organic disease. (c) Although loss of recent memory is not a necessary accompaniment of organic dementia, it is not seen in functional states. If adequate testing can be done, therefore, the finding of a definite recent memory deficit strongly militates against functional disease. The two major exceptions are depressive pseudodementia and malingering. It is rare

for the malingering person to mimic convincingly the type of memory loss seen in those with organic disease. He is more likely to forget everything, including items of remote memory usually retained by truly amnesic persons. (d) Regressive reflexes (see chap. 6) are indicative of organic disease. (e) Urinary incontinence is rarely seen in adults with functional disease.

Depressive pseudodementia presents a difficult clinical problem. These patients, usually elderly, have decreased activity and speech and deficits in intellectual functioning. Depressive symptoms may not be prominent. When there is doubt and the preliminary medical evaluation for dementia is negative, it is sometimes worthwhile to treat these patients for depression (with drugs or, in some intractable cases, shock therapy). Patients with pseudodementia usually respond, and their intellectual functioning returns to normal.

Types of Dementia

Dementia is not a unitary condition. Findings differ greatly among patients, reflecting, to a large extent, the regions of the brain involved or the nature of the biochemical insult. Localization of hemispheric function was discussed in chapter 2.

LOSS OF RECENT MEMORY

Loss of recent memory (as tested by a person's ability to remember three items after five minutes with distraction) in the absence of defects of attention (as tested, for example, by the digit span) is indicative of bilateral lesions in the hippocampi or related structures (fornices, mamillary bodies, dorsomedial thalamus). A limited number of pathologic states, therefore, underlie this type of problem (Table 11–1). Unilateral damage to the hippocampal and adjacent neocortical regions may cause verbal memory defects if the lesion is in the dominant hemisphere. Difficulties learning visuospatial tasks have been noted in persons with dam-

TABLE 11–1.—CAUSES OF SELECTIVE LOSS OF RECENT MEMORY

A. Hippocampal damage
  1. Postanoxic or posthypoglycemic
  2. Posttraumatic
  3. Infectious (herpes simplex encephalitis)
  4. Vascular (posterior cerebral artery occlusion)
  5. Temporal lobe epilepsy (ictal or postictal): transient
  6. Surgery: bilateral temporal lobectomies
  7. Degenerative disease: Alzheimer's disease
B. Fornix (debatable)
C. Mamillary bodies and/or dorsomedial thalamus (bilateral lesions)
  1. Wernicke-Korsakoff disease
  2. Tumors of the third ventricle, hypothalamus, or parasellar region
D. Anticholinergic drugs

age or removal of the right temporal lobe. The defects with unilateral disease tend to be mild and may be temporary in some, whereas bilateral hippocampal-temporal lobe damage leaves devastating recent memory problems.

FRONTAL LOBE DEMENTIA

Persons with frontal lobe lesions may have significant dementia with no abnormality of recent memory. Often intellectual function is intact on routine testing, but the patient's behavior is inappropriate (see chap. 2). Later tests of manipulation of knowledge (calculations, proverbs, similarities) are poorly done. Regressive reflexes are commonly seen at this stage.

CORTICAL DEMENTIA

Cognitive functions such as language, praxis, and visuospatial functions can be impaired by diseases that affect the cortex, e.g., stroke, Alzheimer's disease, and Jacob-Kreutzfeldt disease. Often these diseases affect other aspects of hemispheric function, such as memory and motivation (frontal lobe function).

SUBCORTICAL DEMENTIA

Dementia can result from diseases that affect mainly subcortical structures. Persons with Steele-Richardson-Olchewsky disease (progressive supranuclear palsy, an uncommon disease affecting the midbrain and other subcortical structures) may show a remarkable slowness in performance; tests are performed well only if the patient is given a great deal of time. Often persons with subcortical disease (such as Parkinson's disease) have dementias that resemble frontal lobe dementias. The exact symptoms of many of these conditions have not been adequately described as yet.

CONFUSIONAL STATES

Deficits in maintaining attention may markedly reduce intellectual functioning. Many metabolic dementias (such as hepatic encephalopathy, delirium tremens, and dementias produced by many drugs) are manifested principally by the inability to attend to important stimuli. Lesions affecting the brain stem or thalamic reticular formation, if insufficient to produce stupor or coma, may result in an attentional deficit. In general, these are referred to as *confusional states*.

ORGANIC PSYCHOSES

Diseases affecting the limbic system or related structures may produce a wide variety of psychiatric findings. Persons with temporal lobe epilepsy commonly have behavioral disturbances, and hyposexuality, hyperreligiosity, and even paranoid psychosis have been described as interictal changes. Aggressive behavior can be seen in persons with lesions in the temporal lobes or the medial hypothalamus. Changes in appetite for food and sex may also result from lesions in these locations. Persons with Huntington's chorea may experience episodes that are indistinguishable from acute paranoid schizophrenia or manic-depressive illness. The list goes on. Obviously, the distinction between functional and organic can be difficult. It is, therefore, important to look for other indications of organic disease in these persons (for example, fever, incontinence, seizures, focal neurologic signs, regressive reflexes, movement disorders) before referring them for psychiatric care.

Evaluation of the Demented Patient

After having decided that a person is demented, certain features of the history and examination help determine the subsequent evaluation.

1. Do the mental changes themselves localize the lesion(s)? The important diagnostic points were reviewed earlier in this chapter and in chapter 2.
2. Are there associated focal neurologic deficits such as hemiparesis, visual field defects, or sensory changes?
3. Are there neurologic deficits suggestive of systems degeneration, for example, chorea, parkinsonism, or cerebellar abnormalities? These might suggest a particular type of degenerative disease (such as Huntington's chorea, parkinsonism, or spinocerebellar degeneration) or, less often, a metabolic problem (such as Wilson's disease or chronic hepatic encephalopathy).
4. Is there evidence of increased intracranial pressure?
5. Certain findings on the neurologic examination strongly suggest a metabolic deficit. A prominent confusional state is one. Multifocal myoclonus and asterixis (see chap. 19) are others often associated with uremic or hepatic encephalopathy.
6. Are there associated symptoms or signs indicative of a systemic disease, such as a thyroid disorder, Cushing's disease, collagen vascular disease, malignancy, or infection?
7. Is the course acute or chronic? Most (but not all) irreversible degenerative diseases are chronic. As mentioned, although the chances of finding a reversible etiology are less with the chronic dementias, remediable causes are found

in enough patients to merit a complete evaluation.

The answers to these general questions determine the sort of evaluation required. If the examination indicates a focal brain lesion, the evaluation should aim to document the lesion (skull x-rays, EEG) and to determine its nature (computerized tomography, and, if necessary, arteriography). If the examination suggests a metabolic problem (confusion without focal neurologic signs), an intensive search for metabolic derangements should be made before looking for focal lesions or bilateral degenerative disease. This evaluation includes numerous blood studies and a lumbar puncture (to exclude subarachnoid hemorrhage or infection). In the patient in whom there is no obvious clue to the nature of the underlying disease, the screening evaluation outlined in

Table 11–2 is indicated. Most of the treatable causes of dementia listed in Table 11–3 (on the following pages) would be excluded on the basis of this evaluation combined with a careful history and physical examination.

Following this evaluation, treatable causes of dementia should have been ruled out; however, there is still a large number of persons for whom no diagnosis has been made. In such patients it is possible that there is an intracranial mass that is not producing focal findings, and is not visible on CT scan, such as a low-grade glioma (an invasive tumor that may not produce much mass effect). Vasculitis confined to the CNS may be difficult to diagnose, as can the remote effects of carcinoma. The vast majority of such patients, however, will have degenerative disease, the most common by far being Alzheimer's disease.

TABLE 11-2.—ROUTINE SCREENING EVALUATION
FOR THE DEMENTED PATIENT*

TEST	INDICATION
Complete blood cell count	Anemia, polycythemia, vitamin B_{12} deficiency (hypersegmentation)
ESR	Vasculitis, tumor, infection
Venereal Disease Research Lab Test and FTA-ABS	Syphilis (in tertiary lues the serum VDRL results may be negative and the FTA positive)
Blood sugar	Hypo- or hyperglycemia
Blood urea nitrogen	Renal failure
Electrolytes	Water intoxication, adrenal disease
Calcium, phosphorus	Hyper- or hypocalcemia, hypophosphatemia
Antinuclear antibody	Vasculitis
Serum protein electrophoresis	Hyperviscosity syndrome from paraproteinemia
T_4	Hyper- or hypothyroidism
Cortisol	Cushing's disease
Serum B_{12}	Pernicious anemia, malabsorption, etc.
Folate, ascorbate, carotene	Malnutrition
Cholesterol and triglycerides	Hyperlipidemic dementia
Liver function tests	Hepatic encephalopathy, metastases
Arterial blood gases	Acidosis, anoxia, etc.
Skull x-rays	Increased intracranial pressure, abnormal calcifications, pineal position, etc.
EEG	Slowed in most metabolic encephalopathies; look for focal abnormalities, constant seizure activity, etc.
CT scan	Tumor (neoplasm, subdural hematoma), inflammatory process, stroke, hydrocephalus
Lumbar puncture, protein, sugar, cells, culture, VDRL, fungal titers, gamma globulin, etc.	If not contraindicated, infection, multiple sclerosis, tumor, etc.

*See also chapter 19.

TABLE 11-3.—MAJOR CAUSES OF DEMENTIA

PROBLEM	DIAGNOSTIC CLUES	TREATMENT
I. Infectious		
*A. Acute bacterial meningitis	Fever, stiff neck; purulent CSF, + gram stain	Appropriate antibiotics
B. Viral encephalitis	Fever, confusion; lymphocytes in CSF	Nonspecific: steroid support; antiviral agent (ARA-A) for herpes simplex encephalitis
*C. Tuberculous meningitis	Headache, stiff neck, malaise, weight loss; CSF: pleocytosis (modest, mainly lymphocytes), low glucose, high protein	INH, ethambutol, streptomycin, other antibiotics, and steroids
*D. Cryptococcal meningitis	Headaches; CSF as in tuberculous meningitis; demonstration of organisms or antigen in CSF	Amphotericin B and 5-fluorocytosine
*E. Tertiary syphilis (general paresis of the insane; rarely seen today)	Poor judgment, grandiosity, frontal release signs; Argyll Robertson pupils; cells in CSF; + CSF VDRL	Penicillin
F. Slow virus infections		
1. Jakob-Creutzfeldt disease	Dementia, basal ganglia signs, startle myoclonus, etc.	None
2. Kuru	Cerebellar degeneration; dementia late; acquired by eating victims	None; prevention is easy: improve eating habits
3. Subacute sclerosing panencephalitis; Dawson's inclusion body encephalitis	Dementia, myoclonus: under 20 years old (caused by measles-like virus); high CSF gamma globulin level	None
4. Progressive multifocal leukoencephalopathy	Multifocal hemispheric signs usually in immunosuppressed patient (on immunosuppressive drugs or with malignancy particularly of reticuloendothelial origin)	None
II. Metabolic		
A. Lack of substrate		
*1. Tissue hypoxia		
a. Low blood Po_2	Cyanosis; blood gases	Oxygen, respiratory support; treat infection and spasm
b. Severe anemia	Hemoglobin, hematocrit	Transfusion, etc.
c. Decreased perfusion		
i. Decreased cardiac output	Hypotension; signs of congestive failure	Appropriate cardiac medications or fluids for hypovolemia; treatment of septic shock, etc.
ii. Arterial obstruction	Usually focal signs	Support, anticoagulation if progressive without hemorrhage.
iii. Increased viscosity (polycy-themia)	Hematocrit	Phlebotomy
*2. Hypoglycemia	Varied clinical picture: often	IV glucose

*Indicates treatable conditions.

(Continued)

TABLE 11–3.—(Cont.)

PROBLEM	DIAGNOSTIC CLUES	TREATMENT
	dizziness, syncope; but may have focal signs; Dx: low blood glucose; 5-hour glucose tolerance test to rule out reactive hypoglycemia	
3. Nutritional deficiency		
*a. Vitamin B_{12} deficiency	Pernicious anemia and/or spinal cord involvement (not always present); lab: low serum B_{12} levels; positive Schilling test; achlorhydria (usually)	IM vitamin B_{12} administration
*b. Thiamine deficiency	Wernicke's encephalopathy: confusion, amnesia, truncal ataxia, disconjugate eye movements; fatal if untreated	IM thiamine
	Korsakoff's psychosis (residual of Wernicke's): amnesia, confabulation	Vitamins; treatment is only partially, if at all, effective
B. Endocrine		
*1. Hypothyroidism	Myxedema, hung-up reflexes, hypothermia; low T4, etc.; hyponatremia	Thyroid hormone replacement
*2. Hyperthyroidism	Weight loss, tremor, etc.; high T4, etc.	Thyroid suppressants; surgery
*3. Cushing's disease	Hypertension, diabetes, cushingoid features; hypokalemia; high cortisol	Surgery
*4. Hyperpara-thyroidism	Hypercalcemia (lethargy, etc.)	Treat hypercalcemia; remove parathyroids
*5. a. Hypopara-thyroidism	Hypocalcemia; diffuse, soft tissue calcification; tetany	Vitamin D
b. Pseudohypo-parathyroidism	Hypocalcemia, skeletal abnormalities, basal ganglia calcification, tetany unusual despite very low calcium levels	
C. Electrolyte imbalance		
*1. Hyponatremia (water intoxica-tion), inappropriate antidiuretic hormone secretion, renal sodium wasting	Lethargy, seizures, low serum sodium	Water-restriction; hypertonic saline (sometimes)
*2. Hypercalcemia	Lethargy, confusion; high serum calcium	Lower calcium (phosphate, steroids, mithromycin, etc.); treat underlying condition
*3. Hypomagnesemia	Confusion, seizures; in setting of persistent diarrhea (especially in infants), or of IV therapy without Mg supplements; serum Mg may not reflect deficiency; calcium usually also low	Magnesium sulfate

*Indicates treatable conditions.

PROBLEM	DIAGNOSTIC CLUES	TREATMENT
*4. Hypocalcemia	Confusion; tetany seizures; serum calcium low	Replace calcium; treat underlying condition
*5. Hyperosmolar coma	High blood glucose, severe dehydration with associated electrolyte abnormalities	Fluids, insulin
D. Toxic		
1. Endogenous		
*a. Hypercapnia (pulmonary insufficiency)	Signs of respiratory insufficiency, asterixis	Assist respirations, pulmonary toilet; antibiotics
*b. Hepatic encephalopathy	Lethargy, dementia, asterixis; hyperventilation with respiratory alkalosis (? central); high serum ammonia; high CSF glutamine; if chronic may see dementia plus choreiform movements and dystonia	Treat infections, gastrointestinal bleeding (when present); cleanse bowel (neomycin enemas, acetic acid enemas, lactulose), L-dopa
*c. Renal insufficiency	Multifocal myoclonus, seizures, asterixis; signs of uremia; high BUN, creatinine	Treat primary disease; dialysis
*d. Acidosis	Hyperventilation, low pH	
i. Diabetic ketoacidosis	Hyperglycemia, ketosis	Fluids, insulin, bicarbonate
ii. Lactic acidosis	Acidosis without hyperglycemia, seen with sepsis, shock, idiopathic	Treat underlying cause; bicarbonate
*e. Wilson's disease	Dystonia, choreiform movements; cirrhosis; high liver copper, low ceruloplasm; high urine copper excretion	Copper-binding agent (penicillamine)
*f. Hyperlipidemia	Greatly increased serum cholesterol and triglycerides	Lower serum lipids
g. Limbic dementia (remote effects of carcinoma)	Memory loss, agitation; may have cerebellar or brain stem signs	None
2. Exogenous toxins		
*a. Drugs	Serum levels, history	
i. Hypnotics	Lethargic, comatose	Fluids, respiratory and blood pressure support; dialysis when appropriate
ii. Aspirin	Metabolic acidosis plus respiratory alkalosis	Fluids; alkalinize urine
iii. Anti-convulsants	Ataxia, dementia, lethargy	Reduce dose
*b. Methanol, ethylene glycol, old paraldehyde	Severe metabolic acidosis, blindness with methanol, hippurate crystals in urine with ethylene glycol	Bicarbonate; ethanol for methanol intoxication
III. Vascular disease		
A. Strokes	Focal signs, CT scan positive with completed stroke	Controversial (see chap. 14)
*B. Hypertensive encephalopathy	Papilledema, proteinuria, diastolic blood pressure	Lower blood pressure

*Indicates treatable conditions.

(Continued)

TABLE 11–3.—(Cont.)

PROBLEM	DIAGNOSTIC CLUES	TREATMENT
	usually above 120; headache, cortical visual loss	
C. Vasculitis (lupus, etc.)	Dementia with or without focal signs; may or may not have other systems involved; high sedimentation rate almost always	No effective treatment for most; steroids used and proved effective only for giant cell cranial arteritis of the aged
IV. Mechanical		
*A. Mass lesions		
1. Neoplasms	Focal signs, except in "silent areas" (i.e., frontal lobes); positive brain scan (over 80%); CT scan positive in most	Surgery, steroids, radiation, chemotherapy
2. Subdural hematoma	Often headache, lethargy; mild focal signs; history of trauma (not always); increasing CSF protein; positive brain scan; positive CT scan	Surgery
3. Intracerebral hematoma	Focal signs, usually; if hematoma is subcortical, in a silent area (less than 10% of spontaneous intracerebral hematomas), focal signs may be minimal; CT scan positive	Surgery
*B. Hydrocephalus	If acute: headache, lethargy, increased intracranial pressure If chronic: dementia, gait disorder (frontal "apraxic" and spastic gait), and urinary incontinence; normal CSF dynamics; CT scan with minimal cortical atrophy and enlarged ventricular system	CSF shunt
V. "Degenerative" diseases		
A. Without elementary neurologic findings		
1. Alzheimer's disease, senile and presenile	Memory loss usually prominent early; very common, the usual senile dementia; CT scan positive	None proved effective
2. Pick's disease	Same; not clinically separable from Alzheimer's: can only be separated pathologically; very rare in United States	None
B. Demyelinating disease		
1. Multiple sclerosis	Evidence clinically of lesions separated in time and space; dementia common late in illness; frequently high CSF gamma globulin percentage of total CSF protein	None (steroids as temporary treatment)
2. Schilder's disease	Usually in children; dementia most prominent	None

*Indicates treatable conditions.

PROBLEM	DIAGNOSTIC CLUES	TREATMENT
	sign, but soon cortical blindness, long-tract signs, etc.	
C. Inborn errors of metabolism		
1. Lipid storage diseases	Tay-Sachs, etc.	None
2. Metachromatic leukodystrophy	Dementia, peripheral neuropathy; absent arylsulfatase A	None
*3. Amino acidurias (many of them)	Variable	Restrictive diet for many
D. Prominent basal ganglia or cerebellar signs		
*1. Parkinsonism	Typical basal ganglia signs (see chaps. 4 and 13)	L-dopa (does not help dementia), amantidine, dopamine agonists
2. Huntington's chorea	Dementia may precede chorea; family history (autosomal dominant)	None, genetic counseling
3. Some spinocerebellar degenerations	Cerebellar, posterior column, pyramidal, and peripheral nerve disease depending on which variant (Friedreich's ataxia most common example)	None
4. Myoclonic epilepsy (certain forms)	Progressive form with Lafora's inclusion bodies produces dementia	None; control seizures
5. Parkinson-dementia complex (Guam)	May be associated with ALS	None

*Indicates treatable conditions.

Normal-Pressure Hydrocephalus

Although there is little question that this entity exists, its exact pathogenesis is disputed, and there is no agreement about how to select patients for treatment. The entity consists of progressive hydrocephalus, with normal CSF pressure (as determined by lumbar puncture), producing dementia, gait disorder, and urinary incontinence. Reducing the hydrocephalus with ventriculoatrial or ventriculoperitoneal shunts improves the clinical picture. The majority of such patients have a history of subarachnoid hemorrhage, trauma or meningeal infection. Presumably, blood or proteinaceous fluid has blocked the normal flow of CSF. In a minority of cases, no such predisposition is apparent. The normal CSF pressure is difficult to explain. In some patients, the CSF pressure fluctuates; although a single lumbar puncture may show normal pressure, 24-hour monitoring demonstrates abnormally high pressures some of the time. In other patients, previous brain pathology (strokes, degenerative disease) may reduce the normal resistance of the ventricular walls and allow ventricular expansion with normal CSF pressures.

To make the diagnosis, the examiner should be able to document the presence of hydrocephalus, the absence of severe cortical atrophy, and inadequate reabsorption of spinal fluid. Computerized tomography (CT) will adequately assess ventricular size and cortical atrophy. Two tests are available to assess CSF flow: cisternography and the

CSF infusion test. These are described in chapter 18. Because these tests do not always predict who will respond to shunting, no absolute guidelines are available for patient selection. The appearance of the patient, the tempo of the illness, the history of predisposing causes, and the results of these tests must all be considered and weighed against the possible complications of shunting (infection, embolization, shunt failure, subdural hematoma, and effusion).

REFERENCE

Wells, C. E.: *Dementia,* ed. 2. Philadelphia, F. A. Davis Co., 1977.

12

Infectious Diseases of the Central Nervous System

EDWARD VALENSTEIN

Meningitis

PURULENT MENINGITIS (ACUTE BACTERIAL MENINGITIS)

BACTERIA reach the subarachnoid space via the bloodstream or, less often, from contiguous structures. The infection is usually confined to the subarachnoid space, but toxins (from bacteria or leukocytes), edema, and vascular changes can affect cerebral function. Patients with bacterial meningitis therefore present with changes in sensorium in addition to headache, fever, and stiff neck. Intracranial pressure is increased because of cerebral edema and interference with the flow of cerebrospinal fluid (CSF) by the inflammatory process.

The lumbar puncture is diagnostic. The CSF is usually under increased pressure. There are often more than 1,000 WBCs/cu mm; however, early in the course (especially of meningococcal meningitis) there may be few or no cells. The amount of protein is usually elevated and the amount of glucose low. The fluid should be gram stained (even if there are no cells); often the organism can be accurately identified. Both aerobic and anaerobic cultures should be obtained.

Prompt treatment (without waiting for the results of culture) is essential. The choice of antibiotic may be guided by the appearance of the organism on the gram stain or, if identification is not certain, by the clinical picture. In neonates, group B beta-hemolytic streptococci and enteric gram-negative bacilli are the most common pathogens, accounting for 60%–70% of the cases of meningitis. From the age of 2 months to 10 years, more than 90% of the cases of meningitis are caused by *Hemophilus influenzae,* meningococci, or pneumococci. Hemophilus meningitis is rare after the age of 10. Although other organisms, such as *Listeria* or *Streptococcus,* occasionally cause meningitis in otherwise healthy individuals, the occurrence of unusual organisms should raise the suspicion of an immune deficiency or an unusual source of infection. Table 12–1 summarizes the common intracranial bacterial infections and the recommended initial therapy.

The complications of purulent meningitis are listed in Table 12–2. Cerebral edema may at times be severe and may lead to transtentorial or foramen magnum herniation and death early in the course of meningitis. The inflammatory process causes a vasculitis that affects the smaller arteries and veins. Usually this does not produce focal neurologic signs; but in more severe cases of meningitis, focal signs may develop, often during the second or third week. Arterial occlusion may occur. Cortical vein thrombosis produces

TABLE 12-1.—TREATMENT OF BACTERIAL
INFECTIONS OF THE CNS

INTRACRANIAL BACTERIAL INFECTION	THERAPY
Neonatal meningitis	
Group B beta-hemolytic streptococci	Penicillin
Enteric bacilli (*Escherichia coli, Proteus, Klebsiella*)	Gentamicin*
Listeria	Ampicillin or penicillin
Unknown	Gentamicin* plus ampicillin or penicillin
Meningitis in children and adults	
H. influenzae	Ampicillin or chloramphenicol
Meningococcal	Penicillin (chloramphenicol)†
Pneumococcal	Penicillin (chloramphenicol, erythromycin)
Unknown	Ampicillin
Meningitis under unusual circumstances	
Staphylococcal (penicillinase-positive)	Methicillin
Gram-negative meningitis	Gentamicin* and chloramphenicol
Pseudomonas	Gentamicin,* colistin,* or polymyxin B*
Tuberculous meningitis	INH and streptomycin plus PAS or ethambutol or rifampin
Neurosyphilis	Penicillin (erythromycin, tetracycline)
Brain abscess (organism unknown)	
Staphylococci not suspected	Penicillin and either tetracycline or chloramphenicol
Staphylococci suspected	Methicillin and chloramphenicol

*Should be given intravenously and intrathecally.
†Antibiotics noted in parentheses may be substituted for penicillin in allergic patients.

hemorrhagic infarction of the cortex, with resultant focal signs and (often) seizures. The thrombophlebitis may spread to involve the venous sinuses, resulting in diminished absorption of CSF and raised intracranial pressure. Raised intracranial pressure may also result from a communicating hydrocephalus secondary to arachnoid inflammation. This may occur after the meningitis has been cured. In infants, increased intracranial pressure and continued fever may result from a subdural effusion. These are usually sterile but may be infected (empyema). If subdural effusions are symptomatic, repeated subdural taps are necessary.

There are various systemic complications of meningitis. Inappropriate ADH secretion may result in hyponatremia and water intoxication. Water restriction is usually effective in treating this transient complication. A more serious complication is disseminated intravascular coagulation, which occurs with purpura, cyanosis, pain, fever, and hypotension. This is due to vasculitis with intravascular deposition of fibrin. Adrenal hemorrhage may accompany this, but the symptoms are thought not to be secondary to adrenal insufficiency. Treatment of the underlying condition is probably the only effective therapy, although steroids and heparin have been advocated. Lactic acidosis also occurs and frequently requires therapy with bicarbonate.

Following recovery from purulent meningitis, residual brain damage may be evidenced by cranial nerve palsies, mental retardation, or seizures. The incidence of brain damage varies with the severity of the meningitis and the organism, and tends to be high in neonatal meningitis.

TABLE 12-2.—COMPLICATIONS OF
PURULENT MENINGITIS

A. Cerebral edema (may lead to herniation)
B. Vasculitis
   1. Arteritis (stroke)
   2. Cortical venous thrombosis (stroke, seizures)
   3. Venous sinus thrombosis (increased intracranial pressure)
C. Hydrocephalus
D. Cranial nerve palsies
E. Subdural effusion or empyema
F. Disseminated intravascular clotting
G. Lactic acidosis
H. Inappropriate ADH secretion
I. Diabetes insipidus
J. Residual findings
   1. Cranial nerve palsies
   2. Mental retardation
   3. Seizures

VIRAL MENINGITIS

Although pathologically some cerebral involvement is seen in most cases of viral meningitides, the clinical picture is more often one of pure meningitis: fever, stiff neck, and sometimes lethargy, but with no focal neurologic signs or seizures. When there are signs of cerebral involvement, the process is called *encephalitis*.

The CSF is usually under normal pressure and there is a moderate number of WBCs (usually fewer than 500/cu mm). Initially these cells are often polys, but after a day or two lymphocytes begin to predominate. The amount of protein in the CSF is normal (or slightly elevated); the level of sugar is normal. The illness is self-limited and sequelae are unusual.

Lymphocytic choriomeningitis infections are atypical in that the CSF pleocytosis is more marked (often several thousand cells, with a marked lymphocytic preponderance) and the pleocytosis may take several weeks to disappear. In other respects, they resemble other varieties of viral meningitis, with recovery being the rule.

GRANULOMATOUS MENINGITIS

The most common types of granulomatous meningitis are tuberculous and cryptococcal meningitis. These infections are often subacute and sometimes chronic; their diagnosis may be extremely difficult.

TUBERCULOUS MENINGITIS.—This occurs most often in children and debilitated adults. The meningitis results from seeding from a tuberculoma in the brain or meninges. The tuberculoma, in turn, arises from the hematogenous spread from a primary focus (usually in the lung). The patients present with headache, malaise, and fever. Weight loss may be prominent. A physical examination may show normal results, or nuchal rigidity may be present. The thick basilar meningitis may produce hydrocephalus, cranial nerve palsies, or an arteritis of the small penetrating arteries of the brain stem. The CSF shows a moderate pleocytosis (usually fewer than 300 WBCs/cu mm), mostly lymphocytes. The level of protein is high, and the amount of sugar low (these changes may be mild early in the course). The organism may be demonstrable by acid-fast bacillus (AFB) stains of the CSF sediment, but often it is not. Cultures may take 4 to 8 weeks to grow. The chest x-ray and tuberculin skin test may be helpful, but both can show normal results (the latter is the result of anergy). If the diagnosis of tuberculous meningitis is suspected on clinical grounds, therefore, treatment should be instituted. INH, streptomycin, and ethambutol in combination are presently the drugs of choice. Rifampin is probably also a useful agent. Steroids may be helpful in reducing the inflammatory response, which itself can contribute to the patient's symptoms. Sequelae are common.

CRYPTOCOCCAL MENINGITIS.—*Cryptococcus neoformans (Torula)* often produces an indolent infection; its symptoms occasionally may extend back months or even years before the diagnosis is made. A debilitated state, immune incompetency or suppression, and diabetes mellitus are frequently associated conditions. Headache is the most common symptom, and mental deterioration may occur. Cranial nerve palsies and focal brain stem dysfunction secondary to arteritis can be prominent. The CSF is similar to that seen in persons with tuberculous meningitis. The fungus may be seen on india ink preparations and may grow in culture. It is not rare, however, for the organism not to show itself. Cryptococcal antigen can often be detected in the CSF, providing a valuable aid to the diagnosis. Treatment is with systemic and intrathecal amphotericin B.

SARCOID. — Although technically not proved to be an infection, sarcoid may nevertheless cause granulomatous meningitis. The symptoms may be nonspecific (headache, nuchal rigidity), and the CSF may be identical to that in persons with tuberculous or fungal meningitis. Transient cranial nerve signs as well as evidence of CNS dysfunction can occur. The diagnosis may be suspected if there is evidence of systemic sarcoidosis, but this is not always the case.

Viral Encephalitis

Meningeal involvement is present in most forms of encephalitis; however, the clinical picture is dominated by evidence of brain dysfunction. In addition to headache and fever, patients often have strikingly depressed levels of consciousness, and seizures are common. Behavioral changes and focal neurologic signs are sometimes present. The CSF contains a moderate number of cells. The level of protein is normal or high, and the amount of sugar is usually normal.

The major causes of viral encephalitis are listed in Table 12–3. The arbovirus encephalitides are usually epidemic; the others are usually sporadic. Because the clinical findings are similar in most cases of encephalitis, the diagnosis of the offending agent must rest on laboratory investigations (growing the virus or detecting increasing levels of antibody titers). We briefly discuss three varieties that can be distinctive.

HERPES SIMPLEX ENCEPHALITIS

This is the most common nonepidemic form of encephalitis. Although many encephalitides are seasonal in their appearance,

especially prominent in the summer, herpes simplex occurs any time of the year. It is caused by the type I herpes simplex virus, normally present in cold sores. The portal of entry in many is presumed to be through the nasal mucosa, accounting for the localization of the disease to the orbitofrontal and anterior temporal cortices. The pathologic reaction is unusually severe, with inflammation, edema, necrosis, and hemorrhage. Clinically, patients often have personality changes (secondary to the involvement of the limbic system). They have difficulty with memory (imprinting) because of involvement of the mesial temporal lobe (hippocampi), and a decreased or lost sense of smell (anosmia) because of involvement of the olfactory bulbs. Headache and fever are usual complaints. If edema is severe, papilledema can be seen. The EEG usually shows bitemporal slowing and sharp activity. If the involvement is asymmetric, hemiparesis or aphasia may be present; the brain scan may show focal uptake in one temporal lobe and the arteriogram may demonstrate temporal lobe swelling. This may be difficult to differentiate from a temporal lobe abscess without surgical exploration and biopsy.

Treatment with an antiviral agent (adenine arabinoside) has recently shown some promise. Combating the host inflammatory response with steroids has been considered by some an effective therapy, despite the theoretical risk of exacerbating the infection and the lack of concrete evidence of efficacy. Survivors may show severe mental changes; not uncommonly, there is a specific deficit in recent memory (imprinting) because of bilateral hippocampal destruction.

RABIES

The incubation period after the bite of a rabid animal may be prolonged (as long as one year). The infection attacks neurons in specific areas, particularly the limbic system, hypothalamic area, and brain stem nuclei. There may be little or no meningeal inflammation (the CSF may be normal). Behavioral

TABLE 12-3.—SOME CAUSES OF VIRAL ENCEPHALITIS

A. Arthropod-borne (arbovirus) infections
  1. Group A
    a. Western equine encephalitis
    b. Eastern equine encephalitis
    c. Venezuelan equine encephalitis
  2. Group B
    a. St. Louis encephalitis
    b. Japanese B encephalitis
    c. Yellow fever
    d. Dengue
  3. Arthropod tick-borne encephalitides
    a. Russian tick-borne complex
    b. Colorado tick fever
  4. Miscellaneous
    a. California encephalitis
    b. Others
B. Picorna virus (enterovirus) infections
  1. Poliomyelitis
  2. Coxsackievirus infections
  3. Echovirus meningoencephalitis
  4. Mengo (encephalomyocarditis virus) encephalitis

C. Myxovirus infections
  1. Influenza
  2. Mumps
  3. Measles
  4. Rabies
  5. Rubella
  6. Newcastle disease
D. Herpesvirus infections
  1. Herpes simplex
  2. Herpes zoster and chickenpox
  3. Virus B (herpesvirus simiae)
  4. Cytomegalic inclusion disease
E. Poxvirus infections
  1. Smallpox encephalitis
  2. Vaccinia encephalitis
F. Others

changes, seizures, and painful spasms of the throat musculature are prominent.

POLIOMYELITIS

Encephalitis is usually a minor aspect of this infection, which has a predilection for anterior horn cells and the cells of the brain stem motor nuclei. Spotty asymmetric weakness, reflex loss, and fasciculations are seen after a prodromal illness and a nonspecific viral meningitis.

Brain Abscess

Bacterial brain abscesses can arise either from direct extension from a parameningeal focus of infection (ear and sinus infections) or by hematogenous spread. Pulmonary pathology (especially bronchiectasis) is the most common source of the hematogenous spread. Persons with cyanotic congenital heart disease and pulmonary arteriovenous malformations are prone to develop abscesses. This is because bacteria originating in the bowel and reaching the vena cava and the right side of the heart via the portal system, liver, and hepatic veins are short-circuited to the left side of the heart and system-

ic circulation. Thus they miss filtration by the pulmonary macrophage system. Although subacute bacterial endocarditis may be associated with mycotic aneurysms and meningoencephalitis, it is infrequently the cause of brain abscess. This may be because the bacteria that usually cause endocarditis are aerophilic and therefore unlikely to propagate within an infarct or ischemic zone; the arterial wall is more prone to involvement because of its high oxygen saturation. The pia-arachnoid surface is also highly vascularized and a favorable site for aerobe propagation. In persons who have cyanotic heart disease a marked reactive or secondary polycythemia causes increased blood viscosity, which may lead to areas of arteriolar sludging and cerebral ischemia. It is in these areas of ischemia that abscesses are most likely to occur. It is not surprising that the bacteria that are usually cultured from them are anaerobes or microaerophilic organisms, which are usually found in the bowel and can survive in an ischemic environment. On the other hand, aerobic bacteria are frequently cultured from abscesses that have sinus tracts connecting them to the exterior, i.e., sinus infections, middle-ear infections, and skull fractures.

Abscesses secondary to ear infections are usually in the middle third of the temporal lobe or, less often, in the cerebellum. Abscesses secondary to spread from the paranasal sinuses or from dental infections are more often in the frontal lobes. Hematogenous spread can result in an abscess in any location, and multiple abscesses are not uncommon.

There are two stages in the development of a bacterial brain abscess. In the first stage, the primary infection is often active, and the brain infection is a cerebritis—an inflammatory response with some tissue breakdown. The patient is usually febrile and may complain of headache. The intracranial pressure is usually raised. There may be focal signs, but lesions in the temporal lobes, frontal lobes, or cerebellum can be distressingly silent. The brain scan or CT scan is usually abnormal and the EEG is usually focally abnormal. Arteriography does not show any well-defined mass. The spinal fluid may show a pleocytosis, with a raised level of protein and a normal amount of glucose, but it can be entirely normal. Treatment with antibiotics alone at this stage may produce complete resolution.

In the second stage, the region of cerebritis becomes organized and walled off, and a true abscess forms. Fever often subsides. There may be signs of an expanding mass. The CSF, EEG, and brain scan are as before. A mass is seen on a CT scan or other contrast study. Treatment with antibiotics alone is not effective because the abscess is walled off; surgical drainage is necessary.

Untreated, the brain abscess may cause cerebral herniation or rupture into the ventricles, causing severe (and often fatal) meningitis. The WBC count in the CSF in the latter instance is often more than 10,000/cu mm.

Empyema

Infection may form in the epidural or subdural spaces; it is usually the result of spread from an adjacent infection (in the bone, skin, or sinuses), but sometimes it arises from hematogenous spread. The diagnosis of cerebral subdural or epidural empyema can be difficult unless there is a high index of suspicion. The symptoms of spinal epidural empyema are somewhat more uniform, but the diagnosis is still often missed. The presenting complaint is usually pain over the infected region, and there is usually fever. The patient then experiences pain in the distribution of the spinal nerve roots in the area. Finally, symptoms referable to the spinal cord occur as a result of compression or infarction secondary to thrombophlebitis. If treatment (surgical drainage and antibiotics) can be instituted before the spinal cord is affected, the outcome should be good; otherwise irreversible cord damage and paralysis can result.

Miscellaneous Infections

BACTERIAL

Numerous bacterial infections may be manifested by processes other than acute purulent meningitis or brain abscess. Tuberculous meningitis has been mentioned. Encephalitis symptoms may be present with pertussis, tularemia, typhoid, and other acute infections. Brucellosis may appear as chronic meningitis. The following, although rarely seen in this country today, are nevertheless important.

SYPHILIS.—Syphilis produces an amazing array of CNS disorders, which can mimic infectious, vascular, neoplastic, or degenerative disease. Meningitis (rarely of clinical significance) may occur within 5 years of a person contracting the infection. From 7 to 15 years after contact, an inflammatory vasculitis (meningovascular syphilis) can produce infarction in virtually any area of the CNS. Tertiary syphilis (15–20 years after contact) has two classic presentations: *tabes dorsalis* and *paretic neurosyphilis* (general paresis of the insane). Tabes is an inflammatory process that affects the dorsal root ganglia, producing loss of position and vibration sensation, loss of deep-tendon reflexes, and severe "lightning" pains in the abdomen and legs. Periodic attacks of abdominal cramps and vomiting are common. The Argyll Robertson pupil (small and irregular with light reaction lost and accommodation preserved) is usually present, and bladder dysfunction is common. General paresis consists of an infection of the cerebral cortex, particularly in the frontal lobes, producing a progressive frontal-lobe-type dementia. Pupillary changes, myoclonic jerks, and tremor are also frequently present.

Neurosyphilis may be diagnosed serologically using nonspecific (reagin) tests such as rapid plasma reagin (RPR) or Venereal Disease Research Lab test (VDRL) or specific treponemal antibody tests such as the fluorescent treponemal antibody test (FTA). The former may have normal results in the serum in tertiary syphilis, and therefore an FTA must always be ordered when this form of the disease is being considered. The CSF VDRL is diagnostic of neurosyphilis because false positives occur only when false-positive blood is inadvertently introduced into the CSF by a traumatic lumbar puncture (see chap. 18). Occasionally all these tests are negative. If symptoms and signs are compatible with CNS syphilis, and if CSF pleocytosis or increased concentrations of CSF protein suggest active disease, treatment should be instituted. Penicillin is the treatment of choice.

LEPROSY.—Because the leprosy bacillus can multiply only at temperatures a few degrees below core body temperature, CNS leprosy is rare if it exists at all. Leprosy produces a peripheral neuropathy, which is characterized by the involvement of nerves only in the cooler parts of the body. In persons with tuberculoid leprosy, nerve trunks are involved; the nerves situated immediately subcutaneously are affected (for example, the ulnar nerve at the elbow). In lepromatous leprosy, terminal nerve endings are involved, producing a patchy sensory loss; the cooler areas of the skin (ears, back of the hands) are affected first. Leprosy is rare in the United States, but worldwide it is one of the most important causes of peripheral neuropathy.

RICKETTSIAL INFECTIONS

The various rickettsial diseases may be accompanied by nonspecific meningoencephalitis. In this country, Rocky Mountain spotted fever is the most common of these conditions and may occur in almost any location. The initial symptoms are often neurologic (headache, stiff neck, lethargy). The diagnosis is suggested by a history of a tick bite and the characteristic rash. Treatment with antibiotics (tetracycline or chloramphenicol) is effective and may be life-saving.

FUNGAL INFECTIONS

Most often fungal infections occur in persons who have altered immune mechanisms: the debilitated or those receiving immunosuppressant therapy. Aspergillosis and candidiasis are not uncommon in these persons. Mucormycosis is usually seen in diabetics, and is often associated with ketoacidosis. CNS involvement is usually secondary to spread from the nasal sinuses to the orbit (causing proptosis and ophthalmoplegia) through the cribriform plate into the brain. Coccidioidomycosis and cryptococcosis may occur in the normal host. Granulomatous meningitis is the usual presentation. Various fungi can produce cerebral granulomata or abscesses. Treatment of fungal infections is generally less satisfactory than treatment of bacterial or rickettsial infections, but some improvement is often obtained with amphotericin B or 5-fluorocytosine.

PROTOZOAL INFECTIONS

Amoeba, trypanosomes, malaria, toxoplasma, and other protozoa may affect the CNS. Toxoplasmosis may be acquired in utero, producing underdevelopment of the cerebrum and resulting in microcephaly and mental retardation. Retinal involvement and intracerebral calcifications (seen on skull x-ray) may aid in making the diagnosis. This infection is also becoming more common in immunosuppressed persons, appearing as destructive meningoencephalitis.

HELMINTH INFESTATIONS

Helminth infestations may produce various CNS findings, including meningoencephalitis (trichinosis), vasculitis (filariasis, schistosomiasis), or focal granulomata (cysticercosis). The patient may have a meningitis or encephalitis picture, or the process may be manifested as a mass lesion or seizure disorder.

Slow Virus Diseases of the Nervous System

Two groups of diseases have been described: one caused by agents that have thus far not been characterized either immunologically or morphologically and the other caused by more conventional viruses (see Table 12–4).

ATYPICAL VIRUSES

This fascinating group of uncommon diseases are pathologically similar and have the following characteristics:

1. They are transmissible experimentally.
2. They have a long latent period (up to many years).
3. Pathologically they resemble degenerative diseases; there is neuronal degeneration with astrocytic reaction but no evidence of inflammation.
4. Clinically they produce a chronic or

TABLE 12–4.—SLOW VIRUS INFECTIONS OF THE CNS

A. Atypical viruses
   1. Scrapie (sheep)
   2. Kuru (human, tribes of New Guinea)
   3. Jakob-Creutzfeldt disease (human)
   4. Transmissible mink encephalopathy
B. Conventional viruses
   1. Visna/maedi (sheep)
   2. Subacute sclerosing panencephalitis (SSPE) (human)
   3. Progressive multifocal leukoencephalopathy (PML) (human)

subacute illness, which is steadily progressive.

5. The nature of the infectious agent is elusive.

These diseases therefore provide possible models for degenerative diseases of the nervous system (such as amyotrophic lateral sclerosis and spinocerebellar degenerations). Because Jakob-Creutzfeldt disease (a progressive dementia with myoclonus, extrapyramidal signs, and sometimes cerebellar and anterior horn involvement) has been transmitted experimentally, this model may also apply to other degenerative diseases of the CNS. As yet, however, efforts to transmit other degenerative diseases have not been successful.

CONVENTIONAL VIRUSES

In persons with these conditions, virus particles can be identified pathologically, immunologically, and by culture. Inflammatory reactions can be seen, and inclusion bodies may be present. They resemble the former group in that they cause a subacute or chronic disease after a long latent period.

Subacute sclerosing panencephalitis (SSPE) is a disease that affects children or adolescents; it presents with progressive mental deterioration, myoclonic jerks, and then progressive pyramidal and extrapyramidal involvement, which leads to death within a few years. The CSF may be normal except for a high level of gamma globulin and high measles antibody titers. A measles-like virus can be grown from infected brain tissue. Some of these children have defective immune responses. The disease may result from infection at an early age with a form of measles virus, but the exact pathogenesis is still unknown.

Progressive multifocal leukoencephalopathy (PML) is a disease that occurs almost exclusively in debilitated persons (most often patients with lymphoma). Pathologically there are small areas of demyelination, and inclusion bodies are seen in oligodendroglia (the cells of the CNS that elaborate myelin). Clinically patients have focal cortical signs, and as lesions become more numerous, the clinical course becomes one of progressive deterioration. Death usually occurs within one to two years. Two different papovaviruses have been isolated: One of them (the JC virus) is a virus with which most adults have had contact.

Cerebrospinal Fluid in Infectious Disease and Related Conditions

The CSF findings in persons with the three major varieties of meningitis have been discussed and are summarized in Table 12-5. Although the differences noted are helpful, it is important to realize that there are exceptions to these rules. Patients with viral meningitis may have more than 1,000 WBCs/cu mm. Acute bacterial meningitis may present with few WBCs for a variety of reasons: (1) the patient's immune response may be inade-

TABLE 12-6.—CAUSES OF LYMPHOCYTIC MENINGITIS*

A. Viral meningitis or encephalitis
B. Indolent bacterial meningitis (sugar level often low)
  1. Partially treated purulent meningitis
  2. Tuberculous meningitis
  3. *Listeria* meningitis
  4. *Brucella* meningitis
  5. Syphilitic meningitis
C. Fungal meningitis (sugar level often low)
D. Sarcoidosis (sugar level often low)
E. Various protozoal or helminthic infections
F. Some rickettsial infections
G. Parameningeal infection
  1. Epidural abscess
  2. Subdural abscess
  3. Brain abscess
  4. Venous thrombosis
H. Noninfectious causes
  1. Chemical meningitis (after pneumoencephalography, myelogram, cisternogram, spinal anesthesia, intrathecal therapy, etc.)
  2. Toxins (lead, arsenic)
  3. Tumors
  4. Demyelinating diseases
  5. Vascular diseases
    a. Vasculitis
    b. Stroke
    c. Subarachnoid hemorrhage

*A modest pleocytosis, mostly lymphocytes, with normal or elevated levels of protein and normal or low amounts of sugar.

quate, (2) the leukocyte response may be suppressed by the presence of alcohol in the blood and tissues, (3) the meningitis may have been partially treated, and (4) the tap may have been done early in the course of the disease before cells appeared. In the second and last instances, a repeat tap in two to six hours usually reveals a brisk pleocytosis.

TABLE 12-5.—CSF FINDINGS IN MAJOR CNS INFECTIONS

	PURULENT MENINGITIS (ACUTE BACTERIAL MENINGITIS)	VIRAL MENINGOENCEPHALITIS	GRANULOMATOUS MENINGITIS (TUBERCULOSIS, FUNGAL MENINGITIS, SARCOID, SYPHILIS, *Listeria*, *Brucella*, ETC.)
WBCs	More than 1,000/cu mm; mostly polys	Less than 500/cu mm; first polys; then lymphs	Less than 200/cu mm; mostly lymphs
Protein	High	Normal or slightly elevated	High
Sugar	Low (often less than 20 mg%)	Normal	Low (rarely as low as in bacterial meningitis)

TABLE 12-7.—CAUSES OF LOW
LEVELS OF SUGAR IN THE CSF

A. Sugar level characteristically low
   1. Bacterial meningitis
   2. Fungal meningitis
   3. Sarcoidosis
B. Sugar level occasionally low
   1. Viral meningitis or encephalitis
   2. Chemical meningitis
   3. Subarachnoid hemorrhage
   4. Meningeal carcinomatosis

Many conditions other than viral infections can produce a modest pleocytosis, normal or elevated levels of protein, and normal (or low) amounts of sugar. These are listed in Table 12-6. Finally, a low level of glucose in the CSF is not pathognomonic of infection. Several mechanisms are invoked to explain the low level of CSF glucose in persons with meningitis: The glucose may be metabolized by organisms, by phagocytes, or by the inflamed meninges and brain. In addition, transport of glucose into the CSF is often blocked in cases of meningitis. Some of these mechanisms may also explain the low level of CSF glucose found in persons with other conditions (Table 12-7).

It should be clear, therefore, that although the CSF findings provide important clues to the diagnosis of CNS infections, the definitive diagnosis rests on identifying the causative organism microscopically or by culture. Serologic methods may be useful, but, in general, evidence of rising titers of antibodies to an infectious agent appears after the illness is over. Recent studies indicate that counterimmunoelectrophoresis may be capable of detecting minute amounts of bacterial antigens in the CSF rapidly and thereby enable the rapid and specific diagnosis of meningitis.

REFERENCES

Baker, A. B., Baker, L. H.: *Clinical Neurology.* New York, Harper & Row, 1974, chaps. 14-19.

Dodge, P. R., Swartz, M. N.: Bacterial meningitis—A review of selected aspects. *N. Engl. J. Med.* 272:954, 1965.

Thompson, R. A., Green, J. R. (eds.): *Infectious Diseases of the Central Nervous System.* Advances in Neurology, vol. 16, New York, Raven Press, 1974.

13

Disorders of Basal Ganglia Function

THE BASAL GANGLIA are composed of the *striate nucleus* (caudate and putamen), the *globus pallidus,* and the *subthalamic nucleus.* The *substantia nigra* is an associated structure with important basal ganglia interconnections. The cerebellum and perhaps also the red nucleus play an important role in some abnormalities associated with basal ganglia disorders. Important interconnections of the basal ganglia are the nigrostriatal pathway, the ansa and the fasciculus lenticularis, and the fasciculus thalamicus, which interconnect the globus pallidus and the ventralis lateralis and ventralis anterior (VL-VA) nuclei of the thalamus, the VL-VA thalamocortical fibers, the subthalamopallidal pathway, striatopallidal fibers, and cerebellothalamic interconnections (Fig 13 – 1).

The normal functions of the human basal ganglia have not been defined clearly. The characteristics of dysfunction associated with destructive or irritative pathology have been our major source for analysis of the function of these structures. Although far from ideal in terms of understanding the workings of the basal ganglia, these observations have been useful in both defining certain basic functions and directing appropriate therapy.

In lower vertebrates the basal ganglia are a major motor control system. With progressive evolution of the brain in higher vertebrates, culminating in humans, the basal ganglia are to a large degree superseded by the pyramidal system and the developing neocerebellar cortices. Some of the following evidence indicates that the globus pallidus is the predominant excitatory or effector structure of the basal ganglia and that the striate nucleus, subthalamic nucleus, substantia nigra, and perhaps also the cerebellum modulate this excitatory system mainly by inhibition. It is very possible that these inhibitory influences are an example of the brain's uneconomic evolution, that is, a development of new or an expansion of old inhibitory systems to diminish the effects of previously useful excitatory systems, in this case the globus pallidus. Instead of being discarded to economize space, structures that may have become functionally vestigial are suppressed.

In primates and other neomammalian species, the basal ganglia appear to subserve rather basic automatic motor behavior, such as subconscious postural control, automatic associated movements (e.g., swinging the arms while walking, which also can be considered a posture-stabilizing influence), and possibly emotional motor expression (e.g., smiling, frowning, laughing, crying, etc.), which is attributed in addition to the relatively old limbic cortical structures.

Some deficits observed with basal ganglia disease reflect loss of the preceding functions; however, other and frequently major

147

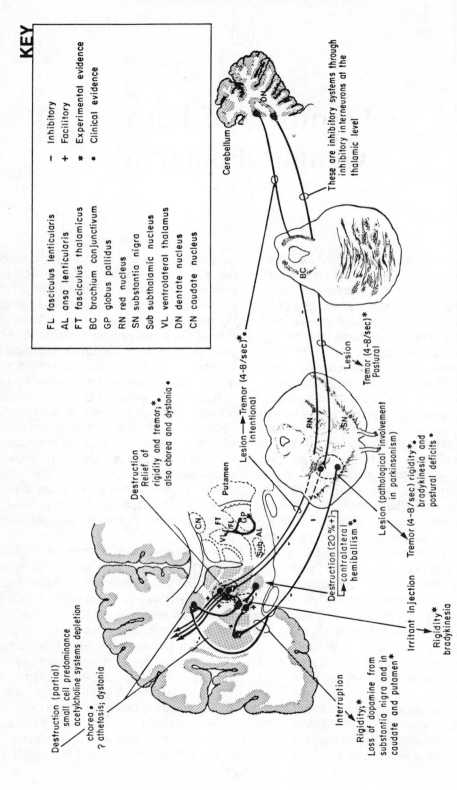

KEY

FL	fasciculus lenticularis	−	Inhibitory
AL	ansa lenticularis	+	Facilitory
FT	fasciculus thalamicus	*	Experimental evidence
BC	brachium conjunctivum	•	Clinical evidence
GP	globus pallidus		
RN	red nucleus		
SN	substantia nigra		
Sub	subthalamic nucleus		
VL	ventrolateral thalamus		
DN	dentate nucleus		
CN	caudate nucleus		

Fig 13–1.—Anatomical schematic illustrating various experimental and clinical evidences for the theoretical bases of basal ganglia disorders.

manifestations fit less easily into a scheme of lost normal function. One can only conclude that they reflect how the remaining normal brain functions when components of the basal ganglia are missing.

There are two major disorder complexes associated with disease of the basal ganglia and related structures: the parkinsonian syndrome and the choreas. Athetosis and the dystonias, also basal ganglia disorders, are much less common, with the exception of spasmodic torticollis and dystonias produced by certain neuroleptic drugs.

Parkinsonian Syndromes

This is a relatively common complex of neurologic abnormalities that has been related to dysfunction in the nigrostriatal dopaminergic systems and possibly also in the cerebellum. A major underlying pathologic abnormality is either a degeneration of substantia nigra neurons, which are the dopamine transmitter system to the striate nuclei, or a suppression by drugs of dopamine effectiveness. The latter is the most common cause of the parkinsonian syndrome today because of the widespread use of certain neuroleptic (tranquilizing) drugs (phenothiazines, butyrophenones, and reserpine). Seen at all age levels, this is an easily reversed complication of drug therapy.

Formerly, most persons affected with parkinsonism were elderly individuals who had progressive degenerative disease of the substantia nigra secondary to the residua of long-past encephalitis, possibly cerebrovascular disease, or idiopathic causes. There are still approximately as many of these patients in absolute numbers as in the past, but, relatively speaking, this number is small. Ameliorative but not curative medical therapy is now available for these patients in the form of dopamine repletion. Rarely is parkinsonism associated with deep-seated neoplasms, which presumably involve the substantia nigra and/or the striatum.

Parkinsonism is characterized by varying degrees of (1) rigidity, (2) bradykinesia, (3) tremor, and (4) postural defects. Dementia, usually appearing late and less severe than the other abnormalities, is also relatively common and considered secondary to degeneration of cerebral cortical neurons.

Rigidity, considered a result of the release of alpha motor neurons from higher inhibition, is plastic in nature and present in all ranges of passive manipulation and active movement. The gamma system probably is not involved because cutting the dorsal roots does not modify the rigidity. The rigidity has a superimposed cogwheel halting character if tremor is part of the syndrome.

Bradykinesia is actually not a slowness of movement so much as an inability to initiate or carry out movements despite the presence of the basic pyramidal-reticular-alpha motor neuron system. An illustration of this presumed dyspraxia is seen in the parkinsonian patient who, frozen with bradykinesia, leaps from his wheelchair and runs with full coordination from a burning house and then safe, settles back to an inability to initiate volitional locomotion. The capability for emotionally driven, well-learned, and relatively automatic behavior is present, but volitional behavior is defective. One can say that if the parkinsonian patient does not have to think about his movements, they are carried out with greater facility. Once movement is initiated, it can sometimes be carried out and more rapidly than normal (a sort of rebound effect). Bradykinesia and rigidity are additive in hindering movement and are usually present together. Bradykinesia is, however, not dependent on or necessarily proportional to rigidity, and vice versa.

Also included by many under bradykinesia is the characteristic depression or loss of associated movements, such as arm swinging while walking and emotional expression— e.g., an immobile face when the patient is happy or sad despite the ability to grimace voluntarily. Facial muscle rigidity can also partly or completely account for the "masked facies."

The *tremor* of parkinsonism is a rhythmic (four to eight per second) oscillation of opposing muscle groups, which is particularly prominent in the distal portions of the extremities. The upper extremities are affected earlier than the lower extremities. The neck and cranial muscles are less frequently involved.

Early in parkinsonism the tremor may begin in one extremity, as may rigidity and bradykinesia as well. Acute generalization to both sides of the body ultimately occurs in most. It has been erroneously considered a tremor at rest, but actually it is a tremor of postural or resting muscle tension. When the patient is completely at rest and relaxed, the tremor disappears, as indeed do almost all types of tremor and adventitious movement disabilities other than seizures. The postural (e.g., arm held in position demanding muscle tone) or resting muscle tension tremor of parkinsonism is to be differentiated from the tremor of neocerebellar involvement, which is not present until the patient directs his limbs into purposeful activity (i.e., intention tremor). Both these tremors, and indeed most adventitious movement abnormalities, are increased by anxiety or any other stress that increases muscle tension; therefore they are reduced to varying degrees by natural or sedative-induced relaxation.

Parkinsonian tremor classically disappears on intention. There is a story, at least partly true, of a skilled surgeon who developed a parkinsonian tremor and continued to operate successfully for some time. As the disease progresses, however, many patients begin to develop an intention tremor, which supports a hypothesis that involvement of the cerebellar system is important in the pathogenesis of parkinsonian tremor.

Postural deficits are less well studied and understood. However, it is characteristic for a person with parkinsonism to have difficulty adjusting to postural change. This can be demonstrated by seating the patient on the edge of a tilt table. When the table is tilted, the normal response is to lean uphill, thus preserving one's balance. The parkinsonian patient tilts with the table without adjusting and topples over (Fig 13-2). If the patient is given a good shove backward, instead of normally catching his balance he tends to fall back like a tree. In some patients this retropulsion can be initiated by simply having the patient attempt to look up or back up. Patients with moderately advanced parkinsonism frequently have a flexed (stooped) posture, which may well be a compensation for the postural imbalance that causes the tendency to retropulsion. Falling is a common problem for parkinsonian patients because of the combination of their rigid/bradykinetic shuffling gait and the postural adjustment deficit. They are unable to make the appropriate kinetic-postural adjustment necessary to prevent themselves from falling. A bizarre but typically parkinsonian fall occurs when the patient is unable to initiate stepping movement with his feet although he has already initiated forward movement of his trunk. To avoid falling on his face, he usually drops to his knees.

Chorea

Chorea is the term for a type of involuntary movement disorder characterized by irregular and fleeting movements of the limbs and/or axial musculature including also the muscles of the face, jaw, and tongue. The intensity of movement varies from very minimal buccolingual chorea characteristic of long-term neuroleptic toxicity to the wild and exhausting limb-flailing chorea called *hemiballism*. Limb tone in persons with chorea is neither rigid nor spastic; it is usually hypotonic or normal.

Degenerative and destructive processes in the striatum and subthalamic nuclei and striatal suppression related to certain classes of drugs are the major pathologic substrates of chorea. Superficially it appears paradoxical that the most common causes of chorei-

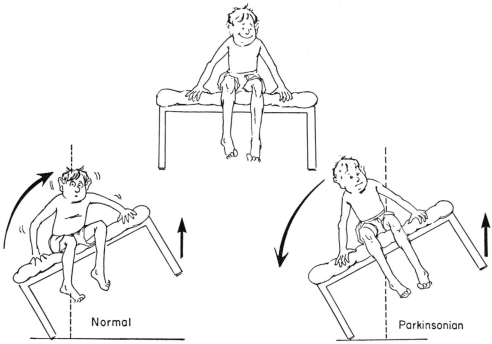

Fig 13—2.—Demonstration of lack of normal response from a patient with parkinsonism to table tilting.

form movement disorders are the same neuroleptic drugs (phenothiazines, butyrophenones, and reserpine) that are the most common cause of parkinsonian disability. Unfortunately the choreiform abnormalities are not so easily reversible and may be permanent in some cases.

The model for choreiform disorders is Huntington's chorea—a rare, inherited (autosomal dominant), degenerative process involving the striatum, particularly the small-cell population (the large-cell neurons are relatively spared), and also the cerebral cortex, giving rise to a combination of progressive limb and axial chorea and dementia. Sometimes early in the disease a parkinsonian syndrome with rigidity and bradykinesia precedes the chorea, presumably because of involvement of the dopamine system of the striatum. This changes to chorea with progression. When this unfortunate process is recognized in a family, genetic counseling becomes paramount as an exercise in prevention, the aim of which is to discontinue the abnormal gene pool.

Sydenham's or rheumatic chorea is a mild, self-limited limb and axial disorder associated with rheumatic fever in children. It is occasionally exacerbated or uncovered in adult women who are pregnant (chorea gravidarum) or taking birth control pills. Because it is reversible and not progressive or fatal, very little is known of the pathophysiology. However, it is presumed that the substrate is striatal dysfunction because the same drugs that to some degree ameliorate Huntington's chorea are also effective against Sydenham's chorea.

Hemiballism is a violent, flailing chorea of the limbs opposite a lesion in the subthalamic nucleus of Luys or, rarely, the striatum. With few exceptions the pathogenesis is infarction, less often hemorrhage, and rarely tumor. Fortunately, in most cases the disease is self-limited because the process (e.g., ischemia) resolves or because the lesion enlarges to involve either the cerebral peduncle or the internal capsule, causing weakness from involvement of the pyramidal system; the chorea, which is expressed through an intact pyramidal system, disappears.

Tardive dyskinesia is the term given to the predominantly axial chorea caused by long-term neuroleptic use, which is seen most often in women. In its mildest form, constant mouthing with protrusion of the lips, mandible, and tongue is seen, not unlike the movements of some very elderly persons and individuals who continually adjust loose upper dental plates. In more advanced stages the trunk muscles are involved and there is a characteristic irregular, incessant pelvic thrusting, which can cause the patient to become a recluse. At present the most successful therapy for this disorder is to increase the neuroleptic dose, producing parkinsonism and thereby ameliorating the chorea at least temporarily (see the following hypotheses).

A variety of metabolic conditions are associated with choreiform movements. Among these are hyperthyroidism, lupus erythematosus (presumably a vasculitis of arteries supplying the striatum), atropine poisoning, anticonvulsant toxicity (e.g., phenytoin, carbamazepine, and phenobarbital), and L-dopa therapy for parkinsonism. Relief coincides with clearing of the metabolic derangement.

Athetosis

Athetosis is a rare movement disorder characterized by involuntary, slow, twisting, writhing movements of the trunk and limbs. It frequently has associated erratic choreiform components. Striatal injury, particularly prominent in the putamen, has been considered the pathophysiologic substrate; however, widespread brain damage is usually present and confounds any clear analysis. The most common cause is perinatal hyperbilirubinemia, which involves the brain

(kernicterus). This leaves the infant with cortical and most prominently basal ganglia damage, with subsequent mental retardation and choreoathetosis.

Dystonias

With one exception the dystonias are uncommon disorders. They are characterized by tortion spasms of the limbs, trunk, and neck. They may be progressive or static and are related to past encephalitis in a few cases but are usually idiopathic. In a few individuals who were well studied post mortem, either no pathology or various combinations of basal ganglia lesions were seen. Spasmodic torticollis is the most common idiopathic form and is characterized by intermittent excessive and involuntary contractions of the sternomastoid muscle on one side (rarely bilateral giving retrocollis).

The one frequently seen dystonia is related to an overdose of neuroleptic drugs and is always reversible when the drug is withdrawn or counteracted by other drugs. Involuntary and occasionally severe tonic contraction of axial muscles is most common, ranging from jaw clenching similar to the trismus (lockjaw) of tetanus to severe opisthotonic posturing similar to that seen in decerebration. Recognition of this easily reversible cause of these otherwise ominous signs is obviously important. A good history can usually clarify the situation, and reversal of the dysfunction with atropinic medication confirms the diagnosis.

It is useful at this point to review some of the many seemingly unrelated experimental and clinical observations that have been made with basal ganglia disorders to suggest some hypotheses and possibly to stimulate further inquiry on your part.

The caudate putamen (striatum) and subthalamic nuclei exert inhibitory influences on the globus pallidus, particularly its medial segment. When these inhibitory influences are suppressed (as with drugs) or destroyed, the globus pallidus is released to hyperexcitability in such a way that, depending on which nucleus or part of a nucleus is involved, a specific movement disorder is manifested. This excessive activity is expressed through the remaining normal motor systems.

Striatal dopamine depletion	→	parkinsonian rigidity and bradykinesia
Striatal small-cell dysfunction	→	chorea, athetosis(?), dystonia(?)
Subthalamic destruction	→	violent hemichorea (hemiballism)

The excessive pallidal activity exerts its effect on the motor system via the ansa and fasciculus lenticularis, which project via the fasciculus thalamicus to the VL-VA thalamic nuclei, which in turn project to the premotor and motor cortex. Predictably, adequate surgical ablation of the globus pallidus or the fasciculus thalamicus relieves to some degree all the preceding movement disorders in the majority of cases (see Fig 13–1). Surgical destruction of the motor cortex, internal capsule, or cerebral peduncle, the last-resort therapies of the past, also give relief but by substituting hemiparesis for the movement disorder.

The rhythmic tremors of neocerebellar involvement and of parkinsonism have a similar rate of four to eight per second. Further correlation is noted late in the course of parkinsonism when the tremor, previously postural in nature, becomes also an intention tremor, as with neocerebellar disease. Interruption of the dentatoneocerebellar output, which projects to the VL thalamus (postulated tremorogenic zone), causes an intention tremor by releasing the latter nucleus. Interruption of the ventrolateral paleoneocerebellar brachium conjunctivum fibers in experimental primates causes a postural tremor similar to that of parkinsonism. Le-

sions of the region that contains these fibers as they pass just above and through the substantia nigra are associated with postural tremor and also may be associated with rigidity and bradykinesia. The rigidity and bradykinesia are related to destruction of the substantia nigra with resultant depression of the putamen caudate inhibitory system.

The most common area of pathologic involvement in parkinsonism is in and around the substantia nigra region. Progressive enlargement of the process could easily extend to involve the proximate neocerebellar systems in and around the red nucleus, causing intention tremor after having already involved the more ventral fibers, destruction of which may cause the typical parkinsonian muscle tension tremor. A destructive lesion where the cerebello-dentato-rubrothalamic pathway impinges on the VL thalamus (i.e., just above the fasciculus thalamicus, the "tremorogenic" zone) causes relief of both cerebellar and parkinsonian tremors in a large percentage of cases (see Fig 13–1).

In summary, it appears that rigidity, choreiform movements, and tremor in a variety of clinical situations are secondary in large part to loss of inhibitory influences on parts of the motor system, i.e., the globus pallidus in rigidity and chorea and the VL tremorogenic zone in tremor. The inhibitory structures include the cerebellum, striate, and subthalamic nuclei.

Dopamine is present in high concentration in the striatum. Substantia nigra endings in the caudate and putamen are dopaminergic. Persons with parkinsonism have degeneration of the substantia nigra and are depleted of dopamine in the striatum. The dopamine precursor, L-dopa, as opposed to dopamine itself, can pass the blood-brain barrier. It is changed by decarboxylase to dopamine, which in high concentrations relieves many symptoms of parkinsonism, particularly rigidity and bradykinesia (also tremor, although in certain cases there is clear-cut dissociation, with relief of rigidity and bradykinesia and very little change in tremor). A reasonable hypothesis based on this information suggests that L-dopa repletes low stores of dopamine in the striatum and causes resurgence of the inhibitory system in these structures. Denervation hypersensitivity in the striatum might explain a nonsynaptic effect of the exogenous dopamine.

You may have concluded that the rigidity and bradykinesia of parkinsonism appear to be counterbalanced by chorea. They cannot exist simultaneously to any significant degree. Chorea can be decreased by giving the drugs (e.g., phenothiazines, butyrophenones, and reserpine) that are complicated by dose-related parkinsonian side effects.

A significant complication of long-term L-dopa administration is the development of choreiform movement, which is relieved in many persons by lowering the dose. This relief is usually at the expense of reappearance of some rigidity and bradykinesia. An interesting parallel exists in the juvenile (or early stage) form of Huntington's chorea, the inherited disorder in which the caudate putamen is the main site of pathology. Rigidity may be the presenting difficulty but it gradually disappears as the disease progresses, to be replaced by the typical choreiform activity.

The acetylcholine system is markedly depleted in the striate nucleus of patients who are dying with Huntington's chorea; dopamine is less so. It is apparent that an equilibrium exists between the effects of acetylcholine and dopamine on the motor system—a relative excess of the dopamine system leads to chorea and a relative depletion to parkinsonian rigidity; a relative excess of acetylcholine leads to parkinsonian rigidity and a relative depletion to chorea. Further evidence of this equilibrium is the appearance of parkinsonian side effects with overdoses of the cholinesterase inhibitor, physostigmine, which raises the level of acetylcholine in the CNS. Atropine poisoning, which blocks the acetylcholine systems both centrally and peripherally, has been reported to cause choreiform activity and is also mildly effective in

nontoxic doses in relieving parkinsonian rigidity.

The neuroleptic drugs (phenothiazines and butyrophenones), among many other effects, deplete or block both dopamine and the acetylcholine systems and usually cause parkinsonian side effects; dystonia is caused by acute overdose. On withdrawing the drugs or decreasing the dose, these difficulties usually clear. Unfortunately, axial and to a lesser degree limb choreiform movements are uncovered in some cases and persist. They can be most disconcerting because they frequently involve the mouth and tongue, and we have seen a number of patients, all elderly women, who have persistent uncontrollable pelvic thrusting. Treating these patients with the same dopamine-blocking neuroleptics is usually successful, presumably on the basis of the reappearance of parkinsonism side effects. Unfortunately, the choreiform-causing changes continue to occur and finally break through the parkinsonian effects so that the dose of the drug must continually be increased. Withdrawing the drug leaves a worse choreiform problem.

It appears that long-term administration of neuroleptic drugs causes a compensatory increase in the number of dopamine receptor sites, thus possibly creating a hypersensitivity. When the drugs are withdrawn, uncovering blocked dopamine receptor sites or increasing dopamine levels toward normal, the total number of active sites may have become so great that there is an excessive dopaminergic response (chorea) to normal levels of dopamine elaboration in the striatum.

We are now looking for agents that will cause parkinsonism without further proliferating dopamine receptors. This might best be accomplished by avoiding dopamine receptor blockers or dopamine depletions. Increasing acetylcholine levels would appear a reasonable approach. Physostigmine, which can, in toxic doses, cause parkinsonian side effects, presumably does not cause destruction in the striatal system; however, in the small nontoxic doses permissible it has not been very effective in preventing chorea. Choline and lecithin, both precursors of acetylcholine centrally and peripherally, show some promise with oral administration. They are natural food substances and not known to be associated with deleterious side effects.

REFERENCES

Calne, D., Chas, J. N., Barbeau, A. (eds.): *Dopaminergic Mechanisms*. Advances in Neurology, vol. 9. New York, Raven Press, 1975.

Carpenter, M. B.: Brain stem and infratentorial neuraxis in experimental dyskinesia. *Arch. Neurol.* 5:504, 1961.

Coleman, J. H., Hayes, P. E.: Drug-induced extrapyramidal effects—A review. *Dis. Nerv. Syst.* 36:591, 1975.

McDowell, F. H., Markham, C. H. (eds.): *Recent Advances in Parkinson's Disease*. Philadelphia, F. A. Davis Co., 1971.

14

Cerebrovascular Disorders

EACH YEAR approximately half a million adults in this country have a stroke. Cerebrovascular dysfunction, occlusive and hemorrhagic, is the third most common cause of death in this country and is very high on the list of disorders causing morbidity. Approximately 2 million people are now disabled from the effects of one or more cerebrovascular events. A great number of these individuals are in the working-age population.

Approximately 80% of all strokes are occlusive. Atherosclerotic thrombotic occlusion and embolic occlusion are the two major categories. A small number of occlusive strokes are caused by inflammatory involvement or spasm of arteries. Rarely is cerebral vein occlusion of etiologic significance.

Although there are no clear-cut data on this point, there is increasing evidence that a major percentage of occlusive strokes are caused by embolism of clot or atheromatous material from cervical carotid or vertebrobasilar atherosclerotic plaques to the intracranial vessels. Complete occlusion of the cervical portion of the internal carotid or vertebral arteries is probably not, as once thought, the most common cause of cerebral infarction, although primary intracranial branch occlusion is still considered a relatively frequent cause of stroke.

Intracranial hemorrhage, excluding traumatic causes, accounts for approximately 20% of all strokes. Primary intracerebral hemorrhage in hypertensive individuals and subarachnoid hemorrhage from congenital or acquired arterial aneurysms or arteriovenous malformations are the major categories.

Occlusive Disease

The brain, in contrast with other organs such as the kidney, is a compactly arranged structure that anatomically segregates functional components in a highly organized manner. Therefore, as opposed to occlusion of an artery supplying a small area of the rather homogeneously arranged kidney, occlusion of an artery supplying a small area of the brain such as the respiratory center of the medulla or the internal capsule has a profound and specific effect. Regeneration of structures or at least functional compensation by the remaining tissue is the rule with most organs. By contrast, significant regeneration does not occur in the brain. Functional compensation does occur, but the margin of safety is not nearly so great as in the kidney or other organs where a large percentage of the organ can be destroyed without gross impairment of function.

The brain makes up only 2% of total body weight but uses more than 10% of the oxygen metabolized by the body, uses almost 20% of the glucose, and receives almost 20% of the cardiac output; these data plus the fact that only three to eight minutes of cardiac arrest result in irreversible brain damage emphasize the striking dependency of the brain on an adequate blood supply for proper functioning.

156

There are well-developed safety factors that help to protect the brain when its blood supply is threatened. The brain vasculature is able to adjust its arterial perfusion over wide changes of blood pressure to keep a relatively constant and adequate blood supply. This self-adjustment or autoregulation causes cerebral vasodilatation when the mean blood pressure drops below normal levels and maintains an adequate blood supply until the mean arterial pressure reaches approximately half the normal levels (50–60 mm Hg); lower pressures are associated with focal and diffuse cerebral dysfunction. This safety factor can be of great importance during systemic hypotension and also at a local level can protect against flow changes caused by increased intracranial pressure or progressive atherosclerotic narrowing of cortical or cerebral arteries.

The cerebral arterial system responds to increasing blood pressure by constriction, thus keeping perfusion within normal ranges and avoiding the possible hemorrhagic consequence of excessive pressures. When mean arterial pressure rises above approximately 150 mm Hg for prolonged periods, however, autoregulation may break down. Segments of cerebral arterioles may dilate to an excessive degree, breaking down internal integrity and the blood-brain barrier and thus allowing focal cerebral edema and dysfunction. This condition has been appropriately labeled *hypertensive encephalopathy* and occurs rarely, probably because extended periods of hypertension of such great degree are unusual.

During systemic hypoxia, the brain is able to extract oxygen from the blood in increasing amounts and thus compensate for arterial hypoxia down to tensions of 50 mm Hg. Beyond this, some vasodilatation probably occurs, possibly on the basis of tissue ischemia and associated local tissue acidosis, which is a strong stimulant of cerebral arteriolar and capillary dilatation. Small changes in the arterial CO_2 partial pressure cause marked changes in cerebral blood flow, presumably by changing the perivascular hydrogen ion concentration. High CO_2 tensions such as occur with pulmonary disease result in a lower pH in tissue and cerebral vasodilatation, which is an indirect protection against the associated hypoxia to which the brain vasculature is less reactive. Low CO_2 partial pressures such as occur with hyperventilation cause a decrease in the perivascular hydrogen ion concentration and subsequent vasoconstriction. This decreases the cerebral vascular bed and may decrease intracranial volume by as much as 2%–3%. During central neurogenic hyperventilation caused by midbrain or pontine dysfunction (see chap. 19), this decrease in volume may have some protective effect against progressive rostrocaudal deterioration.

Collateral circulation is the major safety factor that helps protect the brain from damage caused by occlusion of one or more of its major arterial inputs. In the human there are many potential channels for collateral circulation, but only a few are significant following cerebrovascular occlusion. The circle of Willis (Fig 14–1) is the most important channel for collateral circulation following occlusion of either the internal carotid system or the basilar system. It is occasionally developmentally incomplete, and even when complete is often an unsuccessful collateral channel unless vessel occlusion occurs, gradually giving an opportunity for increased compensatory flow through usually small-caliber posterior and/or anterior communicating arteries. Fortunately a common cause of closure in the major cerebral vessels is gradual atherosclerotic thrombotic occlusion, which often allows time for adequate development of collateral flow to the distribution of the affected vessel. The most frequently occluded major vessel is the internal carotid artery in the cervical region just above the bifurcation of the common carotid artery. Following occlusion and despite frequent anomalous variations in the circle of

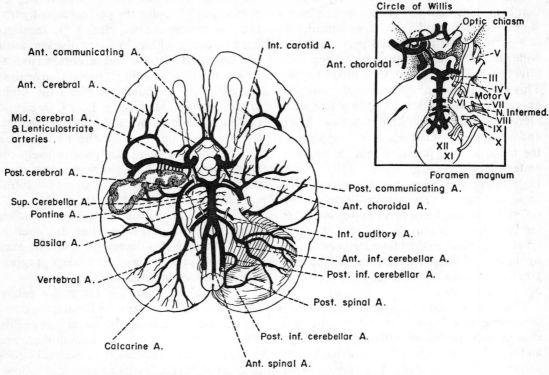

Fig 14—1.—Major arterial branches of the vertebrobasilar and carotid systems and the interconnecting circle of Willis.

Willis, collateral flow is possible in approximately 90% of the population from the opposite carotid system via a patent anterior communicating artery or from the vertebrobasilar system through a patent ipsilateral posterior communicating artery, or from both sources. This rather optimistic view of the compensatory potential of the circle of Willis is somewhat dampened when one notes that at the advanced age associated with cerebrovascular occlusive disease, collateral channels are not immune to sclerotic occlusive changes and therefore may have less potential for meeting increased demands. Also, if embolic occlusion of major cerebral vessels is a common cause of strokes as suggested, and if the emboli as suspected lodge beyond the circle of Willis, for example, in the middle cerebral artery or its branches, then the circle proves useless as

a collateral supply. The rapidity of occlusion with embolism also tends to preclude a useful development of collateral from other sources.

Anastomoses between the main cerebral arteries and the main cerebellar arteries exist at the arteriolar level in the pia over the respective hemispheres, and there are even interconnections between the cerebellar arterial branches and the posterior cerebral artery. These channels are variable and also limited by the same factors that limit the effectiveness of the circle of Willis, i.e., anatomical variability, the rapidity of occlusion, and the condition of the vessels. The penetrating arterial branches that reach the deeper structures of the brain anastomose to some degree at a capillary level with neighboring arterial branches, but this collateral circulation by itself is rarely of functional significance following an occlusion and the penetrating vessels therefore act essentially as end arteries.

The third group of potential collateral channels are connections between the external and internal carotid arteries (e.g., external maxillary-ophthalmic-internal carotid). These potential channels are rarely significant as a sole source of collateral circulation in persons with acute stroke. However, they may give major collateral support and decrease the severity of or prevent ischemia with slowly progressive occlusions of major vessels. Individuals have been described who have minimal symptoms or signs of cerebral ischemia but have complete occlusion of three and even all four major cervical vessels (both internal carotids and vertebral arteries). Arteriograms reveal large collateral channels from the external carotid system that anastomose with the intracranial arterial systems through the orbit and foramen magnum. Very gradual and probably staggered carotid and vertebral occlusion allows these compensatory channels to enlarge and prevent major ischemic destruction.

Closely related to collateral circulation and perhaps of more dependable functional significance is the presence of overlapping blood supply to regions. This becomes clear to you if you review the areas of blood supply, especially of the brain stem and deeper structures of the cerebral hemispheres. With ischemia in the distribution of a single-vessel system (e.g., the middle cerebral, Fig 14−2), these areas of overlap restrict the area of dysfunction and destruction. If flow is affected diffusely, however, as with severe systemic hypotension (shock), these areas, somewhat inappropriately called *watershed areas,* become the regions of greatest damage. This is because they are at the farthest reaches of blood supply and therefore are the first to suffer decreased flow with decreased perfusion pressure.

Almost 50% of persons who suffer a complete ischemic stroke have stenotic or occlusive disease in the cervical vessels. Also,

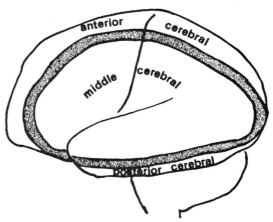

Fig 14−2. — Diagram of the zone of cerebral cortical arterial overlap, the so-called watershed area. With single-vessel occlusion, the overlap helps to preserve cortical integrity within its territory. With systemic hypotension, this zone suffers most because it is at the farthest reaches of the three major arterial supplies.

approximately half of patients with completed ischemic stroke have a history of prodromal symptoms and signs referable to ischemia in the areas supplied by the involved vessels. These episodic signs and symptoms take the form of transient neurologic deficits (transient ischemic attacks, TIAs).

Diagnostic and Therapeutic Considerations

For therapeutic convenience and with some arbitrary delineation, the degree of cerebral arterial occlusive disease has been divided into: (1) transient ischemic attack, (2) stroke-in-evolution, and (3) completed stroke.

TRANSIENT ISCHEMIC ATTACK

The transient ischemic attack (TIA) is defined as a reversible episode of neurologic deficit caused by vascular insufficiency usually lasting no longer than minutes but occasionally persisting for 24 hours and rarely several days. Complete recovery is the major categorical criterion. Approximately half the persons who develop completed ischemic destruction (infarction) of brain tissue have had premonitory transient ischemic attacks, thus underscoring the importance of recognizing the TIA, which represents a stage in the evolution of cerebrovascular disease that is in many instances treatable. Treatment aims at alleviating the attacks and staying or preventing progression to completed infarction.

From 20% to 40% of persons with TIAs progress to cerebral infarction. The prognosis for vertebrobasilar distribution attacks is somewhat better than that for carotid attacks, with approximately 20% and 40%, respectively, developing infarction on long-term follow-up, if untreated.

SYNDROMES OF THE CAROTID SYSTEM.— Transient monocular visual obscuration (amaurosis fugax) referable to retinal ischemia and transient contralateral hemimotor, hemisensory, and hemivisual deficits referable to hemispheric ischemia are the characteristic components of carotid-middle cerebral TIAs. Aphasia is present if the dominant hemisphere is involved. If retinal symptoms are present with hemispheric symptoms or, as is more common, in isolation, internal carotid stenotic or ulcerative disease is very likely. Cerebral symptoms alone may be caused by either cervical carotid disease or hemispheric small-vessel disease. A palpably depressed carotid pulsation is presumptive evidence of stenotic or occlusive disease. However, the pulse frequently is not depressed because of a patent overlying external carotid, because the internal carotid stenosis causes insignificant depression of flow, or because the common carotid pulse may be transmitted to and palpable over a blocked internal carotid segment. The presence of an ipsilateral carotid bruit (usually in early systole and high-pitched) not referred from aortic valvular disease is strong evidence of carotid stenosis; however, almost 75% of patients with radiologically proved carotid stenosis do not have a bruit audible at the bedside. Approximately 10% of adults who have a carotid bruit on routine examination with no history of ischemic disease have normal carotids on angiographic investigation. Therefore, when a nonradiated bruit is heard over the carotids, atherosclerotic disease is present in 90% of cases, whether symptomatic or not.

When is a carotid lesion significant? Before blood flow is obstructed, a carotid stenosis must be at least two-thirds complete; the diameter of the lumen as demonstrated angiographically is usually 1 mm or smaller. As mentioned, approximately 90% of the population can, because of collateral circulation through the circle of Willis, withstand complete occlusion of a single carotid or vertebral artery without ischemic symptoms, barring significant small-vessel occlusive disease beyond the circle of Willis. Rapid occlusion by trauma or thrombus in an otherwise normal carotid is more likely to be associated with cerebral symptoms because of lack of time for collateral circulation to develop to full effectiveness.

Systemic blood pressure must be markedly lowered in persons who have small- or large-vessel stenotic disease before retinal, cerebral, or brain stem ischemia is symptomatic. Because of this and the previous safety factors, it is not surprising that relatively few transient ischemic attacks are caused by hemodynamic failure. Certainly some are but it has been shown now that more transient ischemic episodes are secondary to microemboli arising from atherosclerotic plaques and ulcers in the cervical vessels. Actual visualization of emboli traversing the retinal arterioles during attacks, the proved response of TIAs to anticoagulants, and the cessation of attacks on complete occlusion of the involved vessel (if no major deficit occurs) are the best evidence for this.

It is concluded that any atherosclerotic common or internal carotid lesion, whether significant stenosis exists or not, can cause transient ischemic attacks by embolus formation from platelet aggregates or atherosclerotic ulcer debris. These emboli, particularly the platelet aggregates, typically are broken up rapidly on meeting the small vessels of the retina and brain and then pass distally with subsequent alleviation of ischemic symptoms and signs.

SYNDROMES OF THE VERTEBROBASILAR SYSTEM.—Transient ischemic symptoms referable to the posterior vascular systems are quite variable, which is consonant with the many functional systems represented in the brain stem and posterior portions of the hemispheres. Alone or in various combinations, vertigo, bilateral blurring or loss of vision, ataxia, diplopia, bilateral or unilateral occasionally alternating sensory and motor deficits, and syncope are common manifestations of vertebrobasilar insufficiency. Transient vertigo or ill-defined dizziness is a very common complaint in persons past age 60 and is not necessarily related to ischemia. Indeed the most common cause is benign positional vertigo, a disorder of aging related to macula-otolith dysfunction and occasionally cervical spondylosis (see chap. 3). The associated symptoms noted earlier must therefore be present before a clinical diagnosis of transient vertebrobasilar ischemia can be entertained. Evidences of vertebral insufficiency at the bedside are (1) depression of blood pressure in either arm, suggesting the possibility of subclavian or innominate artery occlusion with reverse flow in the ipsilateral vertebral artery; (2) bruits over the supraclavicular regions in the absence of aortic ejection murmur, suggesting either subclavian or vertebral narrowing; (3) bruits over the posterior triangle of neck, which may be changed on turning the head, suggesting vertebral narrowing; and (4) production of vertebrobasilar ischemia symptoms and signs by flexing, extending, or rotating the neck, suggesting osteoarthritic compression of the vertebral artery in the transverse vertebral foramina.

DIFFERENTIAL DIAGNOSIS.—A broad range of differential diagnostic possibilities does not exist in the age range when one is most susceptible to cerebrovascular disease (45 years and older). Migraine equivalent, focal seizures, benign positional vertigo, Ménière's disease, and demyelinating disease are the most commonly encountered categories. Historical information is usually sufficient to eliminate or implicate these possibilities. Cranial arteritis (temporal arteritis) must be considered in the patient over 50 who has transient amaurosis usually with but occasionally without temporal headache. Such persons almost invariably have an elevated sedimentation rate (rarely less and usually higher than 50 mm/hour), in most cases have a positive temporal artery biopsy specimen, and respond to corticosteroid therapy. Occasionally persons with cranial arteritis have a stroke caused by inflammatory occlusion of major cervical (most often the vertebral artery) or cerebral vessels. Therefore, a test of sedimentation rate should be ordered routinely in all stroke patients. Although the patient with hypoglycemia usually shows evidence of diffuse bilateral cerebral dysfunction, occasionally the presenting picture is one of focal and lateralized difficulty. Hemiparesis, aphasia, and other focal abnormalities of relatively acute onset suggest occlusive or hemorrhagic stroke. It is reasonable therefore to check the blood glucose level early in all apparent stroke patients. Treatment with glucose of the rare patient with hypoglycemic "stroke" usually gives dramatic results.

MEDICAL THERAPY.—It has been fairly well established that anticoagulation with the antithrombin agent coumarin and its congeners (and also heparin) significantly decreases the incidence of transient ischemic attacks. It is likely, though not clearly established at this time, that this type of anticoagulation decreases somewhat the incidence of cerebral infarction. Progression of atherosclerotic arterial occlusive disease is not prevented by anticoagulation; it is the prevention of formation of fibrin-bound platelet clots, potential emboli, at the site of stenosis and/or ulceration that best accounts for decreased transient ischemic attacks. This mechanism presumably also decreases the formation of larger clots that can potentially form larger emboli, and it may therefore account for the claimed beneficial effect of anticoagulation in preventing completed strokes.

Persons with clinical evidence of embolization from sources other than the cervical vessels (e.g., atrial fibrillation, diseased or prosthetic cardiac valves, and infarcted cardiac walls) also benefit from anticoagulation. Following embolic arterial occlusion and infarction of the brain, some hemorrhage into the damaged site frequently results. Nevertheless many now do not consider this to be a contraindication to anticoagulation because major conversion of infarction to expanding hemorrhage does not occur with significantly increased frequency in these individuals when they are anticoagulated.

Acetylsalicylic acid, dipyridamole, and some other medications inhibit platelet aggregability and therefore might be expected to decrease the incidence of TIAs. Prospective study has now demonstrated a statistically significant diminution of transient ischemic attacks by these agents. Some prospective evidence is available that indicates a favorable effect of these medications in preventing embolization from artificial cardiac valves. Our clinical impression to date is that persons with amaurosis fugax as their only symptom do better on aspirin than those with cerebral symptoms. It is possible that larger clots are necessary to depress a functionally significant amount of cerebral tissue, whereas small platelet clump emboli are not reflected at all as dysfunction. The retina does not have the safety factor or redundancy of function of the massive cerebral hemispheres, so small platelet clumps are capable of producing transient visual obscuration. At present we are using aspirin in combination with dipyridamole in patients with TIAs who are not surgical candidates and who cannot be anticoagulated with coumarin medications. Also we routinely give this combination to patients with symptoms of vertebrobasilar

insufficiency. As with the retina, small platelet clump emboli may effectively cause dysfunction in the vertebrobasilar distribution, i.e., the brain stem, where there is much less redundancy of function. Antiplatelet medications have not been clearly proved in preventing cerebral infarction, although recent results of several multiple-institution studies suggest a positive effect. In particular, men with TIA appear to have approximately 50% less chance of going on to have a completed stroke if they take acetylsalicylic acid than if they do not. For unknown reasons, women gain no protection.

SURGICAL THERAPY.—Carotid stenosis on the side of transient symptoms is the most clearly established reason for vascular surgery today. Many feel this is the treatment of choice, despite some evidence favoring anticoagulation, for prophylaxis against further TIAs and, more important, final infarction. Completely occluded carotids are rarely operated on now because of the high risk of hemorrhagic complications and surgical failure. Though not prospectively proved of value, it seems rational to attack stenotic carotid vessels surgically opposite a symptomatic hemisphere when the remaining carotid artery is completely occluded. An increased collateral circulation safety factor is the therapeutic aim. Some preliminary evidence indicates that 5%–10% of patients subsequently occlude an endarterectomized carotid artery. This dampens enthusiasm for endarterectomy in patients who have one carotid artery already occluded.

Vertebrobasilar ischemic disease is not so often surgically approachable. Proximal subclavian or innominate stenosis, proximal vertebral stenosis, and vertebral impingement in the transverse cervical foramina by osteoarthritic spurs are the major indications for surgery at present, and a variety of procedures have proved successful. In some cases of osteoarthritis, moderate immobilization of the neck with a soft orthopedic collar is adequate to enable the person to avoid surgery.

In all patients going to surgery in our institution, especially those with carotid disease, antiplatelet anticoagulation (where not medically contraindicated) is begun prior to surgery to decrease the incidence of operative embolization and is carried on after surgery for one to two months during postoperative reepithelialization of the intima-denuded vessels, which may be prone to platelet clumping and embolus formation.

STROKE-IN-EVOLUTION

Approximately 20% of persons who go on to suffer cerebral infarction and approximately 10% of those who suffer a cerebral hemorrhage have a history of evolution of deficit over several hours to several days and rarely longer. Anticoagulation with heparin is usually considered worthwhile prophylaxis in patients with ischemia-infarction-in-evolution. However, patient selection must be made with care because anticoagulation is contraindicated for persons with cerebral hemorrhage and also for those with severe hypertension. In Table 14–1 are listed some useful points to distinguish hemorrhage from ischemia-infarction.

Differential points that stand out and are the most useful are the history of stepwise evolution with frequent reversal of deficit (TIA) in occlusive disease, the presence of red blood cells in the spinal fluid, and elevated CSF pressure in patients with hemorrhage. There are cases that cannot be clinically differentiated, and then anticoagulation cannot be started before carrying out angiography of the neck and cerebral vessels. Many major centers and more and more smaller medical centers now have computerized axial tomographic x-ray units available, which can rapidly differentiate intracranial hemorrhage from infarction (see chap. 18). Clearly this technique, which is noninvasive and therefore not subject to the potential complications of lumbar puncture and arteriography, has revolutionized the emergency diagnosis of intracranial catastrophe. When immediately available, it is the diagnostic procedure of choice for stroke-in-evolution and

many other conditions (see chap. 18).

Other modes of therapy, which have some rationale but are unproved in efficacy, aim at relatively or absolutely increasing the collateral blood supply or the amount of tissue oxygen to regions of progressing ischemia. Hyperventilation is useful at early stages of experimental occlusion in limiting the extent of infarction. Hyperventilation decreases arterial CO_2, causing an alkalosis that constricts normal cerebral arterioles, thus decreasing the blood flow to normal tissue and possibly shunting blood into the ischemic arterial bed where tissue acidosis has maximally dilated the arterioles. If experimental animals are hyperventilated before or within one hour after arterial occlusion, infarction size is decreased; however, beyond one hour after occlusion, no effect is seen. Obviously this limits the usefulness of hyperventilation to the acute period and possibly to the evolving ischemic stroke, but no prospective proof of its clinical efficacy is available.

Oxygenation of an ischemic brain can be increased in the hyperbaric chamber and stroke dysfunction can be alleviated in some cases by this means. Unfortunately the deficits return when the patient is removed from the chamber. Standard means of oxygenation (e.g., nasal mask or catheter) have not proved useful unless they alleviate a systemic respiratory hypoxia.

The cerebral need for oxygen can be decreased by hypothermia and some depressant drugs (e.g., barbiturates). Experimental evidence in animals with vascular occlusions supports the hypothesis that this might preserve some ischemic neurons from destruction while collateral circulation develops. No prospective clinical data are available to support or refute these findings.

In most institutions surgery is not considered a useful approach to the occlusive stroke-in-evolution. However, if the stroke is stayed spontaneously or by conservative therapy and little neurologic deficit remains, the patient should be considered for evaluation for prophylactic cervical vessel surgery.

TABLE 14-1. — DIFFERENTIAL CHARACTERISTICS
OF INTRACEREBRAL HEMORRHAGE AND
ISCHEMIC STROKE

	ISCHEMIA-INFARCTION	HEMORRHAGE
1. Stepwise progression	Common	Unusual
Reversible episodes	Common	Rare, if ever
2. CSF		
Blood	Rare (occasionally with embolus)	75%
Elevated pressure	Rare	75%
Elevated pressure or blood	Rare	95%
3. Headache	Infrequent	Frequent, severe
Nausea and vomiting	With vertebrobasilar occlusive disease	Common
4. Rapid loss of consciousness	10%	50%
5. Elevated blood pressure by history	50%	90%
6. Fundi: papilledema	Rare	Common; can occur within $\frac{1}{2}$ hour of catastrophe
Subhyaloid hemorrhage	Rare	Common
7. Leukocytosis > 20,000	10%	50%
8. Fever	Uncommon	Common
9. Mortality	20%–30%	75%–80%

COMPLETED STROKE

The completed cerebral infarction is defined in two ways, temporal and anatomical. *Temporal* completion is a fixed, neurologic deficit lasting more than several days. Any recovery that occurs thereafter is related to dissipation of edema, vascular collateralization of surviving but functionally depressed tissue, and functional reorganization of surviving brain. The last, though formerly believed of great importance, has the least significance in recovery except in children. *Anatomical* completion refers to infarction of the entire region of supply of a major cerebral vessel (e.g., the middle cerebral artery). In this sense, infarction in the distribution of one branch of the middle cerebral artery, producing for example an isolated expressive aphasia or monoparesis, is considered incomplete.

No proved therapy exists for reversing the temporally completed infarction, whether anatomically complete or not. A new approach, however, aims at preventing or suppressing the significant cerebral edema, which almost invariably follows infarction and may be clinically significant from eight hours to seven days following the primary insult. This edema, by compressing contiguous vessels, may increase the area of destruction and also can cause secondary brain stem compression by the various routes of herniation of brain substance (e.g., tentorial and foramen magnum herniation; see chap. 19 on stupor and coma). Herniation with brain stem compression is the most common cause of death occurring during the acute phase of infarction and also hemorrhage.

Various measures have been tried to prevent or lessen the edema to decrease both morbidity (size of stroke) and mortality. Corticosteroids, although useful in decreasing the cerebral edema caused by neoplasms and inflammatory lesions, are not effective in decreasing the edema of cerebral ischemia. Hyperosmotic agents (e.g., urea, mannitol, glycerol), which dehydrate normal brain tissue, probably do not affect the edema in an ischemic or infarcted area that does not have access to the agents. They have not been clearly shown to decrease the morbidity of infarction. By shrinking the normal surrounding brain tissues, however, they may prevent herniation and brain stem compression and this probably accounts for the efficacy of these agents in decreasing mortality.

Surgical therapy in persons with anatomically incomplete infarction, as suggested, is considered useful prophylaxis against complete infarction for those with milder deficits who have approachable cervical carotid stenotic or ulcerative disease. A stenotic lesion, if hemodynamically insignificant (i.e., less than 70% occluded with normal distal flow), can be operated on almost immediately; if 70% or more occlusion and decreased distal flow are present, a wait of six to eight weeks is necessary to allow reconstitution of necrotic blood vessels at the site of infarction, which could hemorrhage if a return of full arterial pressure occurs too soon.

PROPHYLAXIS

The major prospectively proved and preventable predisposition to occlusive and hemorrhagic stroke is hypertension. The pulsatile trauma to arteries caused by systemic hypertension presumably initiates the atherosclerotic process and also causes microscopic arterial wall trauma and aneurysmal ballooning in smaller radicles, which is the presumed source of most intracerebral hypertensive hemorrhages. Most authorities now feel that treatment of even mild hypertension is useful prophylaxis against stroke.

Persons with diabetes mellitus are predisposed to atherosclerosis and occlusive stroke. It has not been shown, however, that treatment of the glucose intolerance is useful prophylaxis against generalized atherosclerosis or stroke. Obesity, hyperlipidemia, lack of exercise, and cigarette smoking, although variably implicated as causes of coronary atherosclerosis and insufficiency, have not been shown to predispose to stroke.

For persons with embolization from cardiac valves, fibrillating auricles, or ischemic endocardium, chronic anticoagulation with antithrombin agents is considered the treatment of choice. Some antiplatelet agents appear also to be of use in persons with artificial heart valves. The risk of turning the frequent diapedetic hemorrhagic infarction of cerebral embolism into a frank expanding intracerebral hemorrhage appears less than the risk of repeated systemic embolizations.

Some Uncommon Causes of Occlusive Stroke

Arteritis is an unusual cause of cerebrovascular occlusive or hemorrhagic disease and probably accounts for less than 1% of strokes in adults. The two major causes of inflammation and occlusion of the cerebral arteries are diffuse or focal autoimmune arteritis (e.g., polyarteritis nodosum, lupus erythematosus, giant cell and other cranial arteritides, and Takayasu's giant cell arteritis of the aortic arch vessels) and septic or infectious arteritis, which may be associated with purulent meningitis or direct involvement of arterial walls by fungi (mucormycosis and aspergillosis in debilitated or diabetic individuals) or bacteria seeded to arteries from septic emboli of cardiac origin. Meningovascular syphilis is a rare cause of stroke today. Thrombotic occlusion of or intracranial hemorrhage from diseased and weakened arterial walls may occur with either autoimmune or septic arteritis. Hemorrhage is most commonly seen with fungal and bacterial involvement where the arterial walls may be weakened and balloon out to form aneurysms, which are prone to rupture. Treatment of arteritic stroke is aimed at the primary process (i.e., corticosteroids for autoimmune disease, antibiotics for infectious disease, surgery where possible for aneurysms) and supportive care.

Occlusive strokes in children, in addition to being associated with cervical or cranial trauma, may follow viral illness and are therefore presumed by many to be caused by focal autoimmune processes or direct viral involvement.

Migraine is rarely associated with ischemic stroke, presumably on the basis of prolonged vasospasm or arterial edema. Women taking birth control medications are slightly more susceptible to cerebral arterial occlusion, and this susceptibility is increased if there is a history of migraine. Many neurologists now advise women with migraine not to take birth control pills.

Vasospasm occurs in a significant number of persons with subarachnoid hemorrhage and can be severe enough to cause ischemia and infarction. The spasm is thought to be related to release of vasoactive substances (e.g., serotonin) into the subarachnoid space from extravasated platelets and possibly also basophils. Prophylactic treatment with alpha-adrenergic blockers and other potential arterial relaxing agents such as the antibiotic kanamycin (which depletes serotonin and blocks bacterial production of vasoactive substances in the bowel) has shown some promise.

Hyperviscosity and hypercoagulable states predispose to arterial occlusive disease, and the risk is greatly amplified if arteriosclerotic vessel changes are already present. Hyperviscosity that causes a sluggish blood flow and a predisposition to coagulation is associated with dehydration, hyperproteinemias, and dysproteinemias (e.g., macroglobulinemias, cold agglutinins), polycythemia, leukemia, and sickle cell disease. Thrombocythemia (excessive platelets), thrombotic thrombocytopenia purpura (abnormal platelets), and rare cancer-associated coagulopathies are examples of excessive clotting capacity that predisposes to arterial occlusion.

Symptomatic cerebral vein or venous sinus occlusion is rare. This may be explained in part by the rich interconnections in the cerebral venous system and the lack of valves in the major sinuses. Both contribute to create a collateral circulation safety factor when focal portions of the venous system are obstructed.

When major channels are occluded, such as the posterior portions of the sagittal sinus, a lateral sinus, or the internal cerebral veins, collateral circulation is frequently inadequate and edema and hemorrhagic infarction may occur and cause a stroke-like picture with headache, focal and diffuse deficits, and focal and generalized seizures. Edema may appear rapidly and massively and lead to rostrocaudal deterioration (herniation) and death (see chap. 19).

Some predisposing elements in venous occlusion are severe dehydration, causing hyperviscosity of blood flow and increased coagulability, other causes of hypercoagulable states (discussed earlier), and infection in the bathing cerebrospinal fluid and neighboring structures involving vein and sinus walls (purulent meningitis, chronic otitis media, and chronic sinusitis).

Therapy is aimed at treating the primary process when possible, decreasing edema, and suppressing seizures. If the patient survives the acute period, recanalization of the veins may occur and considerable function may return to the involved cerebral tissue, which has not lost its arterial supply

Hemorrhagic Cerebrovascular Disease

Intracranial hemorrhage falls into two major categories: (1) spontaneous hemorrhage associated with hypertension and with congenital or other arterial aneurysms and arteriovenous malformations, and (2) traumatic hemorrhages into the epidural, subdural, and subarachnoid spaces or parenchyma of the central nervous system. Traumatic hemorrhage is discussed in chapter 17.

Spontaneous intracranial hemorrhage accounts for approximately 20% of all strokes. The primary hemorrhage may be into the parenchyma of the central nervous system or into the subarachnoid space. Parenchymal hemorrhages often dissect into the ventricular system or directly into the subarachnoid space, whereas primary subarachnoid hemorrhages frequently dissect into the cerebral parenchyma.

Intraparenchymal hemorrhages are almost invariably associated with hypertension and are presumed by many to be the result of weakening of arterial walls by the trauma of an excessive pulse pressure. The most common sites of involvement are (1) the region of the putamen-external capsule in the distribution of the lenticulostriate branches of the middle cerebral artery (60%), (2) the thalamus in the distribution of the small penetrating vessels from the posterior cerebral and posterior communicating arteries (10%), (3) the cerebellum in the distribution of the deep penetrating branches of the superior cerebellar artery (10%), and (4) the pons in the distribution of the paramedian branches of the basilar artery (10%). The remaining 10% occur into the white matter of various lobes of the cerebral hemispheres.

Less often primary intraparenchymal hemorrhage is associated with bleeding diatheses such as arteriovenous and capillary malformations, thrombocytopenia, leukemia, and anticoagulant therapy. Massive hemorrhage may occur into rapidly growing malignant neoplasms, which outstrip their blood supply and develop central necrosis.

It is frequently difficult to differentiate intraparenchymal hemorrhage from massive infarction; however, certain aspects of the history and observations are suggestive (see Table 14-1). A history of hypertension, headache, and vomiting at the onset of stroke, signs of rapidly expanding unilateral intracranial mass (e.g., evidence of secondary compression of the brain stem leading to decreasing awareness and coma, progressive pupillary and oculomotor-vestibular dysfunction, and abnormal respiratory patterns of neurogenic origin), papilledema, and acute fundal hemorrhages implicate hemorrhage as the basic pathologic process. If nausea and vomiting with associated occipital headache and ataxia precede cranial nerve dysfunction and depression of consciousness in a hypertensive patient, cerebellar hemorrhage must

be considered because it may be surgically remediable, whereas thalamic, pontine, and putamenal hemorrhages usually are not. If available, as mentioned earlier, computerized axial tomographic radiography (CT scanning) quickly determines the presence and location of intracranial hemorrhage (see chap. 18).

Ninety percent of primary subarachnoid hemorrhages arise from congenitally derived arterial outpouchings (berry aneurysms) that lie at bifurcations of the major components of the circle of Willis. The most common sites are the carotid-posterior communicating and the anterior cerebral-anterior communicating artery junctions. Defects in the elastic membrane and media of the arteries are considered the basis for berry aneurysm formation. They rupture most often in early to late middle life, rarely in childhood, presumably after years of pulsatile trauma have caused them to balloon into a thin-walled sac. The presence of hypertension predisposes to earlier ruptures. Approximately 1%–2% of the population has berry aneurysms as determined in general autopsy series. Of those who have aneurysms, approximately 15% have more than one.

A small number of primary subarachnoid hemorrhages arise from aneurysms caused by bacterial or fungal inflammation and necrosis of arterial walls as described in the earlier section on occlusive disease. Aneurysms associated with bacteria occur most frequently in small arterial branches over the surface of the cerebral or cerebellar hemispheres. With fungal involvement, major arteries at the base of the brain are frequently affected.

Approximately 10% of subarachnoid hemorrhages originate from congenital arteriovenous malformations on the surface of the cerebral hemispheres.

The sudden onset of a severe headache occasionally initiated by a "popping" or "bursting" sensation is typical of a subarachnoid hemorrhage from an aneurysm. The breakdown products of blood cause a chemical meningitis within several hours following the hemorrhage, which is manifested as nuchal rigidity and frequently a low-grade fever. Platelet or basophil lysis or just the mechanical trauma of tearing of the aneurysm wall may cause some vasospasm and ischemia-infarction with focal or diffuse neurologic deficit. Large amounts of subarachnoid blood frequently block egress of cerebrospinal fluid (CSF) from the subarachnoid space by plugging the arachnoid villi or obstructing CSF flow from the basal cisternae over the hemispheres or by both processes. This results in an acute communicating hydrocephalus with diffuse cerebral dysfunction. With partial blocks or the development of a chronic inflammatory response to the presence of blood, a slowly progressive communicating hydrocephalus may develop and appear as progressive dementia with gait abnormality and incontinence. This may become manifest after the patient has been improving from the acute hemorrhagic event.

Focal signs may also be caused by dissection of the subarachnoid hemorrhage into the parenchyma of the brain. This occurs most commonly with anterior communicating aneurysms, which are tightly enclosed between the frontal lobes, and middle cerebral aneurysms, which are tightly enclosed between the operculum and the insula.

In the absence of focal signs, the CSF must be examined by lumbar puncture to determine whether subarachnoid hemorrhage is present. If there are focal signs, the diagnostic procedures of choice are CT scanning to determine the presence or absence of hemorrhage and radiographic opacification of the cerebral arteries (angiography) to find the aneurysm or arteriovenous malformation if surgery is being considered. Lumbar puncture is somewhat risky because it may lead to further hemispheric shift and secondary brain stem compression if there is an expanding hemorrhagic mass (see chaps. 18 and 19).

Aneurysm surgery in the hands of a skilled surgeon is successful in selected cases. Clipping the neck of the aneurysm is generally the procedure of choice.

Arteriovenous malformations may be suspected before hemorrhage occurs because they may give rise to unilateral vascular headaches, sometimes focal seizures, and/or sensorimotor deficits. Some have an audible bruit that can be heard by listening over the skull.

The mortality from untreated subarachnoid hemorrhage is approximately 50%, although this refers mainly to hemorrhage from aneurysm. Arteriovenous hemorrhages tend to occur at a lower pressure head, cause less tissue destruction, and are more likely to arrest spontaneously. The mortality from malformation hemorrhage is approximately 10%. Production of temporary hypercoagulability (e.g., with substances such as epsilon aminocaproic acid) decreases the likelihood of rebleeding from aneurysms, presumably by increasing the likelihood of clotting within the aneurysm and at its rupture site. The rebleeding, which is likely to occur in the first two weeks after the initial hemorrhage, is the major cause of death.

Intraparenchymal hemorrhage causes death in almost two thirds of an unselected series of patients, with the exception of cerebellar hemorrhage, which, when treated by aspiration, may have a mortality in the range of 50%. Lobar hemorrhage may have a mortality of less than 50% with or without surgical treatment. The comatose patient with intraparenchymal hemorrhage at any site rarely survives; the alert and stable patient has a much better prognosis.

CT scanning has recognized many small intraparenchymal self-limited hemorrhages that in the past were evident only as rapid-onset clinical deficits of a focal nature and were presumed to be ischemic strokes. Adding these cases to the total population of persons with hemorrhage has progressively decreased the mortality statistics. Nevertheless, for the clinically catastrophic presentation, the prognosis for survival still remains very poor.

REFERENCES

Hutchinson, E. G., Acheson, J.: *Strokes: Natural History, Pathology and Surgical Treatment.* Philadelphia, W. B. Saunders Co., 1975.

Marshall, J.: *The Management of Cerebrovascular Disease*, ed. 3. Oxford, Blackwell Scientific Publications, 1976.

15

Mass Lesions

NEOPLASMS, BOTH MALIGNANT AND BENIGN, are the most common mass lesions affecting the intracranial and intraspinal contents. Inflammatory masses (i.e., granuloma, abscess, and, rarely, localized hemorrhagic viral encephalitis) and chronic subdural hematomas and subdural abscesses are less common mass lesions, which on occasion must be considered in the differential diagnosis. They are expanding mass lesions and therefore their clinical presentation is much the same as that of neoplasms, except that the inflammatory lesions are frequently associated with some systemic signs of infection. Acute spontaneous intracranial hemorrhage also presents as an expanding intracranial mass lesion unless it is confined to the subarachnoid space.

We use neoplasms as our model in this chapter. Many of the principles concerning the effects of neoplasms also hold for other categories of mass lesions. They are considered further in chapters 12, 14, and 17.

Table 15–1 lists the types of neoplasms that most commonly affect the brain and spinal cord. Central nervous system neoplasms are seen in persons of all ages. Posterior cranial fossa and spinal cord neoplasms predominate in children, whereas middle and anterior cranial fossa tumors are most common in adults. Metastatic neoplasms are common in adults and unusual in children. Breast and lung carcinomas are the most common neoplasms in adults to metastasize to the CNS, and they do so in about one quarter of persons who have these malig-

nancies. The most common primary neoplasms are gliomas, and malignant astrocytoma (glioblastoma multiforme) leads the list.

There is a hereditary predisposition to develop CNS neoplasms in individuals with von Recklinghausen's disease (neurofibromatosis) who have a relatively high incidence of acoustic and other cranial nerve neurilemomas, glial neoplasms, and meningiomas. The same predisposition is seen in persons with tuberous sclerosis and several other rare conditions.

The manifestations of CNS neoplasms are several and depend on a variety of factors. *Ablation* of nervous tissue and loss of function are to a large degree proportional to the rate of tumor growth. Slow-growing neoplasms such as meningiomas and neurilemomas cause relatively little dysfunction until very late because of the ability of the brain (and to lesser degree the spinal cord) to accommodate and compensate in pace with the expanding, compressive process. Rapidly enlarging neoplasms such as metastatic tumors and glioblastomas cause early progressive loss of function. Occasionally, a rapidly growing neoplasm causes sudden loss of function and appears as a stroke. This is usually the result of hemorrhage into the core of the neoplasm, which has become necrotic by outstripping its blood supply. Also, edema may appear rapidly in and around certain neoplasms, most notably metastatic tumors, and cause the rapid appearance of symptoms and signs. Though dysfunction appears rapidly with glioblastomas, it is frequently less than the tumor size would predict because the tumor infiltrates nervous tissue and leaves many neurons functioning. Removal of the tumor therefore almost always increases a patient's neurologic deficit.

Loss of function also depends on the tumor's *location*. Frontal-pole tumors produce few, if any, deficits until they are very large (we have on record a frontal-pole menin-

TABLE 15-1.—MOST COMMON NEOPLASMS TO INVOLVE CENTRAL NERVOUS SYSTEM

LOCATION	TYPE
Cerebral hemispheres	*Primary*
	Glioma
	Glioblastoma
	Astrocytoma
	Oligodendroglioma
	Meningioma
	Secondary
	Metastatic carcinoma
	Lung
	Breast
	Bowel
	Kidney
	Ovary
	Melanoma
Cerebellum	*Primary*
	Glioma
	Gliomas of childhood
	Medulloblastoma
	Astrocytoma
	Hemangioblastoma
	Secondary
	Metastatic carcinoma
	Lung
	Breast
	Other
Pituitary	Adenoma
	Functional
	Eosinophilic
	Basophilic
	Invasive
	Nonfunctional
	Chromophobe
	Craniopharyngioma
Brain stem	Childhood gliomas
	Ependymoma
Cranial nerves	Neurilemoma
	Acoustic—vestibular
	Other nerves
Spinal cord	Ependymoma
	Astrocytoma
	Meningioma
	Neurofibroma
	Neurilemoma
	Metastatic

gioma that was the size of an orange and produced no noticeable loss of function). At the other extreme, very small metastases or primary tumors involving the functionally compact brain stem and spinal cord may cause early dysfunction. Intracranial tumors usually produce focal (segmental) defects by direct compression of nervous tissue, by edema (which on occasion and for unknown reasons can be massive) within nervous tissue in and around the mass, and by ischemia caused by compression of blood vessels supplying the surrounding brain. Some rapidly growing and very vascular neoplasms may cause ischemic deficits by stealing the blood flow from proximate normal brain tissue.

Expanding masses, both supratentorial and subtentorial, create vectors of force that can only be directed toward the major exit of the otherwise closed cranial cavity, the foramen magnum. This gives rise to a frequently lethal secondary effect of mass lesions, tentorial and foramen magnum herniation, or rostrocaudal deterioration, which is discussed further in chapter 19 on stupor and coma. Infants whose cranial sutures are not closed do not show rostrocaudal deterioration until quite late because the cranial cavity can enlarge progressively with widening of the sutures. Papilledema, swelling of the optic nerve head, which is a reflection of increased intracranial pressure, is also late in developing or absent in infants with expansion of the intracranial contents for the same reasons.

Neoplasms involving the pituitary gland, hypothalamus, or both most commonly give rise to ablative dysfunction with *systemic metabolic effects*. Combinations of loss of posterior pituitary function (diabetes insipidus) and anterior pituitary function (hypogonadism, hypoadrenalism, hypothyroidism, and insufficient growth) are seen. Hypothalamic involvement may also cause changes in behavior (hypophagia, hyperphagia, placidity, sedation, low threshold for rage reactions) and autonomic function disorders (Horner's syndrome, disordered temperature regulation with hypothermia from posterior involvement or hyperthermia from anterior involvement). Encroachment on the neighboring optic chiasma leads to visual field defects, classically bitemporal hemianopia (see chap. 3).

Anterior pituitary tumors may produce *positive humoral effects*. Eosinophilic adenomas secreting growth hormone are associated with gigantism in children or acromegaly in adults, whereas basophilic adenomas are associated with Cushing's hyperadrenal syndrome. Anterior pituitary adenomas are frequently associated with excess prolactin production and galactorrhea; this may be more pronounced and is more commonly associated with tumors that have extended beyond the confines of the pituitary fossa.

A more bizarre positive humoral affect is seen with some hemangioblastomas of the cerebellum. An erythropoietin-like substance is secreted, causing polycythemia.

Irritative phenomena commonly are the presenting symptoms and signs of neoplasm. Seizures are the problems that bring approximately one quarter of persons with neoplasms to a physician and localize the tumor to the cerebral hemispheres. If focal, the seizures may localize the tumor precisely. Any patient over the age of 30 who has a recent onset of seizures, particularly focal seizures, is considered a tumor suspect until adequate neurologic workup proves otherwise.

Pain, specifically headache or backache, occurs in a high proportion of persons with rapidly expanding masses, less often with slow-growing tumors, and is a manifestation of increased intracranial pressure and traction on the pain-sensitive structures of the cranium and spine (the blood vessels, meninges, bony envelopments, and dorsal roots, less often central sensory tracts); pain can be significant in localization.

Increased intracranial pressure is characteristic of many intracranial masses and it is related to tumor size, edema, rapidity of growth, ventricular system obstruction (i.e., hydrocephalus), rate of cerebrospinal fluid absorption relative to production, venous obstruction, presence or absence of closed cranial sutures, and other unknown factors. The most common symptom associated with increased intracranial pressure is headache, frequently worse in the mornings after the subject has been horizontal through the night, which presumably causes a slight increase in pressure in the superior vena cava-jugular system and therefore intracranially. Strictly speaking, however, increased intracranial pressure alone does not necessarily cause headache. It is usually the process that has caused the increased pressure that also causes the headache by involving pain-sensitive intracranial structures such as superficial cerebral vessels, dura, and some cranial and upper spinal nerves (see chap. 16). Possibly, increased morning headache is then the result of increased pressure-induced peri- and intratumor edema with accentuation of the tumor's size and traction effects. Nausea and vomiting are also relatively common and considered secondary to traction on lower brain stem emetic centers or a reflection of increased autonomic afferent bombardment of the brain stem caused by traction of blood vessels and meningeal investments.

The most easily observed and most telling sign of increased intracranial pressure on examination is papilledema, swelling of the optic nerve head, which is associated with a loss of retinal venous pulsations and enlargement of the blind spot on visual field testing. (See the section on papilledema in chap. 1.) As mentioned, papilledema may not be manifested in infants whose cranial sutures have not yet closed. Also, older patients who have increased intraocular pressure (glaucoma) do not readily develop papilledema.

A rising or, less commonly, a slowed pulse rate and elevation of blood pressure are occasional and ominous signs of increasing intracranial pressure and imminent or ongoing rostrocaudal deterioration. It is hypothesized by some that rising pulse rate and blood pressure are compensatory autoregulating responses to the decreased cerebral blood flow caused by the raised intracranial pressure. The slowed pulse, when it occurs, appears to be a vagal excitation or release phenomenon. It may be a response of the carotid sinus to the acute rise in blood pressure or a release of the medulla and vagal outflow from diencephalic sympathetic counter forces.

In infants prior to the age of 1½ years, the anterior fontanelle is open and on palpation is usually depressed and pulsatile. With an increase in intracranial pressure, the fontanelle bulges even when the infant is held in an erect position and pulsations may be absent.

False localizing signs are abnormalities found on neurologic examination that are distant and frequently misleading secondary effects of tumor enlargement. The most common are related to expanding supratentorial masses and are: (1) unilateral or bilateral sixth-nerve palsies caused by rostrocaudal displacement of the brain stem with stretching of the already taut abducens nerves; (2) third-nerve dysfunction from compression by herniating temporal lobe as the nerve passes forward at the edge of the tentorium; (3) compression of the contralateral cerebral peduncle against the edge of the tentorium, causing an ipsilateral to mass hemiparesis; (4) posterior cerebral artery compression against the edge of the ipsilateral to mass tentorium, causing ischemia-infarction of the occipital cortex and a contralateral homonymous hemianopsia; and (5) hydrocephalus secondary to tumor compression and occlusion of fourth ventricle, aqueduct of Sylvius, third ventricle, or foramen of Monro, which causes diffuse hemispheric dysfunction (i.e., dementia) that may obscure the local compressive and destructive signs of the mass itself.

It is typical for a person with a neoplasm to have a downhill course interrupted by periods of some improvement. No proved explanation of this phenomenon is available; however, it is speculated that changing levels of edema and vascular integrity around the tumor are important and that circadian changes in circulating cortisol levels may bring about these changes. Variations in absorption and production of cerebrospinal fluid in response to the mass and increased intracranial pressure may also play a role.

In summary, the typical patient afflicted with a rapidly growing brain tumor has a progressive focal loss of neurologic function, with or without seizure activity. He complains of headache, which is frequently worse in the morning and associated with nausea, less often vomiting, and may be generalized or focal. On examination, early or well-developed papilledema may be present and focal signs of neurologic dysfunction are elicited.

In contrast, the person with a slowly growing neoplasm (e.g., meningioma) may develop very little abnormality until the tumor has become very large (may take many years) and accommodation is no longer possible, at which time a relatively acute decompensation may occur.

With spinal cord neoplasm, extrinsic or intrinsic, progressive segmental and long-tract motor and sensory deficits are typical. Focal back, neck, or limb pain is most common, with extramedullary masses affecting spinal roots and the bony encasement.

A thorough neurologic examination utilizing the patient's story to assess the problem usually localizes the neoplasm.

X-rays of the skull, brain scan, and electroencephalography are routine diagnostic procedures to be carried out on all persons suspected of having an intracranial tumor. Computerized axial tomography (CT) scanning is routine where available. By this noninvasive procedure, intracranial lesions that are of different density from the brain can be delineated. Where density differences are too small for visualization, enhancement procedures may be effective (see chap. 18).

Opacification of the cerebral arteries and veins (angiography) is the next step. Distortion of the arteries and veins and ventricular and subarachnoid spaces by mass lesions is sought in these studies. Abnormal tumor vessels can also be delineated with arteriography in some neoplasms. Arteriovenous malformations and giant aneurysms may be manifested as mass lesions and are best delineated by angiography. Angiography is followed if necessary by pneumoencephalography or ventriculography, which is more hazardous because of a finite possibility of precipitating rostrocaudal deterioration. For this reason, these tests are best carried out in cooperation with a neurosurgeon who can intervene rapidly if deterioration occurs. (Where CT scanning is available, these tests have become almost obsolete.)

Lumbar puncture is carried out to study the cerebrospinal fluid after results of the routine diagnostic procedures have proved negative. If preliminary observations indicate a mass lesion or suggest increased intracranial pressure, a lumbar puncture should not be done because of the chance of precipitating rostrocaudal deterioration by the rapid and possibly differential lowering of the CSF pressure in the lumbar subarachnoid space. A lumbar puncture is carried out as a preliminary examination only when (1) CNS infection (in particular, meningitis) is suspected, (2) one is considering immediate anticoagulation in a patient with stroke-in-evolution, and (3) a patient has severe acute headache or other symptoms or a history that suggests subarachnoid hemorrhage in the absence of focal neurologic deficit. In the latter situation, focal deficit demands hospital admission for comprehensive study including arteriography *prior* to lumbar puncture. With neoplasm, elevation of the level of protein in the CSF is the major finding sought, and it is nonspecifically elevated in a majority of persons. Occasionally neoplastic cells are shed into the CSF and can be identified by cytologic techniques; tumor typing may also be

possible. Both metastatic and primary malignant neoplasms are likely to shed malignant cells into the CSF, particularly those tumors located near the subarachnoid or ventricular surface of the brain. Rarely, a meningeal inflammatory response occurs with superficial and especially necrotic tumors. The CSF is infiltrated with predominantly mononuclear white cells. A polymorphonuclear cell predominance may occur, and there may be an acute, full-blown clinical picture of meningitis.

Spine films are routine for persons suspected of harboring spinal neoplasm. Progressive para- or quadriparesis is characteristic of spinal tumor and is a major neurologic emergency. Myelography (opacification of the spinal subarachnoid space by a radiopaque dye or delineation of canal contents by air, see chap. 18) is the definitive study and should be done as soon as possible so that surgical and/or medical treatment can be started prior to final and irreversible compression and infarction of the spinal cord.

Treatment of CNS neoplasms is either palliative (surgical decompression, chemotherapy and radiotherapy, and corticosteroid and hyperosmotic agent decrease of edema) or curative (surgical removal, occasionally radiotherapy and rarely chemotherapy). Palliative therapy is used most for malignant tumors or tumors that are not removable because of proximity to or presence within vital centers. Curative therapy is most often for benign, accessible tumors and rarely for isolated, single metastases.

REFERENCES

Jennett, W. B.: *An Introduction to Neurosurgery,* ed. 3. St. Louis, C. V. Mosby Co., 1977.

Rubinstein, L. J.: *Tumors of the Central Nervous System, Atlas of Tumor Pathology,* 2d Series, fasc. 6. Washington, D.C., Armed Forces Institute of Pathology, 1972.

16

Headaches

EDWARD VALENSTEIN

Introduction

INTRACRANIAL DISEASE can produce pain in only a limited number of ways. With rare exception, stimulation or destruction of the brain itself does not produce pain. The following intracranial structures are pain-sensitive:

1. Meningeal arteries
2. Proximal portions of the cerebral arteries
3. Dura at the base of the brain
4. Venous sinuses
5. Cranial nerves 5, 7, 9, and 10 and cervical nerves 1, 2, and 3

DISTORTION OR TRACTION

Increased intracranial pressure, when it does not result in traction on pain-sensitive structures, does not cause headache. You may raise your own intracranial pressure to abnormally high values transiently by the Valsalva maneuver; this does not cause pain. Conversely, an intracranial mass that distorts the dura or the arteries at the base of the brain causes headache even if the intracranial pressure is normal.

Drainage of spinal fluid with the patient in erect posture causes headache, presumably secondary to traction on the venous sinuses. This is thought to be the mechanism of headache following lumbar puncture, which is relieved when the person lies down.

DISTENSION OF A VESSEL

Distension of extracranial and occasionally intracranial arteries is thought to be the cause of pain in migraine. Increased flow through collateral circulation may produce the headache that sometimes accompanies large-vessel occlusion.

INFLAMMATION

Inflammation in the subarachnoid space, whether caused by infection, hemorrhage, or chemical irritation, results in headache.

REFERRAL OF PAIN

In general, lesions above the tentorium produce pain that is referred to the trigeminal distribution (the forehead or behind the eye), because the dura in this region is supplied by the trigeminal nerve. Lesions in the posterior fossa produce pain in the ear and the back of the head (this part of the dura is supplied by cranial nerves 9 and 10 and the upper three cervical roots). When the first cervical segment has a dorsal root (as in about 50% of individuals), it may, in addition to receiving afferents from the posterior fossa, which refer pain to the occiput and ear, refer pain to the orbit. It has been speculated that this is related to the overlap of the lowermost portion of the spinal nucleus of the trigeminal nerve (somatotopically representing the

175

ophthalmic division) and the uppermost portion of the substantia gelatinosa. Irritation of cranial nerves 7, 9, and 10 may be referred to the ear, because the ear has cutaneous supply from each of these nerves as well as cranial nerve 5.

Although the location of pain may at times be misleading, in general, pain *lateralization* accurately predicts the side of the lesion.

Classification of Headaches

Table 16–1 presents a clinically useful classification of headaches. The clinical evaluation of the person who has headaches should be designed to define a primary cause for headache when possible (categories A and B) and thereby rule out disease that might endanger the patient. When this is not possible, the evaluation should suggest a classification of the headache based on the characteristic symptoms (categories C and D).

DANGEROUS HEADACHES

These represent a small minority of headaches. Fortunately, with a little thought, it is quite easy to rule out most of these conditions on the basis of the history and examination alone. Most of these conditions are discussed elsewhere in this book. The following comments apply to the patient whose chief complaint is headache (i.e., the patient is not comatose or hemiplegic, etc.). This does not imply that isolated headache is the typical presentation for these conditions, but the person who has a hemiparesis or seizure or coma from a tumor or intracranial hemorrhage does not present a problem in the differential diagnosis of headache.

MENINGEAL IRRITATION.—These include subarachnoid hemorrhage and meningitis.

Subarachnoid hemorrhage.—Arterial bleeding in the subarachnoid space from a ruptured aneurysm is almost invariably accompanied by the *sudden* (instantaneous) onset of *severe* pain and frequently vomiting.

The pain persists and the patient usually looks very ill or uncomfortable. Nuchal rigidity is often (but not always) found. The remainder of the neurologic examination *can* be normal. The history of the *sudden* onset of a severe headache that persists, therefore, indicates subarachnoid hemorrhage until proved otherwise. Lumbar puncture is indicated in the absence of neurologic signs other than those of meningeal irritation.

Meningitis.—This diagnosis should not prove difficult because the patient looks ill, and fever and nuchal rigidity are usually present. Remember that in the elderly or debilitated person and in the young child, nuchal rigidity may not be present (see chap. 12).

INTRACRANIAL MASS LESIONS.—This category contains neoplasms, intracerebral hemorrhage, subdural or epidural hemorrhage, abscess, and hydrocephalus.

Neoplasms.—Persons often seek medical advice about their headaches because they are afraid they have a brain tumor. Fortunately, although most persons with brain tumors have headache, the vast majority of patients with headache do not have brain tumors. The headache of brain tumor is often mild and nonspecific; it may be worse in the morning; and on examination, vigorous head shaking may elicit focal pain. If focal symptoms, seizures, focal neurologic signs, or evidence of increased intracranial pressure are present, a full evaluation must be undertaken. In the absence of any of these findings, brain tumor may practically be dismissed as a diagnosis.

Intracerebral hemorrhage.—This is nearly always accompanied by focal neurologic signs or symptoms. Hypertension, trauma, or defects in coagulation are the usual antecedents (see chap. 14).

Subdural or epidural hemorrhage.—Epidural and acute subdural hemorrhage occurs in the context of acute head trauma. The chronic subdural hematoma may manifest itself weeks or months after an injury, and headache may be the most prominent symp-

TABLE 16-1.—CLASSIFICATION OF HEADACHES

A. Dangerous headaches
  1. Meningeal irritation
    a. Subarachnoid hemorrhage
    b. Meningitis and meningoencephalitis
  2. Intracranial mass lesions
    a. Neoplasms
    b. Intracerebral hemorrhage
    c. Subdural or epidural hemorrhage
    d. Abscess
    e. Acute hydrocephalus
    f. Other
  3. Vascular headaches
    a. Temporal arteritis
    b. Hypertensive encephalopathy
    c. Arteriovenous malformations and expanding aneurysms
  4. Cervical fracture or dislocation
  5. Metabolic
    a. Hypoglycemia
    b. Hypercapnea
    c. Anoxia
    d. Anemia
  6. Glaucoma

B. Extracranial lesions
  1. Sinuses (infection, tumor)
  2. Cervical spine disease
  3. Dental problems
  4. Temporomandibular joint
  5. Ear infections, etc.
  6. Eye (glaucoma, uveitis)
  7. Extracranial arteries
  8. Nerve lesions
  9. Other
C. Specific syndromes
  1. Migraine
  2. Cluster headaches
  3. Neuralgias
    a. Trigeminal (tic douloureux)
    b. Glossopharyngeal
  4. Others
D. Nonspecific headaches
  1. "Tension" headache
  2. Posttraumatic
  3. Metabolic
  4. Psychiatric
  5. Other

tom. This headache must be differentiated from the common postconcussion headache. The latter may persist for weeks or months after an injury and may be accompanied by dizziness or vertigo and mild mental changes. All these symptoms gradually subside. When symptoms increase or when there are lateralizing neurologic findings, subdural hematoma must be suspected.

Abscess (see chap. 12).—Focal signs or mental changes are often present. There may be evidence of increased intracranial pressure. The history may suggest some source of infection (ear infection, bronchiectasis, etc.) or a reason to be susceptible to infection (cyanotic congenital heart disease, immunosuppressant therapy).

Acute hydrocephalus.—This may be caused by inflammation, blood, or tumor obstructing CSF pathways. Acute hydrocephalus is accompanied by evidence of brain dysfunction: confusion, lethargy, ataxia, incontinence, and others. The fundi may show evidence of increased intracranial pressure.

VASCULAR HEADACHES.—These headaches include temporal arteritis, hypertensive encephalopathy, and vascular malformations.

Temporal arteritis.—This is a systemic vasculitis with a predilection for the cranial vessels, which rarely occurs in persons less than 50 years old. The clinical picture may include (1) polymyalgia rheumatica—malaise, loss of energy, proximal joint pains, and myalgias; (2) nonspecific headaches, sometimes associated with tenderness and swelling over the temporal arteries; and (3) evidence of arterial insufficiency. The latter may involve the external carotid circulation, producing the unique symptoms of jaw claudication or infarction of the tongue or scalp; or it may involve the internal carotid circulation, producing retinal ischemia and blindness or, less commonly, stroke. The sedimentation rate is usually very high. The disease can be dramatically reversed with steroids. In the person over 50, the ESR should therefore be checked if the history is moderately suggestive of temporal arteritis or polymyalgia rheumatica. If the ESR is high, a temporal artery biopsy often confirms the diagnosis, and treatment can be started without delay. At times, the clinical picture may be sufficiently suggestive so that a trial of therapy may be indicated despite normal test results.

Hypertensive encephalopathy.—Cerebral vasoconstriction occurs in response to systemic hypertension to preserve a constant cerebral blood flow. It is thought that in persons with hypertensive encephalopathy, this cerebral autoregulation fails and segments of arteries dilate despite severe hypertension. This results in edema and hemorrhage. The diagnosis should be considered in patients with severe hypertension (diastolic pressure more than 120 mm Hg) or in previously normotensive patients who suddenly develop less severe hypertension. Retinal changes and renal disease are frequent accompaniments. Milder degrees of hypertension are generally not associated with headache.

Vascular malformations.—Headache from vascular malformations is discussed later in relation to migraine headache.

CERVICAL FRACTURE OR DISLOCATION.— Pain from the cervical region (arising from periosteum, ligaments, nerve irritation, or reflex muscle spasm) is usually felt over the neck and occiput, but can be referred around the temples and into the frontal region. In a person with a history of neck trauma or with symptoms or signs of cervical root or cord compression, cervical spine x-rays must be obtained to rule out a condition that might result in cord compression. Lateral views in flexion and extension are useful to detect excessive mobility of the spine.

METABOLIC HEADACHES.—Headache is often associated with hypoxemia, hypercapnea, and anemia, possibly related to the cerebral vasodilatation that may accompany these conditions.

GLAUCOMA.—Headache may accompany glaucoma, usually the acute, narrow-angle type. Pain is localized in the eye or behind the eye.

From the preceding discussion, a physician can be fairly sure of excluding "dangerous" headaches by the following:

1. There should be no history of serious head or neck injury, of seizures or focal neurologic symptoms, or of infections that may predispose to meningitis or brain abscess.
2. The patient should be afebrile.
3. The diastolic blood pressure should not be greater than 120.
4. The fundi should be normal.
5. The neck should be supple.
6. There should be no cranial bruits.
7. The neurologic examination should be normal; the patient should not be lethargic or confused.
8. In appropriate cases, complete blood cell count, ESR, skull or neck x-rays should be obtained.

The duration of the headache is also significant: headache arising recently in a patient who is not prone to them arouses more suspicions than headache that has been recurrent for years. In addition, the patient's complaints often suggest an alternative diagnosis. A patient with typical migraine or cluster headache need not be evaluated for other causes of headache.

HEADACHES FROM EXTRACRANIAL LESIONS

These are listed in part in Table 16–1. The location of the pain often suggests the site of pathology. Other symptoms may accompany the condition: postnasal drip may accompany sinusitis, and on examination there may be tenderness over the affected sinus. Pain increased by chewing points to dental or temporomandibular joint pathology. Uveitis or glaucoma should not be easily missed. Errors of refraction do not commonly cause headache (despite the popular belief to the contrary). The headaches that accompany cervical spine disease may resemble "tension" headaches, in that both produce spasm of neck musculature.

SPECIFIC HEADACHE SYNDROMES

MIGRAINE.—A migraine attack may consist of an aura and a headache, or either alone. In the absence of the aura, it may be difficult to diagnose migraine with certainty. The following are useful diagnostic features (the most helpful are shown by asterisks):

*1. The headache is episodic; persons can usually tell exactly when a migraine is beginning. The end of the headache may be less well defined, but it is unusual for a migraine to last more than 1–2 days.

2. Onset is often in childhood or adolescence, although it can arise at any age.

3. The headache is often unilateral (but may be bilateral).

*4. The headache is usually severe, throbbing, and often accompanied by nausea (and sometimes by vomiting, diarrhea, and other symptoms).

5. The headache lasts from several hours to two days.

6. Patients often feel like going to bed, and sleep may terminate an attack.

7. There is frequently a family history of migraine.

8. It can sometimes be relieved by taking ergotamine early in the course.

9. Photophobia and an intolerance of loud sounds are common complaints during the headache.

10. There may be a history in childhood of motion sickness or cyclic vomiting.

Physiologically, the headache of migraine is accompanied by vasodilatation of the extracranial arteries, and compression of the carotid (not recommended) or temporal artery on the side of the headache may relieve the pain. Treatment with vasoconstrictors (chiefly ergotamine) may abort a headache.

The *aura* of a migraine is much more specific than the headache, and a diagnosis of migraine may be made on the basis of the nature of the aura alone. As mentioned, the aura is not always present; in fact, migraine without aura (called "common migraine") is much more common than migraine with aura (called "classic migraine"). Being able to define the aura, however, is important not only in diagnosing migraine but also in differentiating this from more serious conditions (seizures or TIAs).

The aura of migraine is thought to be initiated by intracranial vasoconstriction and consequent cerebral ischemia. Treatment with ergotamine sometimes prolongs an aura. Rarely, the aura persists permanently, indicating infarction of the brain. The most common symptoms involve *visual, somatosensory,* and *language* functions.

The visual aura is variable: scintillating scotomata are characteristic, but negative scotomata, or blurring of the visual field, may also be seen. The symptoms are often homonymous (from cortical involvement), but symptoms referable to retinal ischemia (visual loss in one eye only) may also exist. The onset is gradual, and the symptoms usually last from 10 to 60 minutes.

The somatosensory march of migraine is characteristic and can be differentiated from sensory seizures or from the usual form of TIA by the following:

1. The onset is gradual.

2. The march is slow; if it arises in the hand, it may take several minutes to reach the elbow and then the face. (Sensory seizure is more rapid.)

3. It usually clears first in the area that was first involved; that is, if it marched from the hand to the face, it clears first in the hand.

4. The symptoms clear, usually within 10 to 60 minutes.

Aphasia is the third most common feature of the migrainous aura. When all three symptoms appear as part of the same aura, it is characteristic for them to appear successively (e.g., visual, then sensory, then speech) rather than concomitantly (although this can also occur).

The slow march of symptoms has led to the speculation that vasoconstriction and cortical ischemia may initiate the aura but that some other process such as spreading cortical depression prolongs it. The rate of march of spreading cortical depression (a wave of depolarization), to date only demonstrated experimentally, has been calculated to be approximtely the same as the rate of march of migrainous scintillating scotomata across the visual field. Repolarization and normal function occur in the wake of the spreading depolarization wave and might well explain the clearing of the visual or somesthetic effects first in the areas first involved.

Other symptoms sometimes associated with the aura (but seen much less often) are true motor weakness, emotional changes, micropsia or macropsia, and symptoms of basilar artery ischemia (diplopia, coma, vertigo). Ophthalmoplegic migraine is a variant that appears clinically quite distinct. Most commonly, the oculomotor nerve is involved; less often, the abducens nerve. Onset of the problem is usually in early childhood. Often the oculomotor or abducens paresis lasts for many weeks after the onset at the *height* of the headache. It is presumed that internal carotid artery dilatation is part of these patients' migraine, and at its height the carotid compresses either the third or sixth nerve in the cavernous sinus to cause paresis or paralysis. With compression damage, one would expect a prolonged recovery period. These rarer manifestations of migraine are often perplexing even to the experienced clinician.

The migrainous aura usually precedes the headache, but it may accompany it or follow it or occur on its own. The latter is particularly true in elderly persons who have a long history of migraine. The headache is often less severe than in common migraine. The headache may be either contralateral or ipsilateral to the neurologic symptoms (or it may be bilateral). This suggests that the aura and the headache may be caused by changes in different circulatory beds—the aura from intracranial vessels and the headache from extracranial vessels.

The treatment of migraine varies with the patient's complaint. If *headache* is the main complaint, ergotamine (when not contraindicated by pregnancy, hypertension, or occlusive vascular disease) is the drug of choice. Cafergot is the most commonly prescribed medication. If the aura is the main problem, ergotamines are probably best avoided. One of the prophylactic medications (phenytoin, propranolol, methysergide, tricyclic antidepressant) can be used if the headaches are severe and frequent (one headache per week or more). Quite often the person who has classic migraine merely needs the reassurance of a diagnosis and does not require any therapy for his infrequent headaches.

The physician should be familiar with the clinical picture of migraine because migraine is rarely *symptomatic* of an underlying illness. A rare exception is arteriovenous malformation (AVM). AVMs (without bleeding) may cause recurrent unilateral migrainous headaches and (even more rarely) may be accompanied by a migraine-like aura. Listening for a cranial bruit should be routine. It is reassuring for the patient with migraine to have had some headaches on the other side or to have the headache ipsilateral to the aura, because this would not be likely with a structural lesion. If this is not the case, the examiner may consider further evaluation to rule out an AVM (skull x-rays, EEG, and CT scan with and without contrast); however, unless one is prepared to suggest surgery for an AVM whose only manifestation is headache, further tests can be deferred.

CLUSTER HEADACHES.—These are characterized as follows:

1. The headache is brief (15 minutes to 2 hours).
2. It occurs once or twice daily (or more),

often at the same time and often at night.

3. The headache is very severe; persons with the headache are usually agitated and prefer to pace the floor.
4. It is often accompanied by lacrimation and nasal congestion on the same side as the headache. An ipsilateral Horner's syndrome may be present during the headache, and miosis may persist after the headache.
5. The headaches occur in *clusters;* they may occur daily for several weeks or months and then disappear entirely for months or years, only to recur later.
6. Men are more commonly affected than women (10:1).

These headaches, although often classified as a type of migraine, are clinically distinct from common or classic migraine. There is also a chemical difference: Persons with migraine have an increase in the level of blood serotonin at the onset of their headache; persons with cluster headache have no change in serotonin levels but have an increase in blood histamine concentration coincident with their headache. In neither instance is the pathogenesis of the headache understood. Despite these differences, cluster headaches may be helped by prophylactic ergotamine administration, methysergide, or other medications effective for migraine prophylaxis. Cluster headaches are not preceded or accompanied by an aura.

NEURALGIAS.—Neuralgic pain is characteristic; it is very sharp, severe, and brief. There is commonly a "trigger point"—an area of skin or mucosa that, when touched, provokes the pain. *Tic douloureux (trigeminal neuralgia)* usually occurs in the elderly and usually involves the second and third divisions of the trigeminal nerve. It should not be accompanied by sensory loss. If there is sensory loss, a structural lesion must be suspected. Neuralgic pain must be distinguished from dental pain, particularly maloc-

clusions. When present in the young adult, it may be symptomatic of multiple sclerosis.

Treatment with phenytoin or carbamazepine is often effective. In persons who do not respond to medical treatment, transection of the trigeminal sensory root may be necessary.

Glossopharyngeal neuralgia is much less common. In this condition, neuralgic pain is felt in the throat and neck and may be triggered by swallowing.

OTHER VARIETIES OF HEADACHE

Dangerous headaches are rare, headaches caused by definable extracranial lesions are more common, and migraine is probably still more common. The majority of people who have headache, however, have none of these conditions. They have muscle tension headaches.

TENSION HEADACHES.—Most people, when under sufficient pressure, get a mild cervical or bifrontal headache. EMG of the frontalis muscle or of the cervical musculature reveals hyperactivity, and measures directed at relaxing these muscles (diazepam, biofeedback therapy, massage) often relieve the headache. At times tension headaches are quite severe, but generally people are able to continue working with them (unlike the case with many migraines or the usual cluster headache) and rarely are ill enough to seek a physician's aid. The headache may be more prominent when the patient thinks he is more relaxed (in the evening or on weekends).

"PSYCHIATRIC" HEADACHES.—A small number of persons complain of intractable, constant, severe, disabling headache for which no cause can be found. As a rule, these persons are severely depressed or have other serious psychopathology. Their headaches may respond to the same medication as common tension headaches, but often they are resistant to all treatment, even narcotic analgesics. Psychiatric treatment or psychotropic drugs (such as antidepressants) are sometimes effective.

REFERENCES

Dalessio, D. J.: *Wolff's Headache and Other Head Pain,* ed. 3. New York, Oxford University Press, 1972.

Sacks, D. W.: *Migraine: Evolution of a Common Disorder.* Berkeley/Los Angeles, University of California Press, 1970.

17

Cranial and Spinal Trauma

JOHN WOODFORD and ALEXANDER REEVES

Cranial Trauma

VEHICULAR ACCIDENTS are the major cause of head trauma in this country. Of those who die from vehicular accidents, 75% die from the primary and secondary effects of trauma on the vital centers of the central nervous system. Of those who survive major head trauma, defects in CNS functioning, ablative or irritative in nature, may be residual, although surprisingly good recovery is the rule if the person survives the days and weeks after trauma.

This chapter deals mainly with evaluation of the person with suspected or proved head injury. As a preamble, some basic principles and definitions should be discussed.

The major effects of trauma on the brain can be divided into two categories: primary and secondary (or late) effects.

The *primary effects* are those that are caused directly by the head trauma and include concussion, contusion, and laceration of the central nervous system.

Concussion is a reversible state of diffuse cerebral dysfunction associated with a transient alteration in consciousness. Typically, there is loss of recently imprinted events (retrograde amnesia) extending for some seconds or minutes prior to the injury and, rarely, with more severe impact, for days or more. A variable period of inability to learn new material (anterograde amnesia) typically follows recovery of consciousness and may

be dense enough to leave the patient with no memory of early postinjury events. Rarely, some patients tell of being "unconscious" for weeks to as long as several months following head injury. In fact, they were not unconscious but were unable to imprint ongoing events. The retrograde amnesia is presumed to be caused by a mechanical distortion of neurons, probably in the temporal lobes, which consolidate the memory trace. The anterograde amnesia is presumed to be the result of distortion of the mesial temporal-limbic circuits known to be necessary for learning.

The underlying pathophysiology of concussion appears to be a shearing effect. Rapid displacement of the head, in either acceleration or deceleration injury, causes a swirling of the cerebrum within the cranium, and shearing forces play most markedly at the junctions between brain tissues of different density. The major zone of diffuse injury is, therefore, the interface between gray and white matter. It is here that microscopic evidence of ruptured axons is found experimentally. It is not surprising that repeated concussions, such as boxers experience, may lead to dementia.

Penetrating injuries of the cranium, such as bullet wounds, frequently cause only focal cerebral dysfunction without loss of consciousness because no cranial displacement and brain shearing occur.

183

Contusions of the brain are bruises usually associated with more severe trauma than necessary for concussion. They are most prominent at the summits of gyri, the cerebral poles, and portions of the brain stem. All these regions lie close to the bony and dural surfaces of the cranial cavity. They may directly underlie the site of the blow to the cranium or may be opposite the site of impact (contrecoup).

Laceration of the brain usually follows cranial trauma severe enough to cause fracture of the skull and penetrating injury to the brain by skull fragments or foreign objects. However, fracture of the skull need not be associated with laceration or contusion or major concussion. On the other hand, laceration may on occasion occur with severe shearing forces unassociated with fracture. Usually some form of hemorrhage (intracerebral, subdural, epidural) is associated with laceration.

The *secondary effects* of cranial trauma that may further compromise brain function are edema, hypoxia, hemorrhage, infection, and epilepsy. *Edema* may be the result of diffuse shearing of capillary, glial, and neuronal membranes or may be secondary to local contusion or laceration. Edema can compromise both arterial and venous cerebral blood flow, causing ischemia and more edema, a vicious cycle sometimes impossible to reverse. The mass effect of edema, focal or diffuse, can precipitate rostrocaudal brain stem deterioration, a major cause of delayed death from head trauma (see chap. 19). Brain dysfunction and destruction are aggravated by *hypoxia,* the result of compromised respiratory function caused by the following: (1) injury to the chest, (2) aspiration pneumonia in the unconscious patient, (3) respiratory center depression from rostrocaudal deterioration or direct damage to the medulla, (4) pulmonary edema secondary to hypothalamic-septal damage, or (5) status epilepticus. Blood loss from multiple injuries and, as mentioned, brain edema further compromise delivery of oxygen to the brain.

Intracranial hemorrhage, arterial or venous, intra- or extracerebral, is a frequent sequela to cranial trauma and may be great enough to cause rostrocaudal brain stem deterioration and death if not recognized and attended to immediately. Rostrocaudal deterioration, if rapid, may itself cause hemorrhage by downward stretching and tearing of the paramedian penetrating arteries of the midbrain and pons. These so-called Duret hemorrhages usually occur when the clinical course of deterioration has reached the midbrain and upper pons (see chap. 19). It is imperative to terminate rostrocaudal changes at the diencephalic or early midbrain level because Duret hemorrhages in most cases probably herald irreversible deterioration and death or, at the least, severe permanent brain disability.

Subdural and epidural hematomas deserve some comment because both demand surgical intervention, which can be curative if undertaken prior to irreversible brain stem damage. Both types of hematoma are extracerebral. For this reason and because they are soft masses, there tends to be relatively little effect on the underlying and compressed cerebral hemispheres. Secondary rostrocaudal distortion of the brain stem usually gives rise to the major clinical signs (Fig 17–1): depression of consciousness (reticular formation), hemiparesis (cerebral peduncles), eye signs (third and sixth nerves), and respiratory pattern abnormalities (see also chap. 19).

Epidural hemorrhages are most often arterial. They are the result of transection of the middle meningeal artery by a skull fracture that passes through the middle meningeal groove. Therefore, the clots typically lie over the temporal lobes. Less often epidural collections are the results of tears in the venous sinuses or leakage from the diploic veins. These hemorrhages may occur over any portion of the hemispheres or in the posterior fossa. The typical temporal arterial hemorrhage gives rise to an acute (hours) syndrome. Classically, trauma se-

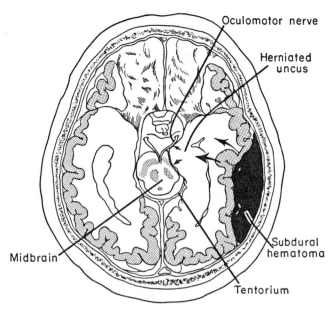

Fig 17–1.—Horizontal section of cranium to show vectors of force *(arrows)* caused by supratentorial mass (subdural hematoma). The right uncus is shown herniating over the tentorial edge and compressing the ipsilateral third nerve and midbrain.

vere enough to cause skull fracture is associated with a concussive loss of consciousness. The patient may awaken from this (lucid interval) only to lose consciousness again from brain stem distortion caused by the clot growth. More often there is no lucid interval. The patient does not have time to awaken from the concussion before compressive brain stem deterioration begins.

Subdural hematomas are typically venous and tend to collect slowly, causing signs and symptoms late (days to months). The hemorrhage is presumed to arise from angular forces that cause the dura to slide on the underlying arachnoid membrane, thus shearing the brain, to venous sinus bridging veins where they pass through the thin subdural space between the two membranes. This space is larger in the aged and others with atrophy of the brain because the subarachnoid membrane is pulled away from the overlying and relatively fixed dura as the brain shrinks. Subdural hemorrhage is more likely to occur in these individuals presumably

because the arachnoid and dura can slide more easily on each other and also because the veins bridging the enlarged subdural space are stretched.

Head trauma that can be so minor that it is not remembered may result in a subdural hematoma under these circumstances. Therapeutic anticoagulation predisposes to subdural hematoma and also intracerebral hemorrhage.

Because subdural venous bleeding is slow to accumulate, gradual shifting of the brain occurs and brain stem distortion can be better accommodated in contrast to the acute brain stem distortions and severe dysfunction caused by epidural and acute subdural hemorrhages. Mild depression of consciousness, difficulty with cognitive function, and chronic headache (from meningeal stretching and increased intracranial pressure) may be the presenting picture. Acute deterioration with a picture of rostrocaudal deterioration of the brain stem function may be superimposed on chronic complaints. The acute change is thought to be caused by fresh bleeding into the subdural hematoma from friable vessels that formed on the surface of the hematoma during the process of organized encapsulation of the clot. In many persons the symptoms of subdural hematoma, especially headache, depression of consciousness, and confusion, wax and wane over hours or days. A similar cyclic picture may be seen with any intracranial mass. No obvious explanation is known for this phenomenon; however, it is speculated that cyclic variations in the levels of cortisol may cause parallel rises and falls in the inflammatory edema associated with subdural hematomas and other masses. Variations in baseline intracranial pressure as determined by cerebrospinal fluid production and absorption may also play a role.

Acute subdural hematomas are seen less frequently. They are usually associated with head trauma severe enough to cause skull fracture and cerebral contusion or laceration. Epidural hematoma and intracerebral hematoma are frequently associated. The mortality is extremely high and the residual dysfunction of survivors is severe.

Dissection of arterial hemorrhage from a ruptured berry aneurysm into the subdural space is occasionally severe enough to cause rapidly progressive rostrocaudal deterioration. When recognized and surgically drained before secondary brain stem hemorrhages occur, survival with little morbidity is possible if the aneurysm itself is ultimately treated successfully.

Intracranial infection is usually the sequela of open injuries and may take the form of diffuse sepsis of the brain coverings (meningitis) or local collections of purulence (cerebral, subdural, and epidural abscess, see chap. 12). Infection of dural sinuses may lead to stasis, occlusion, and infarction (see chap. 14).

The early recognition of posttraumatic meningitis or its prophylaxis in situations with which it is highly associated is critical. Unrecognized and untreated, which is most likely to occur in the unconscious patient, meningitis is a likely cause of death. Depressed fractures that tear the dura and lie under or near scalp laceration are predisposed to infection. Fractures through sinuses (sphenoid, ethmoid, and frontal sinuses) are frequently associated with dural tears and subsequent meningitis or intracerebral abscess. If such fractures lack dural tear, they may be associated with extradural buildup of purulence (epidural abscess). Fracture of the cribriform plate or petrous bone may, if the dura is breached, create a communication between the subarachnoid space and the nasal cavity or external auditory cavities. The former may be recognized by leakage of CSF through the nose (rhinorrhea) and the latter by leakage from the ear (otorrhea). This leakage reflects a potential direct passage for bacteria to travel from the exterior to the subarachnoid space. The presence of glucose in the fluid, if collectible, is diagnostic. These leaks may persist long after recovery from trauma because CSF pressure presumably keeps them open. They may cause recurrent meningitis if not repaired.

Epilepsy may be a sequela of head injury. Seizures, frequently focal motor or focal with major motor generalization, occur in the first week after nonmissile trauma in approximately 5% of patients, but they herald chronic epilepsy in only 25% of those so involved. Seizures appearing weeks to years following injury are much more likely to represent a chronic and recurring disorder. Approximately 5% of persons with nonmissile injuries develop seizures after one week, and the presence of more than 24 hours of anterograde amnesia, a dural tear, or seizures within the first week following injury increases the likelihood that these late seizures will be recurrent. Many authorities suggest a period (up to several years) of prophylactic anticonvulsant therapy for patients with seizures appearing early and late. However, there is no clear evidence that this decreases the incidence of recurrent seizures on termination of the prophylaxis.

General Evaluation

Before any useful or reliable neurologic examination can be performed on a patient with acute head injury, the following other essential systems must be evaluated.

1. An adequate airway and adequate oxygenation must be assured. This can usually be tested by a brief physical examination and/or chest x-ray and by arterial blood gas measurements. Hypoxia is commonly associated with head injury in the immediate posttrauma period because of the frequency of lung contusion and/or emesis with aspiration of gastric contents. The hypoxic patient's neurologic status can often be dramatically improved by establishing adequate oxygenation.

2. Blood pressure and pulse should be noted. Adequate blood volume and pressure are also necessary for adequate cerebral oxygenation. Beware— shock is *not* due to reversible cerebral injury. Shock is from noncerebral causes such as hypovolemia (i.e., from a hidden site of hemorrhage), cardiac failure, or sepsis. Shock that can be produced by cerebral injury is manifest by a loss of peripheral vasomotor tone and is mediated by the medulla. Shock from medullary failure is seldom seen even in the agonal patient.

3. Body core temperature should be noted. Hypothermia secondary to exposure can cause marked neurologic changes. Hypothermia decreases CNS metabolism and tends to decrease the level of consciousness, reflexes, and nearly all motor responses.

4. Baseline blood studies should be done (blood count, electrolytes, and glucose) when the patient is first seen. If the patient is unconscious and a known diabetic, a bolus of intravenous 50% glucose should be administered after the blood glucose is drawn. Immediate treatment of hypoglycemia (quite possible in the diabetic who is unable to eat because of trauma) is necessary to minimize brain damage.

Along with assuring an adequate airway, oxygenation, perfusion, and a normal body temperature, a brief history of the trauma can be extremely helpful. Progression or nonprogression of the patient's level of consciousness from the time of trauma to the time he is being seen by the examiner should be documented if possible. Was the patient immediately unconscious? For how long? Was he awake and talking or walking after the trauma? Did any witnesses observe seizure activity? Did the patient strike his head and then become unconscious, or did he first become unconscious and then strike his head?

If available, a brief history may also be important. Was the patient taking any medication, alcohol, or other drugs? Did the patient have a preexisting illness, seizure disorder, or history of syncope?

Clinical Neurologic Evaluation

BRAIN STEM EVALUATION OF THE PERSON WITH HEAD TRAUMA

The most sensitive and reliable clinical parameter of brain function is the patient's level of consciousness (mediated primarily by the ascending reticular formation of the brain stem, see chap. 19). On the initial and all subsequent examinations, the level of consciousness should be clearly described and recorded. Confusing and ambiguous terms such as "stupor," "lethargy," and "coma" should be avoided unless defined. Decreasing levels of consciousness often follow a logical progression and can be documented in a stepwise pattern (Table 17–1).

After the age of 8 to 11 years, the skull is a nonexpanding bony encasement for the brain. The only direction in which an expanding supratentorial mass can force the brain is through the tentorial opening into the posterior fossa. The midbrain with its segment of reticular activating system normally occupies this tentorial opening. As a supratentorial mass enlarges, it causes transtentorial herniation of the mesial portion of the ipsilateral temporal lobe with compression of the brain stem and reticular activating system. This is first shown clinically in most cases by a decrease in the level of consciousness.

Toward the foramen magnum is the main direction for expansion of a posterior fossa mass. Expanding mass lesions of the posterior fossa can produce foramen magnum impaction by forcing the cerebellar tonsils into the upper cervical spinal canal. This may produce compression of the medulla with sudden apnea and death from asphyxiation.

Direct involvement of the brain stem may occur at several levels. Major occipital trauma causes posterior displacement of the brain stem, which, without complicating fracture, should be tolerated at most levels. If, however, the tentorial notch (incisure) is small (i.e., the tentorial size varies somewhat and its anterior edge may be close to the quadrigeminal plate), the midbrain may be concussed by the rigid leading edge of the tentorium. At the same time, the fourth nerves may become involved by posterior stretching. With a severe linear occipital trauma, especially if a fracture occurs, vertebral arterial compromise may occur with subsequent pontomedullary dysfunction.

Other clinical parameters that help to establish progressing brain stem dysfunction (see also chap. 19) are:

1. *Respiratory pattern.*—Normal breathing progresses to hyperventilation ("central neurogenic hyperventilation") as the midbrain is compressed, and then to an irregular respiratory pattern or apnea as the medulla is compressed.

2. *Pupillary response.*—Equally responsive pupils progress to midposition without response to light as the upper midbrain (the region of the third cranial nerve nucleus) is compressed. No further change is seen even with increased transtentorial herniation and descending brain stem compression.

3. *Oculocephalic reflex.*—This reflex should normally be inhibited in the conscious person and disinhibited in the person with depressed consciousness. It can be elicited by briskly turning the patient's head. If the response is present (disinhibited), the patient's eyes appear to be fixed on an imaginary point as the head is turned. If the reflex is absent, the eyes turn with the head. The movements of adduction first disappear with upper midbrain (third-nerve) compression, and the movements of abduction disappear when the compression progresses to involve the pons (sixth nerve). With downward movement of the brain stem caused by expansion of the supratentorial contents, loss of abduction (lateral rectus function) may occur before parenchymal involvement of the pons. This is caused by stretching of the sixth nerve against the edge of the petrous bone (see chaps. 3 and 19).

4. *Motor response.*—Normal motor strength and tone progress to intermittent decorticate or decerebrate posturing as the midbrain is compressed. The progression is then to flaccid areflexia

TABLE 17–1—PROGRESSION OF DECREASING CONSCIOUSNESS

1. Alert and oriented.
2. Confused and drowsy but awakens to verbal stimuli.
3. Drowsy and awakens to noxious stimuli only.
4. Unconscious but responds appropriately to noxious stimulation by reaching in attempt to remove the stimulus.
5. Unconscious and responds inappropriately to noxious stimulation by random arm and leg movements.
6. Unconscious but responds to noxious stimulation with leg extension and arm flexion posturing (decorticate) or arm extension and internal rotation posturing (decerebrate).
7. No response to even noxious stimulation.

as the pons and medulla are compressed. Decerebrate posturing is manifested by intermittent leg extension along with arm extension and internal rotation. This is seen when descending inhibitory nerve impulses from the cerebral cortex and basal ganglia to the facilitatory areas in the brain stem are physiologically interrupted. The interruption must be at the level of the midbrain or below but at least above the level of the vestibular nuclei to produce this increase in postural tone (see chaps. 4 and 19). Decorticate posturing is similar but manifested by intermittent leg extension along with arm flexion and internal rotation. To produce this type of posturing, descending cortical motor impulses must be interrupted. This interruption must be above the level of the midbrain, leaving the rubrospinal and vestibulospinal motor systems intact and facilitated (see chap. 4).

CEREBRAL HEMISPHERE FUNCTIONAL EVALUATION

Cerebral hemisphere dysfunction after head trauma, unlike brain stem dysfunction, is not clearly correlated with changes in the level of consciousness. Large cerebral hemisphere lesions can be found in persons who are alert, particularly if the trauma did not cause direct brain stem damage and the lesion does not act as an expanding mass and cause transtentorial herniation.

In trauma, two basic mechanisms are responsible for focal cerebral hemisphere deficits:

1. Direct compression of the brain by a mass lesion (hematoma, edematous brain tissue) or by cortical or subcortical brain contusion. Common findings associated with compression or contusion are:
   a. Contralateral motor weakness with frontal lesions
   b. Receptive aphasia of varying degree with left temporoparietal lesions
   c. Contralateral loss of sensation with parietal lesions
   d. Contralateral visual field deficits with temporal, parietal, or occipital lesions
2. Uncal (mesial temporal lobe) herniation secondary to a lateral supratentorial mass lesion. The associated findings are:
   a. Progressive ipsilateral third cranial nerve dysfunction (Fig 17-1). This is caused by direct peripheral third-nerve compression by the herniated uncus at the tentorial incisura. The pupil fully dilates and the extraocular muscle movements of the eye controlled by the third nerve become paralyzed on that side.
   b. Hemiparesis is also seen with the third cranial nerve deficit. If the paresis is ipsilateral to the pupillary dilatation, it is caused by a shifting of the brain and brain stem away from the extracerebral lesion (usually hemorrhage) with pressure of the contralateral cerebral peduncle against the rigid tentorial edge (Kernohan's notch—Fig 17-2). If the paresis is contralateral, it is caused by direct compression or destruction of the cerebral hemisphere and descending fiber tract.

Lesions that produce cerebral hemisphere deficits also act as expanding masses and produce transtentorial herniation. Persons with head trauma who show signs of cerebral hemisphere dysfunction usually have alterations in their level of consciousness that frequently are the result of herniation compression of the brain stem. However, direct traumatic injury to the brain stem may also cause depression of consciousness, particularly following severe trauma. Cranial nerve dysfunction usually belies the presence of direct brain stem involvement, whereas depression of consciousness usually precedes cranial

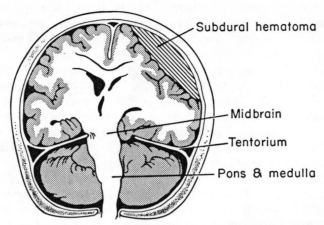

Fig 17–2.—Impingement of the cerebral peduncle against the rigid tentorial edge opposite an expanding high-convexity supratentorial lesion (subdural hematoma) causing hemiparesis ipsilateral to the mass. This occurs in as many as one third of persons who have subdural hematoma.

dysfunction with supratentorial expanding lesions. The exception, low temporal lesions when the third nerve may be involved early, was described earlier (see chap. 19 also).

Neck Injury in the Unconscious Patient

An assumption that should be made in the initial evaluation of an unconscious trauma patient is that he has an unstable neck fracture until proved otherwise by x-ray. Head and neck movements should be minimized during the examination. If moved or turned, the head and body should remain as a unit, en bloc.

The initial evaluation of a person with head trauma to this point has included checking the following:

1. Respiratory airway patency, oxygenation (arterial blood gases) and perfusion (blood pressure and pulse), and body temperature.
2. Brain stem function.—The level of consciousness is the most important parameter.
3. Cerebral hemisphere function.

4. Cervical spine stability.—A lateral cervical spine x-ray showing all seven cervical vertebrae is necessary for identification of cervical spine fracture and/or instability.

Pre-existing Disease Complicating Head Trauma

In the evaluation of an unconscious person, a history of minor head trauma with a disproportionate loss of consciousness should alert the examiner to the possibility of a preexisting reason for the clinical findings. Other possible causes are:

1. Metabolic: endogenous or exogenous, such as hypoxia, hypoglycemia, sepsis, hepatic or renal failure, and medication overdose (see chap. 20).
2. A pre-existing seizure disorder appearing as postictal coma.
3. Other neurologic disease: subarachnoid hemorrhage, vascular occlusive disease, brain tumor, or chronic subdural hematoma.

If a history strongly suggests any of these,

the head trauma may be only an incidental factor in producing the neurologic picture.

Commonly Described Neurologic Signs of Head Trauma

Papilledema is evidence for increased intracranial pressure. Thirty minutes to several hours of increased pressure are required before papilledema becomes clinically apparent.

Papilledema as viewed through the ophthalmoscope probably has several causes. The optic nerve is surrounded by a sleeve of dura, which is continuous with the sclera. Between this sleeve and the optic nerve is a space that communicates with the subarachnoid space. Increased intracranial pressure, which is reflected in the subarachnoid space, is therefore communicated into the optic nerve sleeve, compressing the optic nerve and thus impeding normal axoplasmic flow from the ganglion cells of the retina into the central nervous system. This may well be the earliest mechanism of swelling of the disk. The swelling of the optic nerve fiber compresses and impedes venous outflow from the retina. This secondary vascular stasis and associated capillary leakage around the optic disk are probably the major cause of visible papilledema.

Some patients do not develop papilledema even with marked elevations of their intracranial pressure. A lack of normal spinal fluid (subarachnoid space) communication along the optic nerve is frequent and is thought by some to explain why papilledema does not always develop with marked elevations of intracranial pressure.

If the intraocular pressure is elevated, as in persons with glaucoma, papilledema does not develop. This may explain why papilledema is frequently not seen in older persons with increased intracranial pressure. Increased intraocular pressure prevents capillary leakage of serum components into the retina around the optic disk, which would otherwise take place with increased central retinal vein pressure and normal intraocular pressure.

Battle's sign is an ecchymotic discoloration over the mastoid bone behind the ear without local skin or scalp contusion. It indicates periosteal bleeding, which drains toward the exterior from a basilar fracture and usually does not develop for several hours following the trauma.

Hematotympanum is blood seen through the tympanic membrane in the middle ear. This finding as well as blood draining from the external ear indicates either a skull fracture across the temporal bone (basilar fracture) or severe shearing of the contents of the middle ear. A conductive or sensorineural hearing loss may be associated.

The facial nerve (VII) passes through the temporal bone next to the middle ear and therefore if hematotympanum is noted, facial nerve function should be carefully tested. Peripheral facial nerve contusion or transection at the fracture line causes facial paralysis, which may develop many hours or days after the trauma.

Cerebrospinal fluid leakage may be noted from the nose or ears. This is not necessarily a bad prognostic sign for neurologic recovery but it does indicate a skull fracture. It should alert the examiner to the possible development of meningitis from retrograde passage of bacteria along the leakage tract.

The Cushing reflex is an elevation in blood pressure and pulse pressure associated with bradycardia. It is seen with increased intracranial pressure or an expanding mass lesion in the posterior fossa. When pressure is placed on the lower brain stem, peripheral vasoconstriction ensues with an increase in blood pressure. The carotid sinus in turn causes reflex cardiac slowing by increasing vagal tone. More often than not, however, the carotid sinus reflex is inadequate to overcome the tachycardia that accompanies the central vasomotor response.

X-Ray Evaluation in Acute Head Trauma

Skull and cervical spine x-rays are usually obtained on the person with acute head trauma as soon as this can be done safely. They can be helpful if they show the following:

1. Calcification of the pineal gland.—This is a midline structure, and a shift of the pineal gland from the midline indicates a shift of the brain. If a lesion is clinically suspected, pineal shift greater than 3 mm from midline is strong evidence for a mass.

2. Skull fracture (any type).—This increases the possibility of an intracranial hematoma. If a fracture line crosses large meningeal vessels in the temporal fossa, the possibility of an acute epidural hematoma is greater. If the fracture crosses a large dural venous sinus (superior sagittal or lateral sinuses), the possibility of a venous epidural or subdural hematoma is increased, particularly if the fracture is separated (diastatic).

3. Depressed skull fracture.—This may require surgical elevation to decrease the possibility of posttraumatic seizures or of a growing skull fracture. A depressed skull fracture with overlying scalp laceration definitely requires surgical exploration and debridement to prevent subgaleal, epidural, or even intracerebral abscess formation.

One point that must be emphasized is that the patient's neurologic status best determines the seriousness of his brain injury. The presence or absence of skull fracture on x-ray is *not helpful* in evaluating the extent of brain injury. The following two cases illustrate this point.

CASE 1

A 46-year-old man was closing his shop in the evening when he was struck from behind with a hammer and robbed. He was unconscious for one to two minutes and then woke up and walked approximately 100 yd to his home. He was then brought to the hospital by his family.

On admission, the man had a large depressed skull fracture, but he was wide awake with no neurologic deficit. The patient was taken to the operating room where his scalp laceration and skull fracture were explored. The fracture was elevated and the wound was cleaned of hair and other contaminants. After surgery he was bright and alert and had no neurologic deficit. He was discharged on the seventh posttrauma day.

CASE 2

A 14-year-old boy was brought to the hospital after falling from a horse and striking his right parietal occipital area. He was immediately unconscious and did not respond to verbal or painful stimuli from the time of the accident until he arrived in the emergency room one hour later. When the patient was first examined in the emergency room, he was unconscious and responding only to painful stimuli with extensor thrusting of his arms and legs and with hyperventilation. His pupils were in midposition and fixed to light, and his oculocephalic reflexes were absent. No other injuries were noted.

No fracture was seen on skull x-ray. The patient received emergency arteriography and no intracranial hematoma was found. The patient died two days later and autopsy showed diffuse cerebral edema and cortical brain contusion. No skull fracture was seen even on open examination of the skull.

Other Diagnostic Procedures

Computerized tomography (CT scan), where it is available, has revolutionized the care of head-injured patients (see chap. 18). Hemorrhage and edema are revealed with facility, and surgical intervention is more rationally decided. The arteriogram, an invasive and potentially dangerous procedure, is rarely used to determine the presence or absence of hematomas in persons with head trauma where CT scanning is available.

Spinal tap is indicated only if there is a serious suspicion of bacterial meningitis. Helpful information is seldom obtained from the spinal tap in the evaluation of acute head trauma and it may be hazardous. Transtentorial or foramen magnum herniation can be precipitated by a lumbar spinal tap in the setting of an expanding intracranial mass.

Spinal Cord Trauma

The spinal cord lies protected within the vertebral spinal canal, a channel lined by bone (vertebral bodies and laminae) and ligamentous structures (e.g., posterior longitudinal ligament and ligamentum flavum). The vertebral body laminae and facet fibrous attachments acting together with the preceding two ligaments form a semiflexible tubular structure that subserves maintenance of erect posture and protection of the spinal cord.

Direct and indirect forces applied to the spine may cause injury to the spinal cord. Direct injuries that distort, fracture, or crush the vertebral column may contuse or lacerate the spinal cord, which lies within the narrow spinal vertebral canal. Stab wounds entering through the interlaminar space may sever the spinal cord without bony injury.

Indirect distortion of the vertebral column is by far the most common cause of spinal cord injury. Acceleration-deceleration forces applied to the head or trunk cause distortion of the vertebral column and its contents. Not surprisingly, the most mobile portions of the vertebral column are the most prone to damaging distortion. These are the lower cervical and thoracolumbar junction regions. The rib cage of the thoracic spine makes it the least mobile and therefore the least likely to be distorted by indirect forces.

Flexion and extension distortions of the cervical spine are the most common cause of spinal cord injury. The vertebral bodies may be displaced anteriorly or posteriorly on themselves (listhesis) with or without ligamentous tears causing concussion, contusion, or laceration of the spinal cord. Severe flexion may stretch the spinal cord upward which in conjunction with the bony displacement mentioned earlier adds further injury. If the forces are great enough, or if there is a predisposing fragility of the spine as in the aged with cervical osteoarthritis, fractures may occur and bony fragments contribute to cord damage.

Acceleration and deceleration vehicular accidents are the most common causes of cervical and thoracolumbar spinal column distortion. Swimming pool diving accidents, associated with flexion or extension deceleration distortion of the cervical spine, are also frequent causes of spinal cord injury. The spinal cord may be damaged by direct compression or disruption (bone displacement or fracture, hematoma, extruded disk material, and ligamentous distortion), stretching, secondary edema following concussion, or secondary vascular occlusive and hemorrhagic phenomena. All degrees of cord dysfunction may result, from complete disruption with crush or lacerating injuries to minor symptoms with no objective losses from minor concussing forces.

A typical crush or contusing lesion involves primarily the central gray matter of the cord with early preservation of the surrounding white matter and long-tract motor and sensory systems. Acutely, this differential involvement is not obvious because functional transection with variable degrees of paraplegia-quadriplegia depending on the level of involvement is evident.

Attempts are being made to determine ways to prevent the ensuing white-matter injury that frequently occurs and may be caused by swelling of the central gray matter or by secondary vascular spasm and ischemia-infarction of the outer layers of the cord. Surgical decompression of the segments involved, spinal-cord cooling to decrease metabolic demands, and vasodilator drugs to prevent vasospasm have been used with variable degrees of reported success.

Any therapeutic approach in the acute event is limited by the delay in getting the patient to an appropriate spinal cord trauma facility. Prevention of further injury by immobilizing the spine at the site of the accident probably is the most effective acute treatment.

When paraplegia is established as a perma-

nent baseline, rehabilitative efforts become of major importance. The average paraplegic can be rehabilitated to become an independent and productive member of society. The prognosis for the quadriplegic patient, if he survives for any length of time, is poor.

REFERENCE

Jennett, W. B.: *An Introduction to Neurosurgery*, ed. 3. Chicago, Year Book Medical Publishers, 1977.

18

Neurologic Tests

EDWARD VALENSTEIN

MANY TESTS are used specifically for the evaluation of neurologic illnesses (Table 18–1). The general physician should be familiar with the diagnostic capabilities of all these tests and should be able to interpret the results of some of them (the lumbar puncture and the brain scan).

Lumbar Puncture

TECHNIQUE

The technique of lumbar puncture is learned in the ward, so only a few points are made here. Spinal taps should not be done above the L2–3 interspace because the spinal cord may be present above this level. If the flow of spinal fluid is not brisk, the following check is simple (Fig 18–1): The manometer is tilted horizontally to increase the flow and then brought back to the vertical position so that the fluid falls to the true spinal fluid pressure. If this maneuver fails to increase the flow, the needle is not properly placed or a nerve root has blocked the needle. Fluid should not be aspirated because this may damage nerve roots. If the initial CSF pressure is high (more than 180 mm H_2O), the physician should try to let it fall without removing fluid; the patient should be encouraged to relax, and his neck and legs should, if necessary, be unflexed (thus reducing venous pressure). He should not be asked to hyperventilate (this causes cerebral vasoconstriction and lowers even truly high CSF pressures). He should be reassured, made comfortable, and allowed to rest for one minute (not much more). Even if the pressure is high, enough CSF should be removed for the performance of routine tests (about 3 cc; 1 cc in each tube).

EXAMINATION OF THE FLUID

Cell counts should be made in the first and last tubes. An india ink preparation to help identify cryptococcal organisms can be used if indicated. The fluid is then centrifuged; the supernatant is decanted and examined for

TABLE 18–1.—TESTS FOR EVALUATING
NEUROLOGIC ILLNESSES

Lumbar puncture, cisternal tap, lateral cervical tap
X-rays of skull and spine
Tomography
Radioisotope brain scan
Cisternography
CSF infusion test
Echoencephalography
Electroencephalography (EEG)
Electromyography (EMG)
Nerve conduction studies
Averaged evoked responses (brainstem auditory, visual, somatosensory)
Psychological testing
Others (audiometry, cystometrograms, etc.)
Computerized axial tomography (CT scan)
Arteriography
Pneumoencephalography and ventriculography
Biopsy: Nerve; Muscle; Brain

195

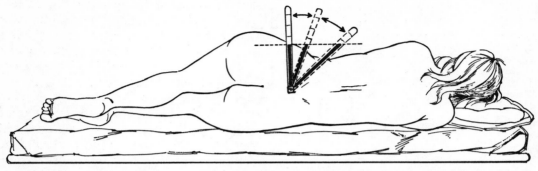

Fig 18–1.—Position for lumbar puncture illustrating the constant level of cerebrospinal fluid in the manometer with tilting, validating correct communication with subarachnoid space.

color (compare with a tube of water against a white background) and then analyzed for protein and sugar. The whole CSF or the sediment can be stained for microorganisms (in appropriate cases). A separate tube (usually tube 2) should be sent for cultures. Fungal and AFB cultures should be requested when indicated. CSF protein electrophoresis can also be obtained when indicated.

INTERPRETATION

CSF PRESSURE.—Although elevated CSF pressure should raise the question of an intracranial mass lesion, intracranial pressure may also increase when there is an obstruction to the flow of CSF or when the intra-

TABLE 18–2.— CAUSES OF RAISED CSF PRESSURE*

A. Intracranial masses (neoplasms, hemorrhages, abscess, or brain edema)
B. Obstruction to the flow of CSF
C. Elevated intracranial venous pressure
  1. Secondary to high systemic venous pressure (congestive heart failure, Valsalva)
  2. Obstruction of venous flow
    a. Poor relaxation (high intra-abdominal pressure transmitted to venous plexuses around the cord)
    b. Obesity (as above; also compression of jugulars by obese neck)
    c. After radical neck surgery (where the major jugular vein, usually the right, has been sacrificed)
    d. Thrombosis of a major venous sinus

*Pressure greater than 180–200 mm of CSF.

cranial venous pressure rises (Table 18–2). Reduced CSF pressure can be artifactual (needle not properly placed, or blocked by a nerve root—check flow) or caused by CSF block (as by a spinal tumor or cerebellar herniation through the foramen magnum), general dehydration, or prior lumbar punctures (the result of CSF leakage through tears in the arachnoid and dura).

XANTHOCHROMIA.—This is usually the result of hemolyzed blood and takes two to six hours to develop after bleeding into the CSF. Initially, the supernatant looks pink; the hemoglobin pigments are then transformed into bilirubin, so that after a day the supernatant looks yellow. The supernatant from a traumatic tap should be clear and colorless. Other causes of xanthochromia are given in Table 18–3.

CELLS (Table 18–4).—Traumatic taps are common, and it is very important to be able to identify them the first time (i.e., without having to repeat the lumbar puncture). The criteria given in Table 18–5 are used.

PROTEIN.—Elevated levels of protein in the CSF have many causes (Table 18–6). Protein electrophoresis may reveal other abnormalities; increased proportions of gamma globulins may be seen in persons with multiple sclerosis, SSPE, or neurosyphilis. The CSF IgG:albumin ratio (using an electroimmunodiffusion method) and the demonstration of oligoclonal IgG bands (using agarose electrophoresis of concentrated

TABLE 18–3.—CAUSES
OF XANTHOCHROMIA

1. Hemolyzed blood
2. Serum (if more than 150,000 RBCs from a traumatic tap, etc.)
3. High level of serum bilirubin
4. High level of serum carotene
5. High level of CSF protein (more than 150 mg% or so, depends on proportion of chromagens)
6. Old age (very slight xanthochromia from increased proportion of chromagens)

CSF) provide evidence of antibody production within the CNS, and are helpful in the diagnosis of multiple sclerosis (but are also positive in chronic CNS infection).

GLUCOSE.—The CSF glucose is normally one half to two thirds of the serum value. For this to hold, ideally the spinal tap should be done under fasting conditions. Changes in CSF glucose lag about 30 minutes behind changes in the serum glucose. The causes of low CSF glucose are reviewed in chapter 12.

STAINS FOR MICROORGANISMS.—When infection is suspected, stains for acid-fast bacilli and gram stains should be obtained, even if there are no WBCs in the CSF. The india ink preparation is useful for detecting cryptococci, but it is difficult to interpret.

CULTURES.—Note that tubercle bacilli may take four to eight weeks to grow out.

OTHER.—Viral cultures and special tests, such as tests for antigens (e.g., cryptococcal antigen), may be useful in special cases.

INDICATIONS

A lumbar puncture must be done if a treatable infection is suspected. It should be done prior to instituting anticoagulation in persons with strokes, because blood in the CSF may

TABLE 18–4.—CELLS IN THE CSF

A. RBC
   1. Traumatic tap
   2. Subarachnoid bleeding prior to tap (trauma, ruptured aneurysm, etc.)
   3. Ventricular leakage of intracerebral hemorrhage
B. WBC (see chap. 12)
C. Tumor cells (must request cytology)

contraindicate anticoagulation. If a CT scanner is available, it can diagnose intracranial bleeding so a lumbar puncture may not be necessary prior to starting anticoagulation. Lumbar puncture is useful for the diagnosis of subarachnoid hemorrhage. It is included in the evaluation of many neurologic conditions (such as stroke and seizures) because abnormalities may point to various possible etiologies. There is usually an indication for doing a lumbar puncture; however, this should be weighed against the possible complications. Often (as in the diagnosis of tumor) better and less risky tests are available and should be tried first.

CONTRAINDICATIONS

Infection overlying the site of lumbar puncture is a relative contraindication. The puncture should be shifted to another level. A spinal tap should be contraindicated by the reasonable suspicion of an intracerebral mass, unless the suspicion of acute infection is stronger and time does not allow for other tests (e.g., CT scanning) to exclude the possibility of a mass lesion. Other contraindications or cautions are listed in Table 18–7.

COMPLICATIONS (Table 18–8)

Posttap headaches are fairly common. Their incidence may be reduced by (1) using a small needle (20 or 22 gauge), (2) having the patient lie prone for three hours after the

TABLE 18–5.—CRITERIA FOR IDENTIFYING
A TRAUMATIC TAP

1. The number of RBCs diminishes greatly between the first and last tubes.
2. The supernatant is not xanthochromic.
3. The CSF white blood cell count is not higher than expected. (When blood has been in the CSF for hours or days, it acts as an irritant and excites a CSF pleocytosis. In a traumatic tap, there should be 1 or 2 WBCs for every 1,000 RBCs if the patient's peripheral blood counts are normal.)

TABLE 18–6.—CAUSES OF ELEVATED CSF PROTEIN*

1. From serum accompanying hemorrhage or a traumatic tap: add approximately 1 mg% protein for every 700 RBCs.
2. Intracerebral hemorrhage (the amount of protein is usually elevated disproportionately to the amount of blood).
3. Many inflammatory conditions.
4. Many neoplasms.
5. Occasionally with degenerative diseases (but usually the level of protein is normal or only minimally elevated).
6. Sometimes with cerebral infarction (usually not greater than 100 mg%).
7. Many peripheral neuropathies.
8. Diabetes mellitus.
9. Guillain-Barré syndrome.
10. Hypothyroidism.
11. Stagnant CSF, as below an obstructing spinal tumor or after a ventricular shunting procedure.
12. Laboratory error.

*Levels greater than 45 mg/dl.

spinal tap, and (3) forcing fluids after the tap. Meningitis is exceedingly rare, as is significant hemorrhage. It is presumed that posttap headaches are caused by leakage of CSF from the puncture in the dura in excess of CSF production, so that a low-volume, low-pressure environment is created in the intracranial space. The headache is typically present only when the patient is in the sitting or erect position, indicating that it is caused by the brain settling against basal structures with stretching of pain-sensitive surface blood vessels and meninges. Rarely, the puncture hole may remain open for long periods (weeks or months) and injection of homologous blood into the site or even surgery may be necessary to stem the leak and alleviate the debilitating headaches.

We presented this information in some detail because the lumbar puncture is an important test that is frequently performed, often by a nonspecialist. Failure to measure pressure, count cells properly, note the presence of xanthochromia, or request the appropriate tests from the laboratory results in inadequate or frankly misleading information. Unfortunately, such failures are common, even in good hospitals. It is therefore important to master the preceding information.

Cisternal Puncture

When CSF cannot be obtained from the lumbar space (and when its analysis is considered essential), a cisternal tap may be required. The needle is placed in the midline, passing just under the occipital bone, into the (usually large) cisterna magna (Fig 18–2). This is technically fairly easy; however, if the needle is advanced too far it can enter the medulla, sometimes causing sudden respiratory arrest and death. The test should therefore be carried out only by experienced physicians (usually neurosurgeons or neurologists). An alternative route frequently used by neurosurgeons and neuroradiologists is

TABLE 18–7.—CONTRAINDICATIONS TO LUMBAR PUNCTURE

PROBLEM	REASON
Infection over the puncture site	May cause meningitis
Intracerebral mass lesion	May cause herniation
Increased intracranial pressure	May be indicative of a mass (see text); if there is no mass, puncture is usually safe
Before planned myelography or pneumoencephalography (7–10 days)	May produce subdural collection of CSF, making studies impossible
Suspected spinal tumor	May produce deterioration; may make myelogram impossible
Coagulation deficit	May result in epidural or subdural hemorrhage, with resulting root and/or cord compression (rare complication)

TABLE 18–8.—COMPLICATIONS
OF LUMBAR PUNCTURE

1. Posttap headache (from fluid leakage through dural tear)
2. Traumatic tap (obscuring the clinical picture)
3. Subdural collection of fluid (may interfere with subsequent studies (cisternogram, PEG, myelogram) or with subsequent lumbar punctures (may show falsely elevated level of protein from stagnation)
4. Herniation with cerebral mass lesions
5. Deterioration of spinal compression with cord tumors
6. Subdural or epidural hemorrhage (in patients with coagulation deficit)

lateral to C-1 with penetration through the large C-1 intervertebral foramen.

The cisternal tap is also used in myelography when the upper margin of a spinal block needs to be defined. It is necessary at times in the intrathecal administration of irritating medications, such as amphotericin B. Medications are diluted more rapidly in the larger and more rapidly circulating volume of the cisterna magna than in the smaller lumbar sac.

Skull X-Rays

Routine skull x-rays are often of little clinical value because the skull is not affected by most intracranial events. Skull x-rays are nevertheless frequently ordered because informative abnormalities are occasionally found (Tables 18–9 and 18–10). In addition, abnormalities in the skull, although not caused by an intracranial process, may help diagnose relevant conditions.

Spine X-Rays

X-rays of the cervical, thoracic, and lumbosacral spine may detect misalignment, fractures, metastatic lesions, degenerative changes, and occasionally enlargement of a foramen or of the walls of the spinal canal from tumors. Considerable discrepancy may exist between the x-rays and the clinical picture; severe degenerative changes in the cervical and lumbar spine may be almost asymptomatic, whereas a protruded intervertebral disk may produce considerable pain or

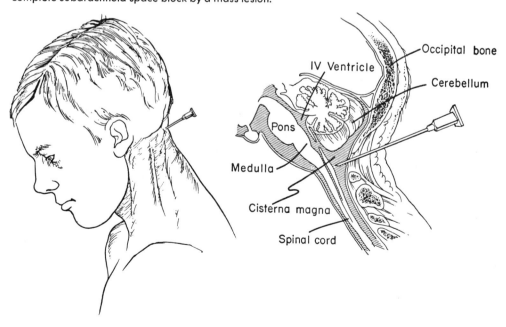

Fig 18–2.—Cisternal subarachnoid puncture, indicated when cerebrospinal fluid cannot be obtained from lumbar space and when myelography is used to determine the upper level of the complete subarachnoid space block by a mass lesion.

TABLE 18-9.—SKULL X-RAYS
IN THE DIAGNOSIS
OF INTRACRANIAL DISEASE

1. Calcified pineal or habenular commissure: this is often shifted with lateralized intracranial masses. Remember, however, that bilateral cerebral masses or masses that are far frontal or occipital may not shift the pineal appreciably.
2. Abnormal calcifications (tumors, aneurysms, arteriovenous malformations, etc.).
3. Increased vascular markings in the skull, when tumors (such as meningiomas) are fed from the external carotid circulation.
4. Sclerosis or erosion from underlying tumors (such as meningiomas).
5. Erosion of the dorsum sellae as a sign of increased intracranial pressure.
6. Enlargement of the sella turcica from an intrasellar mass.
7. Enlargement of the optic foramen or of the internal auditory meatus or canal from tumors of the second or eighth cranial nerves. Erosion of other foramina may also be detected with special views (foramen rotundum, ovale, jugular foramen, etc.).
8. In children, spreading sutures, indicative of increased pressure.

focal neurologic deficit without causing any abnormality on the plain x-ray.

Oblique views of the cervical spine demonstrate the neural foramina. The lateral cervical spine x-ray demonstrates the AP diameter of the spinal canal (Fig 18–3). Persons with congenitally narrow canals are more likely to develop cord compression with trauma or with the degenerative changes that occur with age (cervical spondylosis).

TABLE 18-10.—OTHER ABNORMALITIES
OF SKULL X-RAYS

1. Fractures: A fracture across the course of the meningeal arteries should lead one to suspect an epidural hematoma. Not all fractures can be seen on x-ray, basilar fractures may be particularly difficult to see.
2. Lytic or blastic lesions, indicative of metastatic tumors.
3. Clouding of the sinuses, often indicative of infection.
4. Osteomyelitis.
5. Structural changes, which may result in CNS damage, such as platybasia, basilar impression, or (in children) synostoses.
6. Some systemic diseases: Paget's disease, osteopetrosis, sickle cell anemia, thalassemia, etc.

Tomography

Tomograms are commonly used to define abnormalities in the complex structures of the base of the skull, including the sella turcica and the petrous pyramids (including the internal auditory canals). They are also useful in detecting fractures of the spine, and in other selected instances.

Radioisotope Brain Scan

Intravenous injection of radioactive isotope is followed by scanning to detect radioactivity over the neck and head. This technique was used to detect gross changes in blood flow (the dynamic scan) and to detect localized breakdown of the blood-brain barrier (the static scan), as sometimes occurs in tumors, strokes, and inflammatory conditions. This study has been largely supplanted by the CT scan, which offers similar information about breakdown of the blood-brain barrier, but also visualizes other intracranial structures. The dynamic scan has been replaced by noninvasive methods of detecting flow in the carotid circulation (see below).

Noninvasive Diagnosis of Carotid Disease

Numerous techniques have been developed to help detect stenosis or occlusion of the carotid arteries. Reduced pressure in the ocular circulation secondary to carotid stenosis or occlusion can be evaluated with oculodynamometry and oculoplethysmography. Reversal of flow in the supraorbital artery caused by occlusion of the ipsilateral carotid can be detected with Doppler ultrasonography. Turbulent flow in the carotid artery can be detected using phonoangiography, and by Doppler imaging techniques. B-mode ultrasonography can visualize carotid stenoses, and with increasing resolution may be able to detect ulcerations in the wall

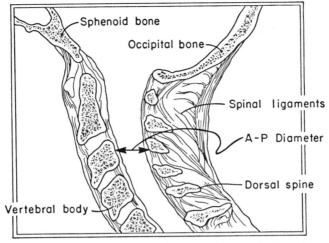

Fig 18–3.—Anterior-posterior diameter of bony spinal canal.

of the carotid artery. Until these tests have been shown to be as good as (or superior to) angiography for the delineation of vascular pathology, angiography will remain the test of choice when the clinical findings indicate that surgery on the carotid artery may be indicated.

Cisternography

The cisternogram provides information about CSF flow. Radioactive isotope is injected (by lumbar puncture) into the subarachnoid space. The patient's head is scanned after 4, 24, 48, and 72 hours. Nor-

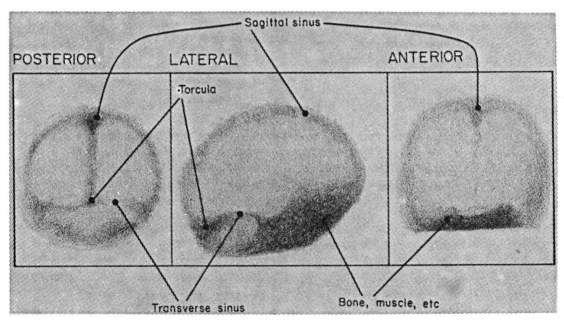

Fig 18–4.—Illustration of normal radionucleotide brain scan. Dark areas represent uptake of radionucleotide by vascular and vascularized structures surrounding the brain.

mally the radioactivity is located in the basal cisternae at 4 hours and over the convexities of the hemispheres at 24 hours, because this is the direction of CSF flow. Subsequent scans show marked diminution of radioactivity due to CSF absorption. When the ventricles are enlarged, some radioactivity may be seen within them. When this enlargement is due to blockage of CSF absorption, the radioactivity remains within the cisternae and ventricles for an abnormally long time.

The cisternogram is used to help diagnose communicating hydrocephalus. It is also useful in detecting CSF leaks (for example, in CSF rhinorrhea). Its principal use is in the evaluation of demented persons for normal-pressure hydrocephalus (see chap. 11). Its usefulness in this regard remains controversial.

COMPLICATIONS

The use of longer-acting radiopharmaceuticals, such as RISA, has been discouraged because exposure may be excessive. Substances with very short half-lives (such as technetium 99m) do not last long enough to produce useful scans. Other substances (indium, for example) are presently being evaluated. Ytterbium has a relatively short half-life and is used by many centers now. Cases of aseptic meningitis were reported with RISA cisternography. Aside from this, the complications are the same as those for lumbar puncture.

CSF Infusion Test

This is also used for the evaluation of CSF flow. Artificial CSF is infused into the lumbar subarachnoid space at a rate equal to twice the rate of CSF production. CSF pressure is monitored continuously. Normally the CSF pressure rises slowly. With a block in CSF absorption, the CSF pressure rises abnormally quickly to abnormally high values. As for the cisternogram, the accuracy of the infusion test in the diagnosis of normal-pressure hydrocephalus is disputed.

Echoencephalography

Ultrahigh frequency sound is applied to the skull and echoes are detected. The sound bounces off the skull and also off CSF-brain interfaces. The most common technique merely locates the third ventricle and is thus a rapid and benign test to detect shifts in midline structures. In practice, it is difficult to perform accurately and so may not be reliable in every institution.

More complex techniques using echoes to detect ventricular size and other intracranial structures have not been reliable enough to gain widespread clinical use.

Electroencephalography (EEG)

The electric activity of the brain can be recorded from electrodes applied to the scalp. The pattern of the EEG varies with age and with the state of attention. In the normal adult, the EEG consists of low-voltage, fast activity when the patient is alert and attentive; alpha rhythm ($8-13$ cps) is more prominent when the eyes are closed and the patient is not concentrating. Slower activity is seen in persons who are drowsy, and specific patterns characterize the different stages of sleep.

Pathologic processes may produce EEG abnormalities (Table $18-11$). Minor abnormalities are seen in a high percentage of brain-damaged persons, but since they are also seen in as many as $10\%-15\%$ of normal persons, they are of little diagnostic value. Conversely, a normal EEG does not rule out serious organic disease affecting the hemispheres.

Special "activating" techniques are used to bring out abnormalities, especially in the diagnosis of seizure disorders. Hyperventilation is used routinely. Photic stimulation may evoke synchronous discharges in normal persons ("photic driving") and may provoke seizures in susceptible individuals. Sleep is useful in bringing out seizure discharges in many persons. Methohexital, an

TABLE 18–11.—MAJOR USES OF THE
ELECTROENCEPHALOGRAM

1. Diagnosis of epilepsy.—Paroxysmal spikes, sharp waves, and/or slow waves may be diagnostic of epilepsy. The EEG can help identify the type of seizure disorder, and it may help localize a seizure focus.
2. Diagnosis of focal structural lesions.—Focal slowing in the EEG may help localize a lesion. The EEG pattern is not specific for any particular type of pathology.
3. Metabolic encephalopathies.—Slowing is seen with most metabolic encephalopathies. Again the EEG pattern is not helpful in diagnosing the type of encephalopathy.
4. Drugs.—Barbiturates and minor tranquilizers frequently produce an excessive amount of low-voltage fast activity.
5. Degenerative disease.—Unusual EEG patterns are seen in a number of degenerative diseases (SSPE and Jakob-Creutzfeldt disease, for example). In the others, the EEG changes are nonspecific and often very slight.
6. Cerebral death.—Two flat EEGs taken 24 hours apart are diagnostic of cerebral death in the absence of hypothermia or drug overdose.

ultrashort-acting barbiturate, has the same effect.

Special placement of electrodes may help diagnose conditions that are not apparent on the routine EEG. Nasopharyngeal electrodes (inserted through the nose, Fig 18–5) record activity from the orbitofrontal and mesial temporal regions remote from electrodes placed on the scalp. These are used principally in the diagnosis of limbic (temporal lobe) epilepsy.

The EEG is attenuated and diffused by the meninges, skull, and scalp. Recording from the extradural space, from the cortex (electrocorticogram), and even from electrodes in the substance of the brain (depth electrodes) may increase accuracy in detecting and localizing abnormal activity. These measures are sometimes used in the evaluation of refractory seizure disorders, especially prior to surgery.

Averaged Evoked Responses (AER)

Electrical responses to sensory stimuli are usually too small to be detected in the routine EEG. By computer averaging responses to repeated stimuli, however, clearcut potentials can be demonstrated to visual, auditory, and somatosensory stimuli. By changing the placement of the recording electrodes, the AER can be made to reflect cortical (as in the case of the standard visual evoked response), brain stem (as in the brain stem auditory evoked response) or spinal cord (as with somatosensory evoked responses) electrical events. Changes in latency or amplitude of specific components of the AER reflect abnormalities in conduction in specific sensory pathways, and thus can help to document the presence and location of lesions. Since areas of demyelination markedly slow conduction velocity, AERs have proved sensitive in detecting subclinical lesions in persons with multiple sclerosis.

Electrodiagnostic Tests

NERVE CONDUCTIONS

Motor and sensory nerve conductions can be determined from peripheral nerves superficial enough to be stimulated transcutaneously. The technique for determining motor nerve conductions is illustrated in Figure 18–6. The muscle action potential is recorded from C, the median nerve is stimulated at B, and the latency (time from stimulus to response) is recorded. Similarly the latency from stimulating the nerve at A is determined. Latency A minus latency B represents the time it takes for the nerve impulse to travel from A to B. The distance from A to B divided by this time is the conduction velocity. The nerve conduction velocity is normal (about 40–70 m/second) as long as there are some fast-conducting fibers left in the nerve. A normal nerve conduction does not, therefore, rule out a peripheral neuropathy. Demyelinating neuropathies (see chap. 8) produce marked slowing of the nerve conductions. Axonal neuropathies may produce some increase in distal latency, but usually the nerve conductions are normal or only

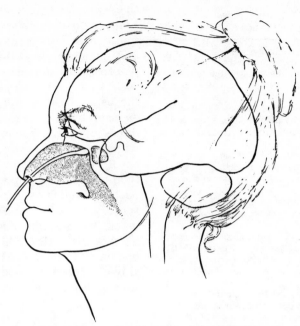

Fig 18—5.—Placement of nasopharyngeal lead for recording the electroencephalogram in proximity to the anterior temporal lobe.

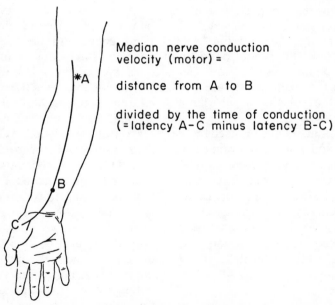

Median nerve conduction velocity (motor) =

distance from A to B

divided by the time of conduction (=latency A–C minus latency B–C)

Fig 18—6.—Skin electrode sites for determining median nerve conduction velocity (see text).

slightly reduced. Focal slowing may be detected in cases of nerve compression.

Sensory nerve conductions are determined by stimulating the skin and recording from the appropriate nerve. The potential recorded is very small, and consequently very mild nerve injuries alter or abolish it.

ELECTROMYOGRAM (EMG)

A needle electrode is inserted in the muscle. Normally there is no muscle activity at rest, but with minimal voluntary contraction, individual motor unit potentials are seen. These represent the summation of the membrane action potentials of many muscle fibers, all innervated by the same anterior horn cell (the motor unit). With increasing contraction, more motor units are recruited, the firing rate increases, and a dense *interference pattern* is seen in which the baseline of the EMG is no longer visible.

CHANGES WITH NEUROPATHY.—When the muscle is partially denervated, there are changes in the excitability of muscle fibers, so that after about three weeks muscle fibers may fire at rest (fibrillations). If denervated fibers are reinnervated by neighboring healthy nerve axons, motor units are formed that are larger than normal. As the number of motor units decreases, the interference pattern seen with maximal contraction becomes less dense, and large polyphasic units are seen.

CHANGES WITH MYOPATHY.—The number of motor units remains normal, and therefore the interference pattern is normal except in the very late stages. The individual units are smaller because some muscle fibers have dropped out. The motor unit potentials are therefore, on the average, smaller in amplitude and shorter in duration. More units must be fired to produce a particular strength of contraction, so the full interference pattern is achieved earlier. Polyphasic potentials are also seen. The EMG picture of *b*rief, *s*mall-amplitude, *a*bundant, *p*olyphasic *p*otentials (BSAPP) is characteristic (although

not pathognomonic) of myopathy. Although usually the muscle is silent at rest, fibrillations can occur, and are often seen in persons with polymyositis, perhaps a result of denervation caused by damage to the intramuscular nerves.

In normal persons muscle activity ceases abruptly with muscle relaxation. In patients with myotonia, repetitive afterdischarges are seen. This correlates with clinical myotonia (see chap. 8) but is more sensitive. Cases of myotonic dystrophy can therefore be diagnosed by EMG before clinically obvious myotonia is present.

NEUROMUSCULAR JUNCTION

Repetitive stimulation of a nerve produces little attenuation of the summated muscle action potential at rates of 3 to 30 per second. In persons with myasthenia gravis, however, this attenuation is marked because neuromuscular transmission is marginal at the start. Conversely, in the "myasthenic" syndrome associated with carcinoma (the Eaton-Lambert syndrome), repetitive stimulation augments the muscle response.

The following three procedures are called *invasive* because air or dye must be injected. In general, they carry a higher morbidity than the foregoing procedures so they are not used as screening tests.

Myelography

Contrast (usually positive contrast, Pantopaque or metrizamide, but air is sometimes used) is introduced into the lumbar subarachnoid space (via lumbar puncture). Because the positive contrast used is heavier than spinal fluid, it can be moved up and down the spinal canal by tilting the patient appropriately. Normally one sees the outline of the spinal canal, the spinal cord, and, to some extent, the nerve roots. The following abnormalities also may be seen (Fig 18–7):

1. Extradural defects (from herniated disks, tumors, etc.).

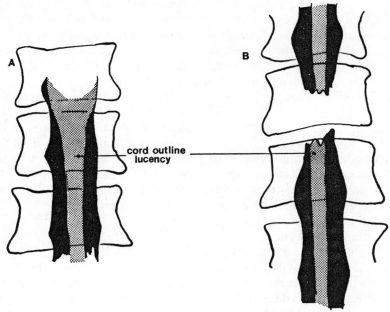

Fig 18–7.—Myelogram showing displacement of subarachnoid space containing radiopaque substance (black). A, intramedullary mass (or midline dorsal or ventral extramedullary, intra- or extradural mass) showing spindle-shaped enlargement of spinal cord. B, extradural mass causing complete block. Substance introduced from lumbar and cisternal punctures to delineate lower and upper extent of block.

2. Intradural extramedullary defects (as from meningiomas or neurofibromas).
3. Intramedullary masses (syringomyelia, ependymoma, glioma, etc.).
4. AV malformations on the surface of the cord may be seen as serpiginous filling defects.

The contrast material may be run up past the foramen magnum to fill the basal cisternae, including the cerebellopontine angles, or (if the patient is supine) the cisterna magnum and the fourth and third ventricles (Fig 18–8). Mass lesions in these locations may be seen with greater accuracy with positive contrast than with air.

Complications are the same as those for lumbar puncture. In addition, a small number of patients (less than 0.5%) develop arachnoiditis of clinical significance from Pantopaque. Metrizamide use occasionally is associated with seizures and encephalopathy if it is allowed to spill into the intracranial subarachnoid space, but because of its water solubility it is absorbed rapidly and arachnoiditis is an unlikely complication.

Pneumoencephalography (PEG)

Air is injected into the lumbar subarachnoid space. Unlike positive contrast (which falls), air rises, so when the patient is sitting, the air rises rapidly to the cisterna magna and then passes into the fourth and third ventricles. X-rays (usually tomograms to blur out the overlying petrous bones) taken shortly after the injection of air show these structures clearly. In addition, by injecting more air and positioning the patient properly, one may see the whole ventricular system and the subarachnoid cisternae. Tomography taken in conjunction with pneumoencepha-

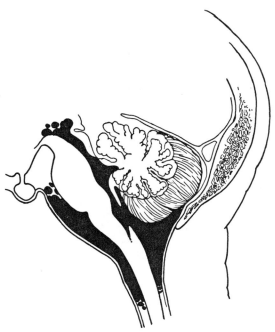

Fig 18—8.—Posterior fossa subarachnoid study with radiopaque substance.

lography can clearly delineate small structures (such as vessels and nerves) that traverse the subarachnoid space at the base of the brain. Since resolution of these structures is better with PEG than with currently available CT scanners, this remains an indication for PEG. The CT scan has replaced the PEG for the evaluation of ventricular size, cortical atrophy, and intracerebral and most intraventricular mass lesions.

Air or positive contrast can be injected directly into the ventricles by advancing a needle through a burr hole. This is called ventriculography, and is sometimes performed to define the site of block in patients with noncommunicating hydrocephalus.

The serious morbidity and mortality of PEG are less than 0.5%. The transient morbidity is 100%; all patients experience severe headache during the procedure, and nausea, vomiting, and transient hypotension are not uncommon. The serious complications include those of lumbar puncture, and the production of subdural hematomas because rapid absorption of air or oxygen in patients with hydrocephalus may cause ventricular collapse.

Arteriography

Contrast material may be injected directly into the carotid arteries (percutaneously) or a catheter may be passed into the aorta (from the femoral artery usually), and one may visualize both carotids and both vertebrals (arch aortogram, four-vessel study) or one may selectively catheterize each of the four vessels.

INDICATIONS

Angiography is the method of choice for visualizing vascular pathology. This includes abnormalities in the extracranial cerebral circulation (the carotid and vertebral arteries and their origins) and intracranial vascular abnormalities (aneurysms, AV malformations, and occlusive disease). In addition, displacement of arteries or veins can be seen with tumors or other mass lesions, or with ventricular enlargement. Extracerebral mass lesions such as subdural hematomas can be clearly delineated.

Although the CT scan can detect ventricular enlargement and mass lesions without the morbidity of angiography, it cannot define vascular disease well. In addition, when mass lesions are defined on CT scan, angiography is still sometimes performed to better localize the lesion and to provide the surgeon with information about its vascular anatomy. Angiography can also define subdural hematomas that may be isodense on CT scan (and hence are not distinguishable from normal brain). The impact of the CT scan has therefore been to decrease drastically the use of radioisotope brain scans and pneumoencephalography, but to decrease only slightly the use of angiography.

COMPLICATIONS

Permanent morbidity or death (usually from stroke) occurs in less than 0.5% to 2% of patients, depending on the experience and skill of the arteriographer and the condition of the patient. Persons with vascular disease (e.g., hypertensives, diabetics) have a higher incidence of complications than other patients. Patients must be selected with some care for this procedure; the benefits must be weighed against the risks.

Computerized Axial Tomography

This new technique is the most significant advance in diagnostic neurology in many years.

TECHNIQUE

A thin beam of x-rays is scanned across the patient's head in one plane (Fig 18–9).

The machine is then adjusted to take a sequence of 180 or more similar scans in the same plane but at different angles. The results, instead of being developed on x-ray film, are fed into a computer, which solves simultaneous equations for each of many thousand points. The computer thereby determines the radiographic density for each of these points. Differences in density that are too small to be detected by plain skull x-rays are demonstrated. The resulting picture consists of a section through the brain in which the subarachnoid spaces, brain, ventricles, and other details of brain anatomy are seen. Tumors, hemorrhages, cysts, hydrocephalus, and other conditions can be identified. The dose of radiation is similar to that of a routine skull series. Intravenous injection of positive contrast material may increase the yield of the procedure by increasing the density of lesions that have a defective blood-brain barrier (some neoplasms, chronic subdural hematomas, abscesses, infarcts, some demyelinating plaques, etc.).

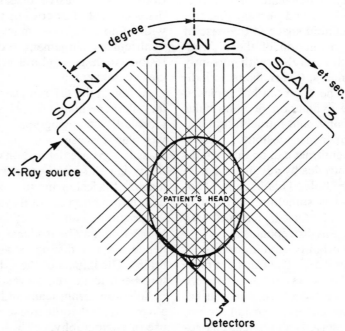

Fig 18–9.—Schematic representation of the principle of computerized axial tomographic x-ray technique.

INDICATIONS

Because computerized axial tomography is noninvasive, it has become an important screening test. It is useful in the diagnosis of infarction, tumor, hemorrhage, hydrocephalus, atrophy, and other processes. It makes the diagnosis of cerebellar hemorrhage, heretofore difficult, relatively easy. It makes it possible to follow ventricular size (and thereby to detect progressive hydrocephalus) without subjecting the patient to discomfort or risk. Water-soluble contrast (metrizamide) injected into the lumbar subarachnoid space can provide adequate contrast so that the shape of the spinal cord and of lesions impinging on the subarachnoid space can be visualized on the CT scan. The CT scan is thus replacing conventional posterior fossa contrast studies. New generations of CT scanners will probably increase resolution and ease of use sufficiently to replace myelography in the assessment of spinal cord lesions.

LIMITATIONS

Some intracranial lesions may be missed. Subdural hemorrhages may be missed because they lie close to the skull, and both blood and bone appear dense. In fact, some chronic subdural hematomas may be of the same radiologic density as the surrounding brain (isodense) and appear only as a shift of brain substance to the opposite side. Vascular lesions, such as aneurysms and AV malformations, are better diagnosed by arteriography. Small irregularities in the ventricular system and some pituitary fossa abnormalities are better detected by pneumoencephalography, because PEG resolution is greater. The brain scan may be superior in detecting multiple lesions or areas of inflammation. Other techniques (such as cisternography or CSF infusion tests) are needed to assess abnormalities in CSF flow. These and other limitations mean that computerized axial tomography complements rather than replaces existing methods.

19

Depression of Consciousness

THE ANATOMICAL SUBSTRATE of consciousness is divided into two regions: the cerebral hemispheres and the reticular formation of the brain stem extending from the midpons through the diencephalon (Fig 19–1). The cerebral hemispheres are the substrate of awareness of self and environment. They embody the sentient functions that define human intellectual existence. The reticular formation supplies crude arousal to the system.

In the absence of hemispheric function, such as following cerebral anoxia from cardiac arrest, the surviving reticular formation and brain stem are capable of supporting a crude sleep-waking vegetative state. In contrast, the cerebral hemispheres cannot function in the absence of reticular activation. Bilateral loss of the reticular formation, for example from ischemic or hemorrhagic transection of the upper brain stem, terminates all sentient cerebral activity.

In this chapter we concern ourselves with processes that depress consciousness by involving the reticular formation alone or in combination with the cerebral hemispheres. Bilateral involvement of the cerebral hemispheres causes varying degrees of loss of cognitive and emotional function, dementia, and was discussed in chapter 11. Late in the course of bilateral cerebral degenerative disease, depressed consciousness may supersede dementia. More often than not, anal-

ysis reveals the presence of one or more metabolic dysfunctions such as hypoxia from the common terminal pneumonitis, sepsis or renal failure from chronic urinary tract infection, or simply malnutrition, all of which depress further the cerebral hemispheres and also the reticular formation.

Definitions

Some definitions are necessary because medical and lay jargon for the various levels of depression of consciousness is legion and loosely applied. The subject's behavior or absence of behavior as determined by careful observation and described in simple terms is most informative.

Coma is a pathologic state of unconsciousness from which a person cannot be aroused to make purposeful responses. As a rule *light coma* is present when reflex motor responses (i.e., decorticate and decerebrate posturing) can be elicited by noxious stimulation. In *deep coma* there is no reflex response.

A patient with decerebrate posturing may be alert on rare occasions. A lesion transecting the lower pons releases the vestibulospinal motor system to respond to noxious stimulation with decerebrate posturing (see chap. 4), and because the upper pons is not affected, this is not associated with depression of consciousness. The decerebrate state usually does not enter into diagnostic considera-

210

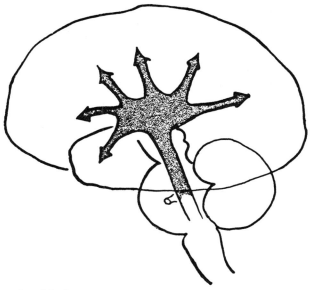

Fig 19—1.—Diagram of the reticular activating system extending from the midpons through the diencephalon to alert the cerebral hemispheres diffusely.

tion during the acute period because spinal shock (see chap. 4) usually precedes the appearance of decerebrate posturing by days to weeks.

Stupor is a state of pathologic reduced consciousness from which the patient can be aroused to purposeful response only with persistent external stimulation. This covers the broad range from persistent drowsiness from which the patient can be aroused by constant stimulation for periods of alert wakefulness to deep stupor from which the patient can be aroused only to poorly directed defense against noxious stimuli.

Sleep is a nonpathologic depression of consciousness from which the subject can be aroused to persistent alert wakefulness with appropriate nonnoxious stimuli. Sleep appears to be an active and reversible suppression of reticular arousal.

Coma-like States

Hysterical coma or stupor is a feigned or subconsciously assumed depression of con-

sciousness differentiated clinically from true coma or stupor by a normal and alert electroencephalogram, the presence of the fast component of nystagmus on caloric irrigation of the external auditory canal (see chap. 3), and the absence of abnormal neurologic signs.

The deefferented state, in which a person has lost most if not all motor behavior, can occur with several conditions. Diffuse neuromuscular dysfunction as with myasthenia gravis (myasthenic crisis or overmedication with cholinesterase inhibitors) and diffuse radiculoneuropathy (the Guillain-Barré syndrome, porphyria) can make a patient behaviorally unresponsive, although he may be perfectly lucid with respiratory support. The history and presentation of these disorders are such that the patient is unlikely to be considered comatose.

When the base of the pons (less often the midbrain) is transected or the lower pons is transected in its entirety by hemorrhage or infarction, a state of deefferentation occurs that renders the patient acutely unresponsive in all motor systems except vertical and convergent eye movement and eye-opening systems, all located in the preserved tegmentum of the midbrain. The auditory system, lying lateral along the brain stem, usually is not affected by the central hemorrhage or infarction, which often arises from involvement of the paramedian vasculature. Thus the patient hears and sees. Unless the clinician asks him to look up or down, the patient may be said to be "locked in," a term aptly applied to this state by Drs. Plum and Posner. Their minimal ability to communicate is often unrecognized, so these patients are usually considered and treated as if comatose.

Table 19–1 lists examples of the more common processes leading to pathologic depression of consciousness.

TABLE 19–1.—PROCESSES LEADING TO PATHOLOGIC DEPRESSION OF CONSCIOUSNESS

A. Reticular formation involvement (common cause of depressed consciousness)
  1. Supratentorial mass lesions that secondarily compress brain stem (e.g., neoplasm, abscess, herpes simplex encephalitis, infarction with swelling, and hemorrhage) (see Fig 19–2)
  2. Subtentorial mass or destructive lesions that compress or directly destroy brain stem (e.g., infarction, hemorrhage—primary brain stem or cerebellar—tumor, abscess)
B. Bilateral hemispheric and reticular formation depression (most common cause of depressed consciousness) (see also Table 11–3), almost always metabolic depression
  1. Oxygen, substrate, or cofactor deficiencies (e.g., ischemia, hypoxia, hypoglycemia, vitamin deficiency)
  2. Toxic
    a. Endogenous—renal failure, hepatic failure, pulmonary failure (CO_2 narcosis), endocrine hyper- or hypofunction
    b. Exogenous (most often diagnosed cause of coma)—sedative drug overdose (e.g., barbiturates, alcohol, tranquilizers, opiates, etc.); acid poisons (e.g., methyl alcohol, paraldehyde, ethylene glycol); enzyme inhibitors (e.g., arsenic, lead and other heavy metals, insecticides, cyanide, salicylates)
    c. CNS infection (meningitis, encephalitis)
  3. Acid-base or ionic abnormalities in CNS environment
  4. Postictal (epileptic) diffuse depression
  5. Traumatic dysfunction without histologic structural change (concussion)

Reticular Formation

Lesions involving primarily the brain stem and reticular formation, for the most part subtentorial, include ischemia-infarction, hemorrhage, neoplasm, abscess, and traumatic disruption.

The brain stem and reticular formation are secondarily compressed by supratentorial processes that take the form of mass lesions such as neoplasms, hemorrhage (intracerebral, subdural, and epidural hematomas), abscess, and ischemia-infarction with a mass effect secondary to edema.

The hemispheric process is unilateral in most instances and contributes focal lateralizing signs and symptoms (e.g., hemiparesis, hemihypoesthesia, dysphasia) that precede secondary brain stem compression and depression of consciousness. Brain stem compression occurs because the vectors of force from an expanding supratentorial mass are ultimately directed toward the tentorial notch, which is the only significant exit from the otherwise closed, rigid-walled, supratentorial space. This progression of events is appropriately called *transtentorial herniation* or, less specifically, *rostrocaudal deterioration*. Progressively, the diencephalon, mesencephalon, and finally the pons and medulla are compromised.

Reticular Formation and Cerebral Hemispheres

The combined depression of the reticular formation and both cerebral hemispheres is almost invariably the result of metabolic abnormality.

Metabolic depression of brain function is the most common cause of stupor and coma but may manifest itself in a number of other ways. The various manifestations of metabolic encephalopathy are discussed in greater detail in chapter 20. Table 19–1 lists the basic categories of metabolic dysfunction associated with depression of consciousness.

Evaluation

It is important to be able to differentiate rapidly between the various causes of depressed consciousness to assure immediate and correct therapeutic management of the patient. At this point, it is useful and expedient to cover the basic neurologic evaluation of the patient with altered consciousness, saving until later some initial evaluation and management problems. As a preview, however, Table 19-2 lists the major steps taken by the physician from the time he reaches the patient's bedside.

The *neurologic evaluation* of the comatose patient can be a relatively rapid and efficient procedure and should enable the examiner, with little difficulty, to differentiate between the two basic causes of depression of consciousness: (1) brain stem reticular formation depression and (2) bilateral cerebral depression and brain stem reticular depression together. It should help to localize further the pathologic process, especially when there is brain stem involvement, and it should aid in determining the specific pathogenesis and evolution of the process. It has been found that careful observation of five categories of neurologic function in most cases is adequate for these purposes: (1) level of consciousness itself, (2) respiratory rate and pattern, (3) pupillary function, (4) oculomotor-vestibular function, and (5) motor function.

Using as a model the process of rostrocaudal deterioration such as would occur with an expanding supratentorial mass (Fig 19-2), let us demonstrate the localizing value of changes in each of the five categories (Table 19-3).

The mass lesion (e.g., right intracerebral hemorrhage) would first manifest itself, not by depressing consciousness, but by the focal signs of *unilateral* hemispheric involvement (i.e., left hemiparesis, left hemisensory defect, left visual field deficit). If we were to see the patient at this time, prior to depression of consciousness, it would not be diffi-

cult to localize and categorize the pathologic process. When expansion of the mass results in *bilateral* pressure on the upper brain stem (i.e., diencephalon), characteristic changes in the parameters we have chosen to examine begin to occur as described in the following outline.

1. *Level of consciousness,* with involvement of:
   a. Upper diencephalon: Persistent drowsiness when strong external stimulation is lacking.
   b. Lower diencephalon: Deep stupor, demanding noxious stimulation* to reach a level of depressed but appropriate responsiveness such as withdrawal from stimulus or feeble attempts to remove stimulus.
   c. Upper mesencephalon: Light coma, noxious stimulation causing only reflex motor response (i.e., decorticate or decerebrate posturing, see Fig 4-1).
   d. Lower mesencephalon through medulla: Deep coma, no response to noxious stimulation.
   e. Selective destruction of the reticular formation below the midpons does not cause depression of consciousness.

2. *Respiration* (see Fig 1-1): Changing patterns are the consequence of release of medullary respiratory centers from various levels of control. Several different patterns of respiration can be discerned and have a general, although not perfectly reliable, relationship to in-

---

*A variety of noxious stimuli are used to elicit behavior in stuporous and comatose patients. Most entail tissue-damaging maneuvers such as forcefully compressing a firm object such as a pen against the fingernail bed, pinching a nipple or testicle, or compressing the supraorbital nerve. More esthetic and usually more effective is irritation of the nares with a cotton wisp. This is a threat to the airway and not surprisingly elicits a large amount of motor activity. If, however, the nares are already stimulated by and accustomed to the presence of an airway or feeding tube, the additional nasal tickle is less effective.

TABLE 19-2.—BASIC EVALUATION OF PATIENT WITH DEPRESSED CONSCIOUSNESS
OF UNKNOWN ETIOLOGY

A. Emergency evaluation.
1. *Establish airway.*
2. *Blood pressure.*—If hypotension is present, determine whether hemorrhage is present; if so, stem and replace lost blood volume. Severe hypertension should be treated by avoiding precipitous drops to hypotensive level.
3. *Temperature.*—If febrile and head trauma and potentially associated cervical spine injury are not factors, chin should be flexed on chest to determine the presence of rigidity of meningeal irritation (meningitis, meningoencephalitis). During chin-on-chest maneuver observe for knee and hip flexion (Brudzinski's sign), which when present confirms meningeal irritation.
4. *Observe and palpate for evidence of head trauma.*—Evaluate tympanic membranes for presence of middle-ear blood (indicates skull fracture) and infection (suggests possible portal of entry for bacterial meningitis). If trauma is evident or suspected, manipulation of the neck should be minimized (head-neck-shoulders fixed with blocks or sandbags if possible) until cervical spine films rule out fracture or dislocation.
5. *Glucose level in blood.*—This can be carried out in several minutes using dip-stick technique, confirmed later by more accurate laboratory analysis. After drawing blood, give 50 gm glucose intravenously to avoid any delay in treating possible hypoglycemia.
6. *Intravenous* (5% dextrose in water) to be started with large-gauge needle also capable of delivering whole blood rapidly.
7. *Indwelling urinary catheter* to be placed in patient who is deeply stuporous or comatose.
8. *History,* if available from relatives, bystanders, or patient himself.
B. Neurologic evaluation.
1. Level of consciousness.
2. Respiratory pattern.
3. Pupil size and function.
4. Oculomotor-vestibular function.
5. Motor function.

C. Laboratory evaluation (as indicated by history, emergency, and neurologic evaluations)(see also chap. 18).
1. *Computerized axial tomography* (CT scan) of cranium if available and indicated. Emergency indications include suspected trauma, stroke, or mass lesion. If not available, echoencephalography may be useful in determining presence of mass lesion causing shift of intracranial structures.
2. *Skull x-rays* to determine presence of fractures, shift of calcified pineal gland or other calcified structures (more reliable than echoencephalogram).
3. *Cervical x-rays* if evidence or suspicion of head trauma.
4. *Blood chemistries.*—Arterial: Po_2, Pco_2, pH; venous: Na, CHl, K, HCO_3, BUN, creatinine, Ca, Mg, liver function tests, drug screen.
5. *Urinalysis.*
6. *Lumbar puncture.*—Only indicated as an emergency in comatose patient if suspect CNS infection; otherwise contraindicated for fear of precipitation of rostrocaudal deterioration with supratentorial and occasionally subtentorial mass lesions.
7. *Electroencephalogram.*—To aid in differentiating true coma (diffuse electric slowing) from hysterical coma (normal pattern). This is not an emergency procedure as a rule. The neurologic examination is adequate to make the distinction. Occasionally comatose patients with destruction of the reticular formation in the pons, midbrain, or lower diencephalon have a persistent alpha frequency (8–13 cps) background rhythm that normally is associated with an alert, sentient state. However, the alpha rhythms of normal individuals disappear on sensory stimulation, while those of "alpha coma" persist. The normal alpha pattern tends to be seen predominantly in the posterior cranial (occipital) leads, while in alpha coma the rhythm is diffusely present. Under any circumstance one should determine with utmost care the presence or absence of the "locked-in" state when an alpha pattern is present by evaluating vertical eye functions (see above and chap. 3) before assuming the presence of alpha coma.

volvement of different levels of the brain stem.
a. Upper diencephalon: Sighing, yawning, accompanying drowsiness.
b. Lower diencephalon: Cheyne-Stokes respiratory pattern. This type of respiration can be seen with

diffuse bilateral cerebral involvement as well and may be most prominent when the patient is sleeping (i.e., presumably when further cerebral depressing mechanisms are in effect). It is also seen during sleep in some normal individuals, and this

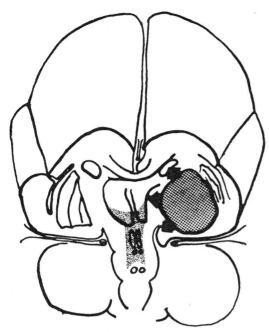

Fig 19–2.—Right cerebral expanding mass (hematoma) originating in the basal ganglia. Arrows represent vectors of force impinging with rostrocaudal progression on the brain stem.

has been reported to be more likely to occur at high altitudes.

c. Upper mesencephalon: Cheyne-Stokes pattern.

d. Lower mesencephalon: Central neurogenic hyperventilation, rapid (20–40 per minute), deep breathing, usually significant enough to cause respiratory alkalosis if no pulmonary compromise is present.

e. Pons: Central neurogenic hyperventilation changing to ataxic respirations (irregularly irregular) that have inconstantly varying rhythm and rate. With primary pontine tegmental involvement, one can see in addition to central neurogenic breathing or ataxic respirations apneustic breaths, which consist of a long arrest of breathing at the end of inspiration and resemble breath holding.

f. Medulla: Depression and final cessation of respiration.

g. When only the medulla remains, the respiratory pattern may change to eupnea (i.e., a normal pattern produced by the intrinsic expiratory-inspiratory rhythm of the medullary respiratory center) or breathing may remain ataxic.

3. *Pupils:* Pupil size and reactivity are mediated through variations in the equilibrium between sympathetic dilation and parasympathetic constriction (see chap. 3).

a. Diencephalon: The pupils are constricted due to suppression of the hypothalamic origins of the sympathetic pupillodilator system; they react to light. However, as the process progresses to involve lower parts of the diencephalon and finally vectors involve the diencephalic-mesencephalic junction at the level of the posterior commissure, the substrate of the afferent arc of the light reflex (pretectal zone) may be compromised, causing a sluggishness of pupillary reactivity when the pupil may still be small.

b. Mesencephalon: If the oculomotor complex of the midbrain or the third nerve is bilaterally and selectively destroyed, the pupils are widely dilated (7–9 mm) because of remaining sympathetic dilator tone and do not react to light. If midbrain suppression is extensive enough to cause depression of consciousness, complete denervation of the iris is likely because of involvement of both the descending sympathetic system, which runs through the reticular formation, and the parasympathetic portion of the oculomotor complex. The pupil would therefore be midposition in size (4–7 mm, varying from individual to individual) and unreactive to light.

c. Pons-medulla: The pupils continue to be midposition and fixed. Selective involvement of the pons or

TABLE 19–3. — ROSTROCAUDAL BRAIN STEM DETERIORATION SECONDARY TO EXPANDING RIGHT SUPRATENTORIAL MASS

ANATOMICAL LEVEL	CONSCIOUSNESS	RESPIRATION	PUPILS	OCULOMOTOR-VESTIBULAR	MOTOR
Upper diencephalon	Drowsy (dull)	Eupnea with yawns and sighs	Small, reactive	Depression of ocular checking and fast component of nystagmus	Left hemiparesis, bilateral paratonia
Lower diencephalon	Coma	Cheyne-Stokes (CSR)	Small, reactive	Loss of above	Left hemiparesis, decorticate
Mesencephalon	Coma	CSR or central neurogenic hyperventilation (CNH)	Midposition, fixed (MPF)	Dysconjugate response; loss of medial rectus function on horizontal gaze; may see loss of lateral rectus function also (see text)	Decerebrate
Upper pons	Coma	CNH or ataxia	MPF	As above	Weak decerebrate
Lower pons	Coma	Ataxia or eupnea	MPF	None	Flaccid, areflexic
Medulla	Coma	Apnea	MPF	None	Same

medulla in the absence of midbrain pathology is expected to cause small, reactive pupils because only the descending sympathetic pathways are damaged. With pontine transection the pupils are frequently 1 mm or smaller. There remains very little potential for further pupil constriction, and for practical purposes at the bedside, the pupils appear unreactive to light unless a very bright light is used and observations are made with a magnifying glass. A similar situation occurs with narcotic overdose, where the pupils may be maximally constricted (pinpoint, 0.5 mm or less) and therefore unreactive to light.

4. *Oculomotor-vestibular function* (see chap. 3).

   a. Diencephalon: Loss of fast or correction component of nystagmus on caloric irrigation of external auditory meatus (to be present, the fast component needs at least diencephalic integrity, possibly basal ganglia integrity is also necessary) and therefore loss of checking on oculocephalic maneuver (i.e., rotat-

ing head horizontally). Tonic conjugate horizontal deviation of the eyes is present with these maneuvers, indicating preservation of brain stem reflex activity.

   b. Mesencephalon: Loss of medial rectus response to caloric and oculocephalic stimulation, lateral rectus function intact. Lateral rectus function may be lost in some patients at this stage or occasionally when compression vectors appear to have progressed no farther than diencephalic levels. This loss is caused by downward displacement of the brain stem and concomitant stretching of the abducens nerve, which courses upward from the ventral pontomedullary junction to turn forward through the dura and over the petrous ridge. It is presumably at this turning point that the stretched nerve is compressed by the rostrocaudal forces. That this can occur without intrinsic involvement of the brain stem is evidenced by the appearance of abducens palsies in pseudotumor cerebri. This is considered by some an idiopathic condition of diffuse interstitial cerebral edema, presumably causing symmetric downward displacement of the brain stem and concomitant abducens palsies, headache, and no intrinsic brain stem dysfunction. Preservation of the *corneal reflex,* a midpons (CN V) to low pons (CN VII) reflex, is adequate evidence that complete loss of horizontal reflex eye movement in our model patient is secondary to mesencephalic third-nerve involvement and extrinsic abducens nerve involvement.

   c. Upper pons: Same as with mesencephalic loss.

   d. Lower pons: Loss of all response to caloric and oculocephalic stimulation because the paramedian reticular formation subserving conjugate horizontal gaze and the sixth-nerve nuclei are affected. No corneal reflex remains.

5. *Motor function* (see chap. 4).

   a. Upper diencephalon: Paratonia is present. It is an active perseveration of position in the limbs when passively manipulated. This appears as a plastic but irregular resistance. It also may be seen with diffuse bilateral hemispheric disease and occasionally has been reported with frontal lobe lesions, occurring contralateral to the site of lesion. The mechanism of this phenomenon has not been elucidated. It is considered by some to represent a primitive and disinhibited conservation of ongoing resting or postural tone.

   b. Lower diencephalon: Decorticate to decerebrate rigidity following noxious stimulation (see Fig 4–1). Early there may be asymmetry in the reflex response. Reflex response may appear first in the already abnormal motor system; that is, the hemiparetic limbs may progress to decorticate and then decerebrate posturing before the less affected descending motor system is involved. In our model (Fig 19–2) left hemiparesis may progress to decorticate posturing while some purposeful response and paratonia may still be present in the right limbs. Decerebrate posturing on the left is paralleled early by decorticate posturing on the right. Finally, decerebrate posturing is present bilaterally and progresses to bilateral flaccid unresponsiveness as lower levels of the brain stem are compromised.

   c. Mesencephalon: Decerebrate posturing with noxious stimulation.

   d. Upper pons: Decerebrate posturing with noxious stimulation weaker.

   e. Lower pons and medulla: No response to noxious stimuli, flaccid. Acute cross-sectional loss of the lower pons almost invariably results in flaccid quadriplegia. If the patient survives, he will progressively develop decerebrate posturing to noxious stimulation and hyperactive reflexes. The flaccid state, as noted in chapter 4, is considered a diaschisis or shock phenomenon and is seen to a greater extent and lasts longer the farther down the neuraxis acute loss of descending motor influences occurs. It is highly unlikely that our model patient would survive the days necessary to regain reflex motor activity. Nevertheless we have cared for patients with primary transection of the lower pons by infarction or hemorrhage who have survived to develop reflex decerebrate posturing while maintaining full consciousness (locked-in state). In our model patient a Babinski response was present initially on the left and then bilaterally at the lower diencephalic level and below. It may be the last remaining limb response to noxious stimulation when the brain stem is failing. Occasionally the Babinski response has been noted at end stage to revert to a tonic flexor response of the large toe.

Summary

Transtentorial-rostrocaudal vectors originating from an expanding supratentorial mass lesion have progressively compromised brain stem functions from the diencephalon through the pons and medulla. Observation of the level of consciousness, respiratory pattern, pupil size and reactivity, oculomotor-vestibular functions, and the motor system allows localization of the process and its progression. In addition, when indicated, the corneal reflex aids in differentiating extrinsic from intrinsic abducens nerve dysfunction.

For didactic purposes, our patient demonstrated a stepwise progression of segmental brain stem loss. For practical purposes, the determination of progressive levels of rostrocaudal determination has prognostic but little therapeutic value when the process has extended beyond the midbrain. When loss of midbrain function is complete in *acute* deterioration, secondary hemorrhages (Duret hemorrhages) develop into the midbrain and pontine tegmentum in most patients. These are presumed secondary to traction and tearing of the paramedian vessels penetrating from the major basal arteries (basilar and posterior cerebral arteries). Irreversible deterioration is the rule at this stage. Therefore it is extremely important to recognize rostrocaudal deterioration early at the diencephalic or preliminary mesencephalic stages. Early therapy to ward off progression may be lifesaving. In *chronically* progressing rostrocaudal deterioration, such as with subdural hemorrhage or neoplasm, secondary tegmental hemorrhages are less likely to occur because vascular and brain stem accommodation may be possible.

Subtentorial processes that affect specific levels of the brain stem are localized equally well with this system. As a rule, subtentorial lesions directly involving the brain stem cause simultaneous cranial nerve dysfunction and depression of consciousness. An exception to this is cerebellar hemorrhage (less often cerebellar infarction with edema), which may initially cause occipital headache, ataxia, and nausea and vomiting before compressing the underlying brain stem. Supratentorial mass lesions, as we saw, first cause focal hemispheric dysfunction and then depression of consciousness followed last by cranial nerve abnormalities.

Metabolic suppression of both hemispheric and brain stem reticular functions initially tends to spare primitive brain stem functions. Thus, despite the presence of coma, brain stem oculovestibular, respiratory, and pupillary functions remain intact until late, and neurologic signs referable to hemispheric depression are symmetrically abnormal. The pupils continue to react to light in patients with metabolic coma even after oculovestibular and respiratory function is lost (mechanical maintenance of respiration is necessary to avoid superimposition of anoxic brain destruction). Chapter 20 will elaborate on the various presentations of metabolic encephalopathy.

We would like to draw your attention to a single important reference for further reading on the subject of stupor and coma. The information in this chapter and also in chapter 20 is considered a basic primer based largely on the text *Diagnosis of Stupor and Coma* by Fred Plum and Jerome Posner. Clarity and completeness of content make their book required reading and reference for all physicians who deal with patients who have depressed levels of consciousness.

REFERENCE

Plum, F., Posner, J. B.: *Diagnosis of Stupor and Coma*, ed. 3. Philadelphia, F. A. Davis Co., 1980.

20

Metabolic Encephalopathy

THE FORMAT OF THIS CHAPTER is different from the preceding ones. We use case reports and their analyses to create a more realistic problem-solving environment. It is assumed that most readers use this text as a primer for clinical neurologic science and have read each chapter in turn. This background gives a fuller understanding of each case problem and its ramifications.

For practical purposes we define metabolic encephalopathy as a potentially reversible abnormality of brain function caused by processes of extracerebral origin. The primary cerebral degenerative disorders are considered only insofar as they must be part of the differential diagnosis for diffuse cerebral dysfunction (see chap. 11).

Persons with metabolic encephalopathy may present in several ways depending on the magnitude and temporal course of the abnormality, the individual's age and neuronal reserve (i.e., his capacity to compensate dysfunction), to a lesser degree the specific metabolic abnormality, and other factors that are not well defined. Depression of consciousness (stupor and coma), progressive loss of intellect (dementia), hyperexcitable states such as agitated dementia (delirium) and seizures (multifocal and generalized myoclonus, generalized tonic-clonic seizures), and less often focal abnormalities of brain function may be the behaviors of metabolic encephalopathy either alone or in combination.

In general, the preceding presentations are not etiologically specific. However, there is usually good evidence on the basis of neurologic examination that metabolic encephalopathy exists. A general physical examination and a reliable medical-neurologic history further delineate the diagnostic possibilities. Appropriate laboratory tests should then define the etiologic factor or factors.

Table 20–1, modified from Plum and Posner, is a comprehensive listing of the major processes capable of producing metabolic derangement of brain function. Analyses of examples of the various presentations of metabolic brain dysfunction follow. The plan is to give you a general approach to the diagnosis and management of metabolic encephalopathy.

Depression of Consciousness

CASE 1

A 54-year-old single man was brought to the emergency room by ambulance. He had been found unresponsive in his apartment. He was last seen 24 hours earlier by friends at a social gathering where his behavior was apparently normal. No medical or neurologic history was known.

EMERGENCY ROOM FINDINGS AND MANAGEMENT.—The following were the initial findings:

1. Mucous membranes were dusky and

219

TABLE 20-1.—EXTRACEREBRAL CAUSES OF METABOLIC ENCEPHALOPATHY*

A. Deprivation of oxygen, substrate, or metabolic cofactors
 1. Hypoxia [interference with oxygen supply to the entire brain—cerebral blood flow (CBF) normal]
  a. Decreased oxygen tension and content of blood
    Pulmonary disease
    Alveolar hypoventilation
    Decreased atmospheric oxygen tension
  b. Decreased oxygen content of blood, normal tension
    Anemia
    Carbon monoxide poisoning
    Methemoglobinemia
 2. Ischemia (diffuse or widespread multifocal interference with blood supply to brain)
  a. Decreased CBF resulting from decreased cardiac output
    Stokes-Adams, cardiac arrest, cardiac arrhythmias
    Myocardial infarction
    Congestive heart failure
    Aortic stenosis
    Pulmonary infarction
  b. Decreased CBF resulting from decreased peripheral resistance in systemic circulation
    Syncope: orthostatic, vasovagal
    Carotid sinus hypersensitivity
    Low blood volume
  c. Decreased CBF due to generalized or multifocal increased vascular resistance
    Hypertensive encephalopathy
    Hyperventilation syndrome
    Hyperviscosity (polycythemia, cryoglobulinemia or macroglobulinemia, sickle cell anemia)
  d. Decreased CBF due to widespread small-vessel occlusions
    Disseminated intravascular coagulation
    Systemic lupus erythematosus
    Subacute bacterial endocarditis
    Fat embolism
    Cerebral malaria
    Cardiopulmonary bypass
    Sickle cell crisis
 3. Hypoglycemia
    Resulting from exogenous insulin
    Spontaneous (endogenous insulin, liver disease, etc.)
    Alcohol consumption, prolonged with no carbohydrate intake
 4. Cofactor deficiency
    Thiamine (Wernicke's encephalopathy)
    Niacin
    Pyridoxine
    Cyanocobalamin

B. Diseases of organs other than brain
 1. Diseases of nonendocrine organs
    Liver (hepatic coma)
    Kidney (uremic coma)
    Lung (CO_2 narcosis)
 2. Hyperfunction and/or hypofunction of endocrine organs
    Pituitary
    Thyroid (myxedema-thyrotoxicosis)
    Parathyroid (hypoparathyroidism and hyperparathyroidism)
    Adrenal (Addison's disease, Cushing's disease, pheochromocytoma)
    Pancreas (diabetes, hypoglycemia)
 3. Other systemic diseases
    Cancer (remote effects)
    Porphyria
C. Exogenous poisons
 1. Sedative drugs
    Barbiturates
    Nonbarbiturate hypnotics
    Tranquilizers
    Bromides
    Ethanol
    Anticholinergics
    Opiates
 2. Acid poisons or poisons with acidic breakdown products
    Paraldehyde
    Methyl alcohol
    Ethylene glycol
    Ammonium chloride
    Salicylates
 3. Enzyme inhibitors
    Heavy metals
    Organic phosphates
    Cyanide
    Salicylates
D. Abnormalities of ionic or acid-base environment of CNS
 1. Water and sodium (hypernatremia and hyponatremia)
 2. Acidosis (metabolic and respiratory)
 3. Alkalosis (metabolic and respiratory)
 4. Potassium (hyperkalemia and hypokalemia)
 5. Magnesium (hypermagnesemia and hypomagnesemia)
 6. Calcium (hypercalcemia and hypocalcemia)
E. Diseases producing toxins or enzyme inhibition in CNS
    Meningitis
    Encephalitis
    Subarachnoid hemorrhage
F. Disordered temperature regulation
    Hypothermia
    Heat stroke
G. Postepileptic (postictal) depression
H. Traumatic dysfunction without histologic structural change (concussion)

*Modified from Plum and Posner.

respirations were shallow at 10 per minute; within minutes the rate fell further. Nasotracheal intubation was achieved and respiration was supported mechanically.

2. Blood pressure was 110/70, pulse 88 and regular, rectal temperature 36.0 C.

3. Blood glucose was drawn and an intravenous started with 5% dextrose and water; 50 gm glucose was given by vein.

4. There was no evidence of head trauma; that is, there was no soft-tissue swelling or depression of the cranium and no contusion or lacerations over the face or scalp. There was no blood behind the tympanic membranes.

5. The ocular fundus had flat disks, and venous pulsations were present.

6. The patient's neck was supple to flexion.

7. An indwelling urinary catheter was placed.

Neurologic evaluation was carried out simultaneously and revealed the following:

1. No response to noxious stimulation (irritation of the nares with a cotton wisp and supraorbital pressure).

2. No spontaneous respiration off the respirator for one minute.

3. Pupils 1 mm in diameter and constricted to bright light.

4. Eyes in neutral position and immobile; no oculocephalic or cold caloric oculomotor-vestibular response.

5. No reflexes or motor responses of any type observed or elicited.

Two diagnoses should be entertained for this dramatic picture. Acute transection of the pons and medulla by hemorrhage or infarction and, less likely, trauma could explain all the findings. Severe metabolic depression of hemisphere and brain stem (reticular formation) function is a much more likely diagnosis. Even if these conditions were equally common, one should approach the problem primarily from a therapeutic viewpoint and consider metabolic disorder the working diagnosis.

Table 19–2 is an outline for the basic emergency room evaluation of patients with depressed consciousness of unknown cause. The emergency measures and laboratory studies are standard and straightforward. The neurologic examination, as formulated by Plum and Posner, is brief but comprehensive enough to tell the examiner whether the depression of consciousness has been caused by a process involving the contents of the supratentorial, infratentorial, or both compartments. Repeated examinations determine the evolution of the process. Last, the examination, when supplemented by selected laboratory studies, helps determine the specific diagnosis.

Let us further analyze our patient and determine why, on the basis of the neurologic examination alone, we should consider his condition typical of metabolic coma. The specific diagnostic possibilities can then be discussed and the laboratory procedures for making the final diagnosis reviewed.

CONSCIOUSNESS.—Alone, stupor or coma (particularly the latter) provides very little to differentiate metabolic from structural involvement of the reticular formation and cerebral hemispheres.

RESPIRATIONS.—Excessive sighing and yawning, Cheyne-Stokes respirations, hyperventilation, hypoventilation, and apnea are nonspecific presentations of bilateral brain stem involvement whether it be structural or metabolic. On the other hand, ataxic respirations and apneustic breaths are seen uncommonly, if at all, with metabolic disease; if present, they indicate structural disease of the pons or medulla.

Our comatose patient, who has progressed from hypoventilation to apnea, must have bilateral involvement of the reticular formation of at least the mesencephalon or upper pons. Involvement of the diencephalic reticular formation alone would more likely be reflected as stupor, whereas involvement of the reticular formation of the lower pons and/or medulla in isolation would not cause depression of consciousness. The apnea reflects loss of function of the medullary reticular formation containing the respiratory center. Therefore we have evidence for involvement of at least the midbrain or pons and the medulla. If the involvement of this extensive amount of brain stem tegmentum is destructive or compressive, we would expect to see evidence for involvement of cranial nerve systems that lie therein. Specifically in our examination we should look for abnormalities of the oculomotor, abducens, and vestibular systems. Metabolic depression first depresses the reticular formation and consciousness. Cranial nerve and vital function (respiration and cardiovascular support) abnormalities tend to occur late. Let us proceed with the examination.

PUPILS.—The pupils of our patient were small (1 mm) and reacted to light. There is very little constriction possible from a resting size this small; therefore, it is necessary to use a strong light and at times a magnifying glass (an otoscope lens is handy) to confirm reactivity. With the exception of a few rare conditions (e.g., the Argyll Robertson pupils of tertiary syphilis), 1-mm pupils react to light. The narcotized pupil is usually maximally constricted (less than 1 mm) and cannot constrict further. Occasionally the pupils are maximally constricted following transection of the pons because of loss of the descending sympathetic systems and presumably a disinhibition and possibly an active facilitation of the Edinger-Westphal complex in the midbrain.

As a rule the last major reflex system lost with metabolic encephalopathy is the light reflex. The parasympathetic system is quite resistant, whereas the sympathetic system, an integral part of the reticular activating system, is depressed early in parallel with depression of consciousness. Small pupils are the rule with metabolic involvements, with the exception of toxicity from drugs that excite the sympathetic system (e.g., amphet-

amine) or depress the parasympathetic system (e.g., atropinics, meperidine, glutethimide).

A destructive lesion transecting the diencephalon could cause the pupillary abnormality in our patient, but it is likely that he would be stuporous and not comatose and it is highly unlikely that respiration would be lost. This would have to be caused by a separate lesion involving the medulla and sparing the midbrain. Midbrain transection causes loss of both sympathetic and parasympathetic systems, thus leaving the pupils in midposition (approximately 4–7 mm) and unreactive to light. Rarely, intraventricular dissection from an intracerebral arterial hemorrhage causes a skip picture. The hemorrhagic mass compresses the diencephalon, depressing consciousness, while it is hypothesized that the intraventricular hemorrhagic pressure wave causes depression of medullary functions when it is reflected against the floor of the fourth ventricle after passing down the ventricular channel. The midbrain and pons might then be initially spared. Acute respiratory arrest from medullary dysfunction is the most likely cause of sudden death associated with intraventricular hemorrhage.

Transection of the pons and the medulla could cause the changes in respiration, consciousness, and pupillary function observed in our patient. It is reasonable to leave this unusual possibility for a diagnosis of exclusion and consider the diagnosis metabolic until proved otherwise. It is statistically much more likely and is amenable to therapy.

OCULOMOTOR-VESTIBULAR SYSTEMS. — With metabolic encephalopathy the basic oculomotor-vestibular reflex system (see chap. 3) first becomes disinhibited as cerebral hemispheric and reticular formation influences are lost. The saccadic or checking component of the oculocephalic response is lost and therefore the fast or checking component of nystagmus elicited by caloric irrigation is also lost. This leaves, in both instances, tonic conjugate deviation of the eyes away from the facilitated horizontal vestibular canal. Ultimately the relatively resistant brain stem reflex system is suppressed, and there is no oculomotor-vestibular response. On occasion bilateral medial rectus function is lost first. In this instance the pupils are not involved, and one can conclude that the medial longitudinal fasciculus is suppressed (internuclear ophthalmoparesis) or that the extraocular segment of the oculomotor nucleus is particularly susceptible to metabolic suppression. The oculomotor-vestibular system is completely suppressed with metabolic disease at about the same time as respiration, with some individual variation. For example, we have seen patients overdosed with barbiturates who have fully disinhibited oculomotor-vestibular responses and no spontaneous respiration, others with spontaneous respiration and absent oculomotor-vestibular response, and others with both respiration and oculomotor-vestibular response lost simultaneously.

Our patient had no oculomotor response at all, which is compatible with destruction of the medulla or pons or severe metabolic suppression.

MOTOR SYSTEMS.—As a rule the motor abnormalities of metabolic encephalopathy are symmetric. Diffuse paratonic perseveration of motor tone, then diffuse weakness, and ultimately flaccid quadriplegia parallel depression of consciousness from stupor through deep coma. Decorticate and decerebrate reflex posturings with noxious stimulation are commonly seen with progressive metabolic suppression of any type. An excellent model for observing these motor changes is the patient undergoing general anesthesia. For that matter, the anesthetized patient is an excellent model for observing all the changes so far mentioned.

During the stages of stupor or during delirium or chronic dementing encephalopathy of metabolic origin, there may be some motor signs that are relatively specific for metabolic encephalopathy. Tremulousness, asterixes

(usually symmetric, irregularly episodic loss of maintained motor tone of the limbs, less commonly of the axial muscles), multifocal myoclonus (diffuse, asynchronous twitching of portions of muscles often strong enough to cause movement at the joints, of larger magnitude than fasciculations), and generalized myoclonic jerks that may or may not lead to major motor seizures should all alert the examiner to the presence of metabolic disorder.

Our patient was flaccid, areflexic, and unresponsive to noxious stimulation, which is compatible with the motor shock state produced by acute transection of the pons or medulla or severe metabolic suppression of the brain stem. A supratentorial lesion with secondary compression and rostrocaudal deterioration of the brain stem would not be possible. The pupils were small and reacted to light.

Recapitulating, the neurologic examination showed a patient who was flaccid, areflexic, and unresponsive to noxious stimulation, who was apneic off the respirator, and who had no oculomotor-vestibular response. His pupils were small and reactive. Although his pons and medulla may have been transected by a destructive lesion, the statistically likely and therapeutically oriented working diagnosis is metabolic encephalopathy. The former diagnosis can wait until we have disproved metabolic disease. Even if the picture were more abnormal—with the blood pressure needing exogenous pressor support and the pupils midposition and unreactive—one would still assume severe metabolic depression until proved otherwise. If secondary to a known destructive process, these last findings would indicate brain death. Metabolic depression of brain function can be complete, meeting the criteria for brain death including a flat electroencephalogram, and with physiologic support complete recovery is possible.

What metabolic categories must be considered for our patient? Table 20–1 gives essentially all the possibilities that might cause brain depression of this degree. Reviewing quickly the major categories of metabolic disease that might cause depression of consciousness, we should be able to narrow the possibilities for our patient and carry out the laboratory tests necessary to define a specific cause.

BASIC SUPPORT SYSTEMS. — These include oxygen, substrate, and cofactors.

Oxygen. — Cardiorespiratory insufficiency caused by acute cardiac arrhythmia with spontaneous reversal might have occurred. Progressive subsequent deterioration with no good evidence for midbrain involvement (i.e., pupils remain reactive and small) to implicate rostrocaudal deterioration and good evidence (normal disks and venous pulsations) against progressive postanoxic cerebral swelling essentially rule out this possibility. Blood gases drawn on the respirator with room air revealed normal pH, Po_2, and Pco_2. An electrocardiogram showed only mild, nonspecific abnormalities and a regular rhythm.

Substrate (glucose). — Hypoglycemia seems an unlikely possibility; there is no history of insulin-dependent diabetes. It must be remembered that it is quite possible to become severely hypoglycemic during prolonged alcohol drinking (days) with no intake of carbohydrates. Glucose and finally glycogen are depleted, gluconeogenesis from protein-amino acid sources is blocked by ethanol, and the blood glucose progressively drops and may reach low enough levels to cause encephalopathy. An insulin-secreting tumor is also a rare cause of severe hypoglycemia.

Hyperglycemic, nonketotic coma is usually preceded by days of progressive deterioration but must be considered a possibility as well as late-stage (i.e., depression severe enough to depress the respiratory center), hyperglycemic, ketotic coma.

A blood glucose determination was carried out on blood drawn prior to the infusion of glucose. A dip-stick test done within minutes showed a level of approximately 200 mgm%.

The laboratory value, available one hour later, was 180 mg%. The normal pH ruled out significant ketosis along with other major causes of metabolic acidosis severe enough to cause depression of consciousness (lactic acidosis, uremia, and exogenous acid poisoning).

Cofactor deficiency. — We have been unable to determine the alcohol intake history of our patient. Wernicke's encephalopathy, a condition caused by thiamine deficiency and usually seen in chronic malnourished alcoholics, could cause this level of depression but seems unlikely because no obvious illness was noted by friends at a cocktail party 24 hours before.

Nevertheless, a multivitamin preparation was added to the glucose infusion because the history was inadequate, and because glucose infusion can precipitate Wernicke's encephalopathy in alcoholics or other malnourished individuals with borderline thiamine stores. The glucose initiates Krebs cycle activity, which presumably ties up residual thiamine stores and deprives the brain of certain poorly understood thiamine-dependent metabolic systems.

DISEASES OF ORGANS OTHER THAN THE BRAIN. — Significant renal and pulmonary failure have been ruled out by pH and blood gas determinations. Hepatic failure with secondary shunting of large-bowel-produced toxins into the systemic circulation must be considered. In a child, Reye's syndrome (parainfectious hepatic insufficiency and secondary brain failure) might appear this rapidly, and fulminant hepatic necrosis, toxic or infectious, in a child or adult could result in acute cerebral depression. Hepatic necrosis is unlikely to occur without significant jaundice, and 24 hours from alertness to this deep coma would seem unlikely. The condition of a patient with chronic cirrhotic liver disease and portal hypertension with significant portal-systemic shunting could rapidly deteriorate under certain stresses. Particularly liable to cause acute deterioration would be hemorrhage into the bowel (e.g., from varices or acute gastritis), causing a massive presentation of protein to large-bowel bacteria.

No stigmata of chronic liver disease were seen, there was no jaundice, and the liver was not palpably enlarged or small to percussion. No stool blood was detected, a nasogastric tube aspirate showed only mucus, and the hematocrit was reported to be normal.

A clue to the presence of chronic portacaval shunting and encephalopathy in less severely depressed patients is respiratory alkalosis secondary to chronic mild hyperventilation, possibly driven by intracellular acidosis at the medullary level. Elevation of the level of blood ammonia or cerebrospinal fluid glutamine, a reflection of elevated amounts of blood ammonia, are usually present to confirm the diagnosis.

Other than abnormalities of glucose metabolism, endocrine disease is unlikely to present as acute coma. Our patient's hypothermia was not low enough to consider deep coma caused by hypothyroidism. Also, a long history of progressive dementing deterioration would be likely. Mild hypothermia is nonspecific for deep-coma states. With lesser depression of brain stem function, this degree of hypothermia is probably most commonly seen with sedative intoxication, particularly the barbiturates.

The remote effects of cancer cause a chronic, occasionally subacute depression of brain function. Porphyria is unlikely to present primarily as depression of consciousness unless, as with other acute neuromuscular disorders (e.g., Guillain-Barré syndrome, occasionally myasthenia gravis), respiratory failure supervenes to cause hypoxia. These categories are unlikely in our patient, who did not lose independent respirations until after arrival in the emergency room and after respiratory support was established.

ABNORMALITIES OF IONIC AND ACID-BASE ENVIRONMENT OF THE BRAIN. — Significant abnormalities of the acid-base environment have been ruled out by pH determination.

Relative hyponatremia secondary to excess water accumulation from excess intake of water or inappropriate secretion of antidiuretic hormone is the only ionic abnormality likely to cause this rapid and severe neurologic deterioration. Electrolyte values were available within an hour from admission and were all normal.

INFECTIOUS DISEASE AND SUBARACHNOID HEMORRHAGE. — Meningitis or encephalitis could cause depression of brain stem function this severe. One might expect fever and possibly some nuchal rigidity; however, by the time these processes cause deep coma, both the fever and nuchal rigidity are likely to be lost. Encephalitis would be the least likely of the two possibilities because severe cerebral swelling would be expected to have compressed the midbrain and caused pupil enlargement and loss of the light reflex. The presence of normal venous pulsations and flat optic disks, reflecting normal intracranial pressure, also rules strongly against this possibility.

Bacterial meningitis so severe would also be unlikely for these reasons, although bacterial toxin could suppress brain function unusually without causing major cerebral swelling or acute communicating hydrocephalus.

Subarachnoid hemorrhage may cause depression of consciousness to the level of stupor, but unless it dissects into the cerebral hemispheres and causes secondary compression of the brain stem, deep coma is unlikely in the acute stage. Evidence for increased intracranial pressure would be expected. Involvement of the midbrain (midposition and fixed pupils) would have occurred as part of the rostrocaudal process with the exception of the rare intraventricular hemorrhage phenomenon described earlier.

To rule out the distant possibility of bacterial meningitis and with the security of a normal optic fundus (a skull x-ray revealed no fracture and the pineal gland was not calcified), a lumbar puncture was performed. The opening pressure was 140 mm cerebrospinal fluid (CSF). The fluid was clear and colorless. Three red cells were present in the first collection tube, none in the third; no white blood cells were present. No organisms were seen on gram stain (individuals with alcohol in their blood or who have for other reasons a poor white blood cell response to bacterial invasion may have a delayed CSF pleocytosis, but bacteria should be demonstrable on gram stain). The level of CSF glucose was 100 mg% and the protein level was 45 mg%.

DISORDERED TEMPERATURE REGULATION. — This is unsupported by findings.

POSTSEIZURE (POSTICTAL) DEPRESSION. — This is unlikely because of too severe depression, and it is progressive in the absence of apparent seizure activity. However, unchecked major motor status epilepticus could result in this severe brain dysfunction because of a mixture of associated metabolic dysfunctions. Hyperthermia, hypoxia, lactic acidosis, and prolonged excessive neuronal activity probably all contribute to brain depression and damage caused by major motor status. If our patient's seizures had arrested spontaneously some hours before he was discovered, these metabolic abnormalities might have cleared. The lack of seizure history, although sedative (ethanol) withdrawal must be kept in mind, and the lack of evidence of expected brain edema make this possibility unlikely.

EXOGENOUS POISONS. — In a busy hospital emergency room, this is the most common diagnosis for patients admitted with coma of unknown etiology. The most common single subgroups are the sedative drugs and aspirin.

For the various reasons given earlier, this major category would be strongly suspected by exclusion in our patient and a serum drug screen carried out. The general serum barbiturate level was determined and found to be in the high toxic range.

Management of the patient with metabolic coma should support vital systems — respiratory and cardiovascular — and, if possible and necessary, remove the metabolic abnormality or allow for its natural dissolu-

tion as with sedative excess. One of the major complications of prolonged coma is pneumonitis. It can usually be avoided by diligent pulmonary toilet. Another complication to be avoided is pulmonary embolism, and therefore pressure stockings should be used routinely.

The patient in this case made a full recovery, subsequently admitting to a reactive depression for which he had taken an overdose of Nembutal, a relatively short-acting barbiturate. Hemodialysis is rarely necessary for treating overdoses of short- and even long-acting barbiturates. If careful physiologic support is continually available, the mortality from barbiturate or other sedative overdose should be less than 1%. With massive overdose of phenobarbital and other long-acting sedatives, the coma may be so prolonged (many days) that physiologic support is strained to the utmost, and then dialysis can shorten the period of critical care. The complications of hemodialysis appear minor enough now to warrant this aggressive approach.

Delirium and Dementia

CASE 2

A 60-year-old married woman in an agitated, confused state was brought to the hospital by her husband. She had been ill with fever, chills, and muscle aches and pains for about a week and confined to bed, treated symptomatically with aspirin for "influenza." Her husband reported her to have been rational until early in the morning of admission, when she awakened and appeared agitated and frightened. She resisted her husband's attempts to take her to the hospital. There was no past history of significant medical illness. She had been taking no regular medications, although her husband claimed she occasionally took chlordiazepoxide for insomnia. She smoked one pack of cigarettes a day and was considered a social drinker, consuming one or two drinks of wine or beer per day in the company of others.

HOSPITAL FINDINGS AND MANAGE-MENT.—Initial findings were as follows:

1. Blood pressure was 160/90; pulse was 110 per minute and regular; temperature was 38.5 C; respirations were 20 per minute and regular.

2. General physical examination was resisted by the patient, who insisted on leaving, more than once walking toward the door wearing only her nightgown. She was disheveled, agitated, and frightened. As best could be judged there were no stigmata of chronic illness. Skin and mucous membrane color was normal. Nuchal mobility was irregularly limited in all ranges in keeping with diffusely present paratonia. No grimacing or Brudzinki's sign was elicited on neck flexion.

3. Neurologic examination revealed her to be confused about where she was, the time of day, and the day of the week. She was unable to remember the examiner's name and did not recognize him when he returned after stepping out of the room for several minutes. Essentially she was unable to imprint new information. Her attention span was shortened, reversals (e.g., saying days of week and spelling WORLD in reverse) were impossible, and she was unable to interpret proverbs at all. She appeared to be episodically actively hallucinating, pointing to and identifying moving objects that were not present. Physical signs of diffuse cerebral dysfunction included the presence of diffuse paratonia (gegenhalten), disinhibited regressive feeding reflexes (snouting, sucking, and rooting), bilaterally disinhibited palmomental responses, loss of checking on oculocephalic testing, and a bilateral forced-grasp response on palmar stimulation. The upper extremities were tremulous when outstretched, and asterixes were noted at the wrists when extended. The deep-tendon reflexes were symmetrically 3+ No other abnormalities were elicited.

Acute and agitated dementia (delirium) is almost always a reflection of metabolic disorder. This presentation and also acute quiet or apathetic dementia may be caused by most of the categories listed in Table 20-1 and is most likely to occur in the early stages of acute metabolic dysfunction. Frequently periods of agitation alternate with periods of apathy and depression of consciousness, ultimately culminating in stupor and coma if the dysfunction magnifies. Sedative (including alcohol, barbiturates, benzodiazepines, etc.) withdrawal states, hypoglycemia, hypoxia, hypermetabolic states including sepsis and hyperthyroidism, hypocalcemia, hypomagnesemia, and hepatic failure appear to be more commonly associated with a hyperexcitable state than other conditions. The excited stage of general anesthesia is a fair model of agitated dementia.

Underlying progressive degenerative brain processes such as Alzheimer's disease can emerge acutely as a florid dementia, agitated or quiet, under the influence of only mild metabolic stress, which alone is not enough to cause cognitive or emotional defect in a normal brain. This is true also for the aged brain, which under normal stress is able to function adequately. The 80-year-old with a temperature of 39 C is much more likely to be confused than the young adult whose neuronal safety factor (numbers of active neurons) is greater. Elderly patients admitted to the hospital on medical or surgical services are frequently seen in consultation for defective cognitive function. CT scans reveal atrophic changes that are compatible with the patients' age but have not been well correlated with studies of cognitive function. Mild metabolic dysfunctions are frequently found such as minimal renal dysfunction, anemia, low-grade fever, mild sedative intoxication (e.g., from tranquilizers and sleeping medications), mild hypoxia from chronic pulmonary disease, and congestive heart failure, usually in various combinations. Correction of the disorder or disorders frequently leads to an improvement in cognitive function.

We have several clues from the history and examination of our patient. She has had a febrile illness and continues to be febrile. A temperature of 38.5 C is inadequate alone to cause clinically obvious cerebral dysfunction. Central nervous system infection, encephalitis or meningitis, could produce this picture. The absence of Brudzinski's sign or behavioral evidence for pain on neck flexion does not support meningeal irritation but does not rule it out. A lumbar puncture should be done when there is (1) suspicion of infection, (2) suspicion of subarachnoid hemorrhage in a patient with no focal neurologic defect, and (3) a patient with an evolving stroke in whom anticoagulation is being considered to rule out hemorrhage. Lumbar puncture in our patient revealed normal pressure, no cells, normal protein and glucose levels, and normal results from gram stain and india ink preparations. The absence of a cellular response does not rule out meningitis or encephalitis but makes both very unlikely, as do normal pressure and normal CSF protein and glucose levels. Routine studies of blood revealed a white blood cell count of 15,000 with a shift to the left—i.e., predominance of neutrophils and their precursors. Further fever workup included urine evaluation and culture, blood cultures, and chest x-ray, all of which showed normal results. Routine blood chemistries including glucose, electrolytes, BUN, Ca^{2+}, Mg^{2+}, liver function tests, and a screen for sedative drugs were normal.

The patient's husband was questioned closely concerning her use of chlordiazepoxide. The possibility that she could be physiologically dependent was emphasized, with the present picture being one of sedative withdrawal delirium (delirium tremens). He had been ministering to her illness during the week and was sure she had not had any sleeping medication. On our instruction he returned home and on careful searching found three partly empty bottles of 25-mg chlordiazepoxide capsules secreted in various parts of the house. They were prescribed by three different physicians: a general practitioner that the husband did not know, the patient's gynecologist, and their family physician. Each prescription had been filled at a different drugstore. This circumstantially confirmed the suspicion of withdrawal delirium, a hypermetabolic condition that appears to be rebound hyperexcitability in a nervous system compensated for chronic sedative depressant affects.

Treatment consisted of sedative replacement; in this case, diazepam was given intravenously until it had a calming effect. Gradual withdrawal was then undertaken, decreasing the drug dose by 10% each day. An uneventful recovery occurred, and subsequently the patient described how she had gradually become dependent on chlordiazepoxide. It is of some interest and instructive that the delirium occurred approximately one week following withdrawal. Sedative withdrawal states, which include hyperirritability, seizures, hallucinosis, and frank delirium tremens, usually appear within 96 hours but sometimes delirium may emerge as late as 14 days after terminating or diminishing intake.

CASE 3

A 65-year-old married man was referred to the neurology clinic for evaluation of his progressive loss of cognitive ability. His wife had noted forgetfulness, carelessness in dress and daily hygiene, and an increasing lack of spontaneity for at least six months.

Examination revealed evidence of diffuse cerebral dysfunction with difficulties in all aspects of cognitive function, and there was an imprinting (recent memory) deficit that was out of proportion to past memory and other cognitive defects. This is rather nonspecific because both degenerative and metabolic processes may affect the limbic cortex earlier and more severely than neocortical regions. Multiple regressive reflexes were easily demonstrated including forced grasping, disinhibited oculocephalic responses, snouting and sucking responses to labial stimulation, and a disinhibited glabellar blinking response. Diffuse mild paratonia was also present. No asterixis or myoclonus was present.

Approximately 80%–85% of persons with progressive dementia are shown to have a degenerative process, most often Alzheimer's disease. On the basis of their clinical profile, it is frequently difficult to differentiate the other 15%–20%, who are more important because they have potentially treatable disorders. There are some clues, however, and with the aid of laboratory screening most can be ferreted out. If the patient is younger than 50, his chances of having a treatable disorder are probably greater. If the disorder is of recent onset and rapidly progressive and if there are frequent fluctuations in the level of function, chances are higher that a treatable disorder is present. If motor stigmata such as tremulousness, asterixes, and multifocal myoclonus are present, it is very likely that a metabolic problem is, at least in part, responsible for the dementia. Focal signs are not characteristic of metabolic disorders, and if they are present with the signs of diffuse dysfunction, they should suggest the possibility of a mass lesion, which may be amenable to therapy.

Although our main purpose is to discuss metabolic disorders that cause brain dysfunction, it is hardly realistic or practical to isolate only metabolic causes of dementia from the other treatable causes. Table 11–3 lists the major causes of dementia. An asterisk marks the treatable categories, which are numerous. Some diagnostic clues and approaches to therapy are also listed.

Our patient appeared to have had a recent onset of his dementia, which leads one to believe there is a fair chance of finding a treatable disorder. However, it is reasonable to equivocate about the time of onset of his dementia because family members may not notice a slowly dementing process until some obviously unacceptable disinhibited social behavior or blatant confusion occurs. The man was 65 years old at the time of admission. He had taken early retirement at age 62 and had been relatively inactive with few hobbies or outside interests for the past three years. Business or work associates are more likely to notice dementia in a compatriot because it may affect his productivity early (but a fairly routinized job may be accomplished effectively by a person well into the dementing process). The inactivity of retirement can easily veil deteriorating brain function, and therefore it is reasonable to suspect that deterioration of our patient's mental capacity may have been occurring for as long as three years. Even if this were sure and made the chances of finding a reversible process less likely, a screening battery to find treatable disorders would be carried out. A comprehensive battery should include at least the following:

Test	To Rule Out
Complete blood count (CBC)	General
Erythrocyte sedimentation rate (ESR)	Vasculitis (collagen disease), infection, occult tumor
BUN	Renal insufficiency
Serum calcium	Hyper- or hypocalcemia
Liver function tests	Hepatic insufficiency; metastatic tumor
Thyroid function tests	Hyper- or hypothyroidism
Serum B_{12} levels and/or Schilling test	B_{12} deficiency
Serum folate	Nutritional deficiency
VDRL	Tertiary syphilis
Lumbar puncture	Increased number of cells (hemorrhage, infection), high level of protein (tumor, etc.), low level of sugar (infection, etc.), increased pressure (tumor, etc.), + VDRL (syphilis)
Chest x-ray	Lung tumor or other metastasized malignancy, diffuse pulmonary disease
Skull x-ray	Skull metastases; intracranial masses (signs of increased pressure, deviated pineal, if calcified, calcified tumor); evidence of trauma
Brain scan or CT scan if available	Mass, hydrocephalus, atrophy, infarctions
EEG	Metabolic encephalopathy; focal lesions; seizure activity; EEG of metabolic encephalopathy is liable to

have diffuse slowing in the delta-theta frequencies, while degenerative disease may cause little (some theta slowing diffusely) or no abnormality

Frequent runs of diffuse delta activity were seen on our patient's EEG, making a metabolic disorder highly suspect. A CT scan showed dilatation of the lateral, third, and probably also the fourth ventricles; no cortical atrophy was evident. A lumbar puncture showed an opening pressure of 160 mm CSF, 10 lymphocytes, a protein of 130, and a glucose of 40 with a concomitant fasting blood glucose count of 100. Although an india ink preparation showed no cryptococci and the organisms did not grow on CSF culturing, cryptococcal antigen was detected in the spinal fluid. A course of treatment with amphotericin B was given, and within three weeks the spinal fluid protein and glucose levels had returned to normal and no cells were detected. Some improvement in the patient's dementia had occurred after two months, but a repeat CT scan showed a continued hydrocephalus. A ventriculoperitoneal shunt was placed and further improvement in mentation followed.

Focal Neurologic Abnormality

CASE 4

A 62-year-old married man was brought to the emergency room on January 3 by ambulance, accompanied by his wife. He had been noted to be weak and uncommunicative that morning. Preliminary examination by emergency room personnel revealed hemiparesis on the right side and aphasia. The neurology consultant was called to evaluate the presumed stroke. The findings were confirmed. The patient was severely dysphasic; his communication was limited to a few perseverated and unintelligible jargon words. He appeared to have a right-sided hemianopsia to threat, responded poorly to noxious stimulation of the right extremities, and had a

right-sided hemiparesis including the right lower facial muscles. The right deep-tendon reflexes were hyperactive and a Babinski response was present on the right.

General examination revealed an otherwise healthy-appearing individual. No evidence of arterial disease was present. A sweetish odor of the breath was present and this prompted the examiner to think of the possibility of metabolic disorder, specifically hyperglycemia with ketosis. The patient's wife volunteered that the previous January a similar event had occurred under the same circumstances, partying over the New Year. He had been found "blacked out," seen at another hospital, "sugared up," and sent home no worse for wear. He had not been nor was he being treated chronically for any illness. Within ten minutes after the patient was first seen, a dip-stick analysis of blood glucose was available. A blood specimen was sent to the laboratory for more accurate evaluation. The dip-stick value for glucose was less than 40 mg%. Fifty grams of glucose were given intravenously, and within thirty minutes the patient was sitting up in bed conversing normally with only minimal residual evidence of right hemiweakness, which subsequently cleared. A laboratory glucose level was available within an hour and was 24 mg%.

It transpired that the patient was a once-a-year heavy drinker, and that this and the previous year he had avoided eating anything over the three days that he was continually drinking hard liquor. As noted, progressive depletion of glucose and glycogen stores would be expected and symptomatic hypoglycemia would ultimately occur because gluconeogenesis from amino acids is blocked by ethanol.

Focal signs of apparent ablative disease are unusual neurologic manifestations of metabolic disease. Hypoglycemia, hepatic encephalopathy, and hypoxia are the most frequently diagnosed conditions producing this confusing picture. Because hypoglycemia is easily treated early, because when prolonged it can cause permanent neurologic defects, and because it can present as coma, stupor, delirium, dementia, generalized and rarely focal seizures, and focal ablative disease, it is reasonable to demand that a blood glucose determination be made early in the evaluation of patients with these symptoms. In patients with coma, stupor, or delirium of unknown etiology, it is reasonable to give 25–50 gm glucose intravenously after drawing blood for glucose evaluation. In patients having a stroke picture or seizures, early determination of the glucose level would appear adequate and could be coupled with an intravenous containing 5% dextrose and water. If a dip-stick determination shows hypoglycemia, 50 gm glucose should be given.

Why do patients with metabolic disorders develop focal loss of function? Some have underlying structural disease such as old areas of infarction or contusion, borderline adequate focal blood supply, or neoplasms. It is presumed that neurons that are defective but functional within or surrounding these structural lesions are depressed early by metabolic stress. This uncovering of focal dysfunction by metabolic stress is relatively nonspecific and has been used by some to help diagnose structural disease of the cerebral hemispheres. A short-acting barbiturate (e.g., amytal) given to toxicity (demonstrated by the presence of nystagmus on forward gaze) may reversibly amplify deficits from small focal cerebral lesions.

There are some patients, however, in whom there is no evidence of an underlying focal lesion and, particularly with hypoglycemia and hepatic encephalopathy, the focal abnormalities may shift during the same or other episodes. If shifting does occur, it makes a metabolic problem seem more likely. No good explanation for this asymmetric metabolic suppression of brain function is available.

CASE 5

A 56-year-old married white man who was previously well was admitted to the hospital in a stupor with clonic twitching of his left extremities and face. He had been feeling ill for several days and his wife had noted him to be lethargic on the morning of admission. At about 8 A.M., when she went to check on him, she noted that his left side was intermittently twitching.

Examination in the emergency room showed respirations were 20 per minute and regular, temperature was 38.5 C, blood pressure 150/90, and pulse was 90 and regular. He was stuporous with appropriate withdrawal responses on the right, and he had continuous clonic twitchings of the left extremities and face, which were synchronous. No other pertinent findings were noted on the remainder of the neurologic examination. On general examination the only feature of note was dryness of the mucous membranes, decreased skin turgor, and myoedema, a bulging of subcutaneous and muscle tissue on percussion, suggesting dehydration. The major laboratory finding was hyperglycemia (blood glucose 1,100 mg%) in the absence of ketosis. In the absence of a history of diabetes mellitus, which is typical for persons developing nonketotic hyperglycemic coma, it was elected to treat him with small doses of insulin and fluid replacement with careful attention to electrolyte levels. Some patients like this are found to be extremely sensitive to insulin and others fairly resistant. Therefore it is important to begin therapy with small doses of insulin to avoid a precipitous drop in the blood glucose level, which may result in rebound cerebral edema. This complication probably occurs because of a buildup of polyols (sorbital, fructose, etc.) or other osmotically active substances intracellularly in the brain in the presence of prolonged hyperglycemia. When the amount of blood glucose is rapidly dropped, causing decreased serum osmolality, the polyols are only slowly metabolized and do not readily diffuse into the extracellular or intravascular space. This creates a relative intracellular hyperosmolality and water is imbibed by the cells, causing edema and dysfunction. The glucose level was gradually reduced over two days. When the level reached approximately 500 mg% at the end of the first day, the focal seizures ceased and the stupor cleared. Mild left-sided hemiparesis and confusion persisted for some hours after the seizures stopped. Twenty-five mg diazepam stopped the seizures only transiently when given intravenously in divided doses. Diphenylhydantoin was given intravenously in a dose of 750 mg over the first day and had no obvious effect on the seizures. However, no generalization to major motor status occurred. No maintenance anticonvulsant was given. It is typical for focal status epilepticus of metabolic origin to be poorly responsive to anticonvulsant medication. As a rule the best therapy is to clear the metabolic abnormality if possible.

Focal status epilepticus (epilepsia partialis continua) has been associated with multiple metabolic abnormalities. Nonketotic hyperglycemic hyperosmolar coma is one of the more common underlying disorders, but we have seen it with uremia, hepatic encephalopathy, hypoxia, hypoglycemia, hyponatremia, encephalitis, meningitis, and theophylline excess, and it has been reported associated with others. It appears to be a rather nonspecific and unusual manifestation of metabolic disorder. It has also been associated with structural lesions, particularly infarction, neoplasms, and other masses unaccompanied by systemic metabolic abnormality.

As with ablative dysfunctions of a focal nature, irritative dysfunctions appear in some cases to be associated with minor subclinical cerebral lesions such as old areas of encephalomalacia (ancient infarcts or hemorrhages) and neoplasms. Presumably damaged but viable neurons surrounding such lesions have a relatively low threshold for group synchronization and seizure formation, and this threshold is breached by metabolic stress. In other cases, postmortem examination has shown no obvious structural defect to account for the focal seizures.

In summary, we have given case examples of the various cerebral manifestations of metabolic disorders. Depression of consciousness, progressive loss of intellect, hyperexcitable states such as delirium and seizures, and less often focal abnormalities of brain function may be the behavioral presentations of metabolic disorders either alone or in combination, and they may alternate in any one patient.

REFERENCE

Plum, F., Posner, J. B.: *Diagnosis of Stupor and Coma,* ed. 3. Philadelphia, F. A. Davis Co., 1980.

GENERAL REFERENCES

Brodal, A.: *Neurological Anatomy in Relation to Clinical Medicine,* ed. 2. New York, Oxford University Press, 1969.

DeJong, R. N.: *The Neurologic Examination,* ed. 4. New York, Paul B. Hoeber, Inc., 1979.

Eliasson, S. G., Prensky, A. L., Hardin, W. B.: *Neurological Pathophysiology,* ed. 2. New York, Oxford University Press, 1978.

Jennett, W. B.: *An Introduction to Neurosurgery,* ed. 3. St. Louis, C. V. Mosby Co., 1977.

Monrad-Krohn, G. H., Refsum, S.: *The Clinical Examination of the Nervous System,* ed. 12. London, H. K. Lewis & Co., 1964.

Spillane, J. D.: *Atlas of Clinical Neurology,* ed. 2. New York, Oxford University Press, 1975.

Vichy, N. A.: *Grinker's Neurology,* ed. 7. Springfield, Ill., Charles C Thomas, Publisher, 1976.

Vinken, P. J., Bruyn, G. N. (eds.): Disturbances of nervous function, in *The Handbook of Clinical Neurology,* vol. 1, New York, John Wiley & Sons, 1969.

Vinken, P. J., Bruyn, G. N. (eds.): Localization in clinical neurology, in *The Handbook of Clinical Neurology,* vol. 2, New York, John Wiley & Sons, 1969.

Walton, J.: *Brain's Diseases of the Nervous System,* ed. 8. New York, Oxford University Press, 1977.

Index

233